Bone Densitometry in Clinical Practice

CURRENT ◊ CLINICAL ◊ PRACTICE

Bone Densitometry in Clinical Practice: *Application and Interpretation,* by *SYDNEY LOU BONNICK,* 1998

Diseases of the Liver and Bile Ducts: *Diagnosis and Treatment,* edited by *GEORGE Y. WU AND JONATHAN ISRAEL,* 1998

The Pain Management Handbook: *A Concise Guide to Diagnosis and Treatment,* edited by *M. ERIC GERSHWIN AND MAURICE E. HAMILTON,* 1998

Sleep Disorders: *Diagnosis and Treatment,* edited by *J. STEVEN POCETA AND MERRILL M. MITLER,* 1998

Allergic Diseases: *Diagnosis and Treatment,* edited by *PHIL LIEBERMAN AND JOHN A. ANDERSON,* 1997

Osteoporosis: *Diagnostic and Therapeutic Principles,* edited by *CLIFFORD J. ROSEN,* 1996

Bone Densitometry in Clinical Practice

Application and Interpretation

Sydney Lou Bonnick, MD

Texas Woman's University, Denton, TX

Foreword by

Paul D. Miller, MD

Colorado Center for Bone Research, Lakewood, CO

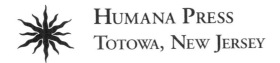

Humana Press
Totowa, New Jersey

999 Riverview Drive, Suite 208
Totowa, New Jersey 07512

For additional copies, pricing for bulk purchases, and/or information about other Humana titles, contact Humana at the above address or at any of the following numbers: Tel.: 973-256-1699; Fax: 973-256-8341; E-mail: humana@humanapr.com, or visit our Website: http://humanapress.com

Cover design by Patricia F. Cleary

Cover illustrations: Figures 3-3 and 10-2A.

This publication is printed on acid-free paper. ∞
ANSI Z39.48-1984 (American National Standards Institute) Permanence of Paper for Printed Library Materials).

Printed in the United States of America. 10 9 8 7 6 5 4 3 2 1

Library of Congress Cataloging-in-Publication Data

Bonnick, Sydney Lou.
Bone densitometry in clinical practice: application and interpretation/by Sydney Lou Bonnick.
p. cm.—(Current clinical practice)
Includes bibliographical references and index.
ISBN 0-89603-513-1 (alk. paper)
1. Bone densitometry. I. Title. II. Series.
[DNLM: 1. Absorptiometry, Photon—methods. 2. Bone and Bones—radionuclide imaging. 3. Bone Density—physiology. 4. Data Interpretation, Statistical. WE 141 B724b 1998]
RC930.5.B68 1998
616.7'1075—dc21
DNLM/DLC
for Library of Congress 98-12447
CIP

FOREWORD

Precision and accuracy are terms that are used in quantitative scientific fields to describe the reproducibility of a measurement or the capacity of a measurement to quantify the actual biological matter present. Precision and accuracy are also important applications in the quality control and quality assurance of the performance and interpretation of bone mass measurements.

Precision and accuracy also reflect the values and qualities of the author of this important text in the clinical application of bone densitometry. The is the first textbook of its kind devoted entirely to the proper use of this technology in the practice of medicine. Dr. Sydney L. Bonnick has devoted a majority of her career helping to define excellence in this exploding area and in doing so, has earned the respect and admiration of the international bone densitometry community.

Confusion abounds in this field due to the proliferation of bone densitometry devices, including the various models that can measure many skeletal sites, the different normative data bases used, and the establishment of diagnostic categories of low bone mass. Dr. Bonnick's authoritative and carefully referenced text will certainly clarify and broaden the knowledge of those physicians who currently perform bone densitometry. This text is designed to be utilized by a wide range of medical specialists: endocrinologists, rheumatologists, gynecologists, radiologists, orthopedic surgeons, and nephrologists. This book will also prove to be an invaluable resource for the technologists who perform the scans, in working closely with their physicians to provide quality care for their patients. The overwhelming problem of osteoporosis detection will never be accomplished without bone mass testing being addressed at the primary care level; therefore, *Bone Densitometry in Clinical Practice* is an important textbook for internists and family physicians as well. Dr. Bonnick's text will help guide competent use of bone densitometry for, as she correctly points out, there is wide room for misuse and misinterpretation by the uneducated in this field

Dr. Bonnick, Research Professor at Texas Woman's University, Denton, Texas, has, with great care and sensitivity, included a chapter on statistics for clinicians that even the author of this foreword can comprehend. She clearly defines how vital it is to have a basic understanding of statistical terms in order to provide the most competent bone densitometry performance and interpretation. Her approach is refreshing and kind.

Dr. Bonnick's chapters on the calculation of precision, the interpretation of serial changes in bone mass, and the reference population database issues should be read and reread by all of us who value the responsibility of this profession.

For those of us who have lived through the years of bone densitometry development, enduring some skepticism along the way, and who have contributed to improving its science and acceptability, Dr. Bonnick's book is very welcome and timely. For those of us who still carry the passion for competent clinical interpretation of bone mass measurement reports, this book will greatly guide that mission.

I have had the privilege of knowing and working closely with Dr. Bonnick for may years and have learned much from her. My own densitometry performance is more accurate and precise because of what she has taught me. This textbook is symbolic of her excellence and is a text that all densitometrists should have, not only on the shelf, but more importantly on their densitometry table and desktop.

Paul D. Miller, *MD, FACP*
Clinical Professor of Medicine
University of Colorado Health Sciences Center
Medical Director
Colorado Center for Bone Research
President
International Society for Clinical Densitometry

PREFACE

Bone densitometry is a fascinating field of medicine. Even in its earliest phases of development, densitometry incorporated aspects of imaging, physics, quantitative analysis, statistics, and computer technology that were applied in the diagnosis and management of multiple disease states. This extraordinary combination of attributes, however, left densitometry without a well-defined niche in clinical medicine. Imaging has traditionally been the purview of the radiologist. Quantitative analysis, however, is more familiar to the pathologist. Metabolic bone disease has been the concern of the internist, rheumatologist, or endocrinologist, and occasionally the nephrologist and orthopedist. And of course, physics, statistics, and computer technology have been left to those hardy souls who enjoy such things.

In 1988, when X-ray based densitometers began to rapidly replace isotope-based densitometers, the door was opened for any medical specialty to perform densitometry. And yet, without a well-defined niche, without a specialty to champion the technology, there were no physicians who, by specialty training, were immediately expert in the utilization of the technology.

In 1983, when I began working with dual-photon absorptiometry, the manufacturers provided four hours of inservice instruction at the time of machine installation along with a brief operator's manual and the promise of technical support whenever it was needed. There were no ongoing programs of continuing education in the performance of densitometry or in the interpretation of the data that it generated. There was no supply of trained densitometry technologists. Conferences on osteoporosis were infrequent and lectures on densitometry were decidedly rare. As a clinical tool, densitometry was viewed with skepticism. None of the notable fracture trials had yet been published. Indeed, these would not come for approximately 10 years. Clinicians, unable in the past to noninvasively measure bone density, saw little need for the ability to do so. The one disease in which densitometry seemed most applicable, osteoporosis, was largely viewed as an unalterable component of aging, making the measurement of bone density superfluous.

Certainly much has changed in recent years. With the ability to measure bone density, many disease states have now been found to be characterized, at least in part, by demineralization. Suddenly, it is not only osteoporosis for which the technology can provide information crucial to disease management. And osteoporosis itself is certainly no longer viewed as unassailable. The fracture trials are published. The therapeutic and preventive efficacy of several drugs has now been documented. And the disease itself is now defined based on the measured level of bone density.

The technology itself is still properly viewed as a quantitative analytical technique rather than an imaging technique. Imaging with densitometry is progressing so rapidly, however, that it is not difficult to foresee the time when some aspects of skeletal radiography may be superseded by morphometric densitometry measurements.

So to whom in medicine does densitometry belong? To no one specialty in particular and to every specialty in general as long as the physician and technologist are committed to learning the unique aspects of this technology and the proper interpretation of the data that it generates. The technology itself is superb. Bone density can be measured with superior accuracy in virtually every region of the skeleton. The machines are capable of the finest precision of any quantitative technique in use in clinical medicine today. But the machines will perform only to the level of the expertise of those who operate them. And the data that they generate will only be as useful as the clarity of the interpretation that is provided by the densitometrist.

In 1990, at the urging of Len Avecilla, who is now the director of certification and site accreditation for the International Society for Clinical Densitometry, I and Paul Miller, MD, independently began teaching courses in bone densitometry for the physician and technologist. The physicians who attended these courses came from all specialties. The technologists were RTs, MRTs, RNs, PAs, and nursing assistants. All of the physicians and technologists who attended the courses shared a common characteristic. None was adequately prepared by their training or experience to operate a densitometer and interpret the results. Like those courses, *Bone Densitometry in Clinical Practice* is written for all who wish to become proficient in the application and interpretation of bone densitometry.

The first five chapters of this book deal with technical issues in the performance of bone densitometry. Chapter 1 reviews the wide variety of equipment available and some of the technical specifications of each. Chapter 2 looks at skeletal nomenclature and the unique aspects of skeletal anatomy in densitometry. The effect of skeletal artifacts on the measurement and interpretation of BMD is discussed. Chapter 3, which deals with statistics, is intended as an overview only. Although most clinicians are familiar with such statistical concepts as the mean, standard deviation, and significance, there are few if any areas of clinical medicine in which the application of statistical principles has assumed such a prominent role as in bone densitometry. Chapter 3 is not intended to replace a review of more thorough statistical texts, but it is intended to ease the pain that the contemplation of such texts can engender. Chapter 4 continues the statistical theme, reviewing the critical performance of precision testing and how the outcome affects the interpretation of serial measurements of bone density. Finally, Chapter 5 reviews issues of machine quality control, which are often underappreciated in clinical settings, but which profoundly affect the validity of the data generated by the densitometers.

The last five chapters address the application and interpretation of the data that are generated. Chapter 6 discusses the variety of ways in which densitometry data can be used to predict fracture risk, whereas Chapter 8 looks at the reference databases to which the patient's data are compared. In interpreting densitometry results in a variety of disease states, the densitometrist must know which skeletal sites are affected and the anticipated rates of change in bone density in those disease states. This information, however, is difficult to acquire in part because of the rapidly changing knowledge base in this field, but largely because of the dispersion of this information across a wide variety of specialty medical journals. In Chapter 7, I have attempted to pull together much of what is known about the effects on bone density of age, disease, and drugs. This information is presented in the form of summaries of articles in the literature rather than simple statements of fact because the information continues to be so volatile. Chapter 9 summarizes and compares the clinical guidelines published by several different medical societies for the application of densitometry and the diagnosis of osteoporosis. Finally, Chapter 10 contains real cases from real patients, bringing to bear all the information in the first nine chapters on the interpretation of the bone density data.

In a few circumstances in this text, data have been incorporated from published abstracts, rather than from peer-reviewed articles. This was done in the interest of providing information rapidly. The reader should be cautioned that data presented in abstract form might change slightly when finally published in a peer-reviewed journal. Some data presented in abstract form are never published in a peer-reviewed journal for a variety of reasons.

Bone densitometry is an extraordinary clinical tool. It provides a safe, noninvasive window to the skeleton. Through that window a physician can obtain vital clinical information that enhances the management of the patient that cannot currently be obtained in any other way. But densitometry as a technology is only as good as the physicians and technologists who operate these machines and interpret the numerical data that come from them. It is hoped that *Bone Densitometry in Clinical Practice* will be useful in helping the densitometrist fulfill the potential that the technology holds for contributing to the highest quality of patient care and disease prevention and management.

Sydney Lou Bonnick

ACKNOWLEDGMENTS

My sincere gratitude is extended to the following individuals who have contributed to this work:

Dr. Paul Miller, of the Colorado Center for Bone Research, Lakewood, CO and President of the International Society for Clinical Densitometry;
Dr. Ken Faulkner, of the Oregon Osteoporosis Center, Portland, OR and Trustee of the International Society for Clinical Densitometry;
Dr. Clifford Rosen, of the Maine Center for Osteoporosis, Research and Education, Bangor, ME;
Dr. Richard Wasnich of the Hawaii Osteoporosis Center, Honolulu, HI; and
Dr. David Nichols, Texas Woman's University, Denton, TX

I would also like to thank James Hanson of Lunar Corp., Mardi Sawyer of Hologic, Inc., Patricia Ito of Dove Medical Systems, and Annette Mollgaard and Tina Gunther of Osteometer MediTech A/S for their assistance and support. I owe a special debt of gratitude to Joyce Paucek of Norland Medical Systems, Inc. for her assistance in a variety of areas dealing with the production of this book., I also owe a special debt of gratitude to Mary Melton, MD, of Merck, Inc. for her initial encouragement and support in the development of the manuscript.

My gratitude is extended to the publishers and authors who permitted me to reproduce excerpts of their work in this volume in the interest of continuing eductaion.

This work was supported in part by an unrestricted educational grant from Merck, Inc.

To Pauline Beery Mack, PhD,
Martha Helen Hale, MD,
and The Pioneers of Texas Woman's University

LIST OF COLOR PLATES

Color plates 1–12 appear as an insert following p. 78; color plates 13–20 appear as an insert following p. 174.

CONTENTS

1 Densitometry Techniques in Medicine Today

Contents

The field of bone densitometry has grown rapidly, particularly in the past 15 years. Many techniques are now available from which the physician may choose. Although the clinical application of these technologies is relatively recent, the history of densitometry began over 60 years ago.

PLAIN RADIOGRAPHY IN THE ASSESSMENT OF BONE DENSITY

Some of the earliest attempts to quantify bone density utilized plain skeletal radiography. When viewed by the unaided eye, plain skeletal radiographs have never been useful for quantifying bone density. Demineralization becomes visually apparent only after 40% or more of the bone density has been lost *(1)*. Beyond that general statement, no quantification of the bone density can be made. Plain radiographs have been used for qualitative and quantitative skeletal morphometry, and were also used to assess bone density based on the optical densities of the skeleton when compared to simultaneously X-rayed standards of known density. With the advent of photon absorptiometric techniques, most of these early methods have fallen into disuse. Nevertheless, a brief review of these techniques should enhance the appreciation of the capabilities of modern testing, as well as provide a background for understanding modern technologies.

QUALITATIVE SPINAL MORPHOMETRY AND THE SINGH INDEX

Qualitative Spinal Morphometry

Qualitative morphometric techniques for the assessment of bone density have been in limited use for over 50 years. Grading systems for the spine relied on the appearance of the trabecular patterns within the vertebral body, and the appearance and thickness of the cortical shell *(2)*. Vertebra were graded from IV down to I, as the vertical trabecular pattern became more pronounced with the loss of the horizontal trabeculae and the cortical shell became progressively thinned. The spine shown in Fig. 1-1 demonstrates a pronounced vertical trabecular pattern. The cortical shell appears to be outlined in white around the more radiotranslucent vertebral body. These vertebrae would be classified as Grade II.

The Singh Index

The Singh Index is a qualitative morphometric technique that was similarly based on trabecular patterns, but based on those seen in the proximal femur *(3)*. Singh and others had noted that there appeared to be a predictable pattern to the disappearance of the five groups of trabeculae in the proximal femur in osteoporosis. Based on this order of disappearance, radiographs of the proximal femur could be graded 1 through 6 with lower values indicating a greater loss of the trabecular patterns normally seen in the proximal femur. Studies evaluating prevalent fractures demonstrated a good association between Singh Index values of 3 or less and the presence of fractures of the hip, spine, or wrist. Figure 1-2 shows a proximal femur with a Singh Index of 2. Only the trabecular pattern known as the principle compressive group, which extends from the medial cortex of the shaft to the upper portion of the head of the femur, remains. This patient was known to have had osteoporotic spine fractures, as well as a contralateral proximal femur fracture. Subsequent attempts to demonstrate a strong correlation of Singh Index values and bone density of the proximal femur, measured by dual-photon absorptiometry, have not been successful *(4)*. These qualitative morphometric techniques were highly subjective. In general, the best

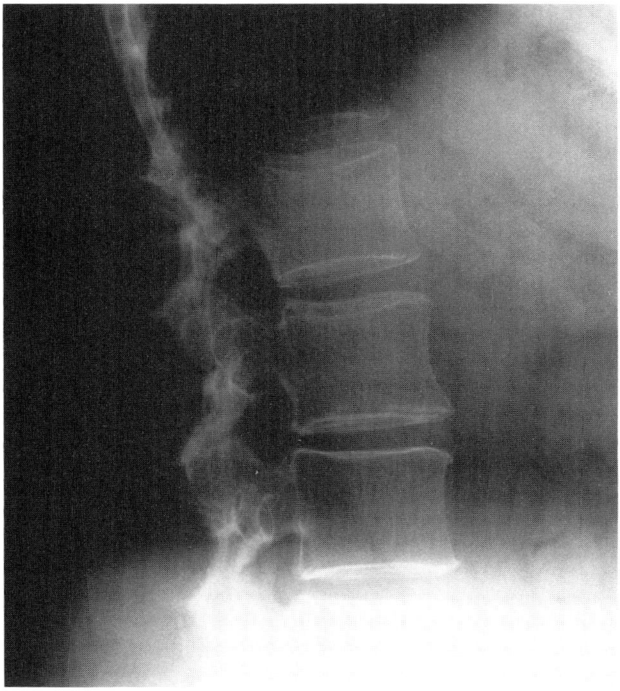

Fig. 1-1. Qualitative spinal morphometry. The vertebrae on this lateral lumbar spine film exhibit marked accentuation of the vertical trabecular pattern and thinning of the cortical shell. This is a Grade II spine.

approach required the creation of a set of reference radiographs of the various grades to which all other radiographs could be compared.

QUANTITATIVE MORPHOMETRIC TECHNIQUES: *CALCAR FEMORALE* THICKNESS, RADIOGRAMMETRY, AND THE RADIOLOGIC OSTEOPOROSIS SCORE

Calcar Femorale Thickness

A little-known quantitative morphometric technique involves the measurement of the thickness of the *calcar femorale*. The *calcar femorale* is the band of cortical bone immediately above the lesser trochanter in the proximal femur. In normal subjects, this thickness is >5 mm. In femoral fracture cases, it is generally <5 mm in thickness *(5)*. The arrow seen in Fig. 1-2 is pointing to the *calcar femorale*. This patient had previously suffered a femoral neck fracture. The thickness of the *calcar femorale* measured 4 mm.

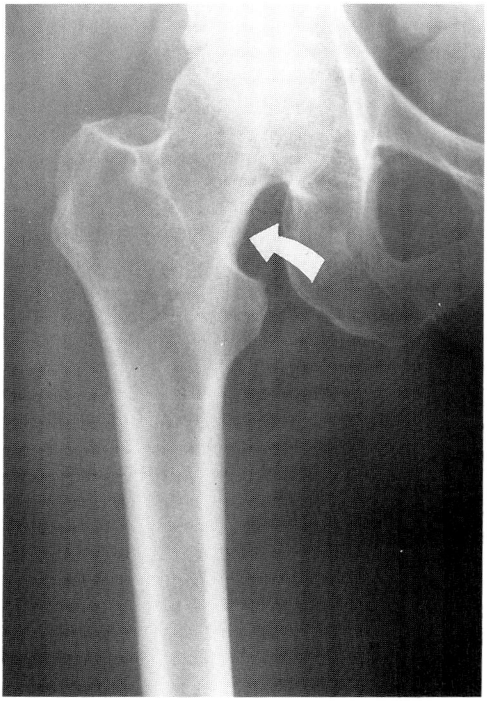

Fig. 1-2. The Singh Index and *calcar femorale* thickness. A Grade 2 Singh Index would be assessed here indicating the presence of osteoporosis. The arrow points to the *calcar femorale*, which measured 4 mm in thickness. Values <5 mm are associated with hip fracture.

Radiogrammetry

Radiogrammetry is the measurement of the dimensions of the bones using skeletal radiographs. Metacarpal radiogrammetry has been in use for over 30 years. The cortical width of the metacarpal was measured in one of two ways. Using a plain radiograph of the hand, and fine calipers or transparent ruler, the total width and medullary width of the metacarpals of the index, long, and ring fingers were measured at the midpoint of the metacarpal. The cortical width was calculated by subtracting the medullary width from the total width. Alternatively, the cortical width could be measured directly. A variety of different calculations were then made, including the metacarpal index (MI) and the hand score (HS). The MI is the cortical width divided by the total width. The HS, which is also known as the percent cortical thickness, is the MI expressed as a percentage. Measurements on the middle three metacarpals of both hands were also made, and used to calculate the six metacarpal hand score (6HS).

Other quantities derived from these measurements included the percent cortical area (%CA), the cortical area (CA), and the cortical area to surface area ratio (CA/SA). The main limitation in all of these measurements is that they were based on the false assumption that the point at which these measurements were made on the metacarpal was a perfect hollow cylinder. Nevertheless, using these measurements and knowledge of the gravimetric density of bone, the bone density, bone ash, and bone calcium could be calculated. The correlation between such measurements and ashed bone is good, ranging from 0.79 to 0.85 *(6,7)*. The precision of metacarpal morphometry is quite variable, depending on the measurement used.* The measurement of total width is very reproducible. The measurement of medullary width, or the direct measurement of cortical width, is less reproducible, because the delineation between the cortical bone and medullary canal is not as distinct as the delineation between the cortical bone and soft tissue. Precision has been variously reported as excellent to poor, but, in expert hands, it is possible to achieve a precision of 1.9% *(8)*.

Although metacarpal radiogrammetry is an old technique, and is somewhat tedious to perform, it remains a viable means of assessing bone density in the metacarpals. Metacarpal radiogrammetry demonstrates a reasonably good correlation to bone density at other skeletal sites measured with photon absorptiometric techniques *(9)*. The technique is very safe, because the biologically significant radiation dose from a hand X ray is extremely low, at only 1 mrem.

Radiogrammetry can also be performed at other sites, such as the phalanx, distal radius, and femur *(10–12)*. Combined measurements of the cortical widths of the distal radius and the second metacarpal have been shown to be highly correlated with bone density in the spine as measured by dual-photon absorptiometry *(10)*.

The Radiologic Osteoporosis Score

The radiologic osteoporosis score combined aspects of both quantitative and qualitative morphometry *(12)*. Developed by Barnett and Nordin, this scoring system utilized radiogrammetry of the femoral shaft and metacarpal, as well as an index of biconcavity of the lumbar vertebra. In calculating what Barnett and Nordin called a peripheral score, the cortical thickness of the femoral shaft divided by the diameter of the shaft, and

*Techniques are often compared on the basis of accuracy and reproducibility. Both are usually described with percent coefficients of variation (%CV). The %CV is the standard deviation (SD) divided by the mean of replicate measurements expressed as a percentage. The lower the %CV, the better the accuracy or reproducibility. Precision, accuracy, and %CV are discussed in detail in Chapters 3 and 4.

expressed as a percentage, was added to a similar measurement of the metacarpal. A score of 88 or less was considered to indicate peripheral osteoporosis. The biconcavity index was calculated by dividing the middle height, usually of the third lumbar vertebra, by its anterior height, and expressing this value as a percentage. A biconcavity index of 80 or less indicated spinal osteoporosis. Combining both the peripheral score and biconcavity index resulted in the total radiologic osteoporosis score, which was considered to indicate osteoporosis if the value was 168 or less.

RADIOGRAPHIC PHOTODENSITOMETRY

Much of the development of the modern techniques of single- and dual-photon absorptiometry and dual-energy X-ray absorptiometry actually came from early work on the X-ray-based method of photodensitometry *(13)*. In photodensitometry, broad-beam X-ray exposures of radiographs were obtained and the density of the skeletal image was quantified using a scanning photodensitometer. The effects of variations in technique, such as exposure settings, beam energy, and film development, were partially compensated by the simultaneous exposure of a step wedge of known densities on the film. An aluminum wedge was most often used, but other materials, such as ivory, were also employed *(11)*. This technique could only be applied to areas of the skeleton in which the soft-tissue coverage was less than 5 cm, such as the hand, forearm, and os calcis, because of technical limitations caused by scattered radiation in thicker parts of the body, and beam hardening, or the preferential attenuation of the softer energies of the polychromatic X-ray beam as it passed through the body. It was also used in cadaver studies of the proximal femur *(14)*. Such studies noted the predictive power for hip fracture of the density of the region in the proximal femur known as Ward's triangle* 30 years before the prospective studies of Cummings et al., using the modern technique of dual-energy X-ray absorptiometry in 1993 *(15)*. The accuracy of such measurements was fairly good, with a %CV of 5%. The correlation between metacarpal photodensitometry and ashed bone was high, at 0.88 *(6)*. This is a slightly better correlation than that seen with metacarpal radiogrammetry. The precision of photodensitometry was not as good, however, ranging from 5 to 15% *(16)*. By comparison, the 6HS was superior *(2)*. Radiation dose to the hand was the same for metacarpal radiogrammetry and radiographic photodensitometry. In both cases, the biologically significant radiation dose was negligible.

*Ward's triangle was first described by F. O. Ward in *Outlines of Human Osteology*, London, Henry Renshaw, 1838. It is a triangular region created by the intersection of three groups of trabeculae in the femoral neck.

Radiographic photodensitometry was developed and used extensively by researchers Pauline Beery Mack and George Vose *(17)*. Many of the original studies of the effects of weightlessness on the skeleton in the Gemini and Apollo astronauts were performed by Mack and her colleagues at Texas Woman's University *(18)*.

RADIOGRAPHIC ABSORPTIOMETRY (RA)

Radiographic absorptiometry (RA) is the modern-day descendant of radiographic photodensitometry *(19,20)*. The ability to digitize high-resolution radiographic images, and to perform computerized analysis of such images, has largely eliminated the errors introduced by differences in radiographic exposure techniques and overlying soft-tissue thickness. As performed in the United States, RA of the hand requires two X rays of the left hand using nonscreened film, each taken at slightly different exposures. The initial recommended settings are 50 kVp at 300 mA for 1 second and 60 kVp at 300 mA for 1 second. The exact settings will vary slightly with the equipment used, and are adjusted so that the background optical density of each of the two hand films matches a sample film supplied by the RA analysis facility. An aluminum alloy reference wedge, also supplied by the analysis facility, is placed on the film prior to exposure, parallel to the middle phalanx of the index finger. The developed films are sent to the RA analysis facility for analysis. The X-ray images are then captured electronically with a high-resolution video camera. The average density of the middle phalanxes of the index, long, and ring fingers is reported in RA units. Figure 1-3 illustrates the X-ray appearance of the hand and aluminum alloy reference wedge. Other manufacturers are employing updated RA techniques, such as the Bonalyzer (Teijin, Tokyo) and the Osteoradiometer (NIM, Verona, Italy).

In cadaveric studies, the accuracy of RA for the assessment of bone mineral content of the middle phalanxes is very good *(21)*. The correlation between the RA values and the ashed weight in the phalanxes is excellent, with $r = 0.983$. The accuracy was 4.8%. The authors of this study did note that increasing thicknesses of soft tissue that might be seen in very obese subjects could potentially result in an underestimation of RA values. The short-term reproducibility of these measurements is also excellent, at 0.6%.

The ability to predict bone density at other skeletal sites from hand RA is as good as that seen with other techniques, such as single-photon absorptiometry, dual-photon absorptiometry, dual-energy X-ray absorptiometry, or quantitative computed tomography of the spine *(19,22)*. This does not mean that RA hand values can be used to accurately predict bone density at other skeletal sites. Although the correlations between the different sites, as measured by the various techniques, are correctly said to be

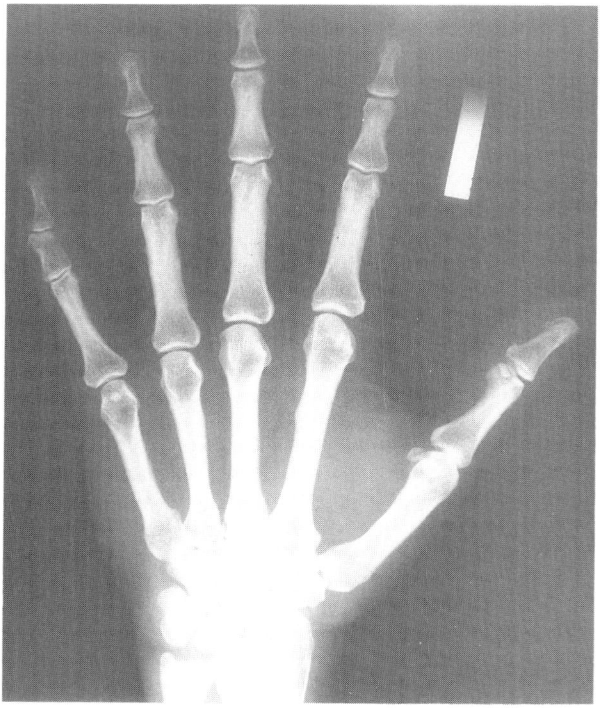

Fig. 1-3. Radiographic absorptiometry. The aluminum step wedge is seen, positioned adjacent and parallel to the middle phalanx of the index finger.

statistically significant, the correlations are too weak to allow clinically useful predictions of bone mass or density at one site from measurement at another.

The utility of modern-day RA in predicting hip fracture risk is suggested by a recent analysis of data acquired during the first National Health and Nutrition Examination Survey (NHANES I, 1971–1975). During this survey, 1559 hand radiographs of Caucasian women were obtained with the older technique of photodensitometry, using the Texas Woman's University wedge *(23)*. During a median follow-up of 14 years, which extended through 1987, 51 hip fractures occurred. Based on radiographic photodensitometry of the second phalanx of the small finger of the left hand, the age-adjusted relative risk for hip fracture per SD decline in bone density was 1.66. These films were reanalyzed using RA, with some compensation for the differences in technique. This reanalysis yielded an increase in relative risk for hip fracture per SD decline in RA bone density to 1.81. A technique such as RA has the obvious advantages of ease of performance and wide-spread geographic accessibility, since standard X-ray equipment is used. The costs of RA include the costs of the X-ray film, the aluminum alloy reference wedge, which is reusable, the performance of two hand films, and postage to, and analysis costs from, the RA analysis facility. In general, these total costs will approach or equal the average cost of bone-density testing with single-photon, dual-photon, or dual-energy X-ray absorptiometry.

PHOTON ABSORPTIOMETRY TECHNIQUES

In radiology, attenuation refers to a reduction in the number and energy of photons in an X-ray beam, or its intensity. To a large extent, the attenuation of X rays is determined by tissue density. A difference in tissue densities is responsible for creating the images seen on an X ray. The more dense the tissue, the more electrons it contains. The number of electrons in the tissue determines the ability of the tissue to either attenuate or transmit the photons in the X-ray beam. The differences in the pattern of transmitted or attenuated photons creates the contrast necessary to discern images on the X ray. If all the photons were attenuated (or none were transmitted), no image would be seen, because the film would be totally white. If all of the photons were transmitted (or none were attenuated), no image would be seen, because the film would be totally black. The difference in the attenuation of the X-ray photon energy by different tissues is responsible for the contrast on an X ray, which enables the images to be seen. If the degree of attenuation could be quantified, it would be possible to quantitatively assess the tissue density as well. This is the premise behind photon absorptiometry and the measurement of bone density.

Single-Photon Absorptiometry (SPA)

Writing in the journal *Science* in 1963, Cameron and Sorenson *(24)* described a new method for determining bone density in vivo by passing a monochromatic or single-energy photon beam through bone and soft tissue. The amount of mineral in the path transversed by the beam could be quantified, based on the difference between the beam intensity before and after passage through the region of interest. In the earliest single-photon absorptiometry (SPA) units, the results of multiple-scan passes at a single location, usually the midradius, were averaged *(25)*. In later units, scan passes at equally spaced intervals along the bone were utilized, so that the mass of mineral per unit of bone length could be calculated. A scintillation detector was used to quantify the photon energy after attenuation by the bone and soft tissue in the scan path. The photon source and the detector are both highly collimated, which means that the size and shape of the beam are restricted. Both move in tandem across the region of interest on the

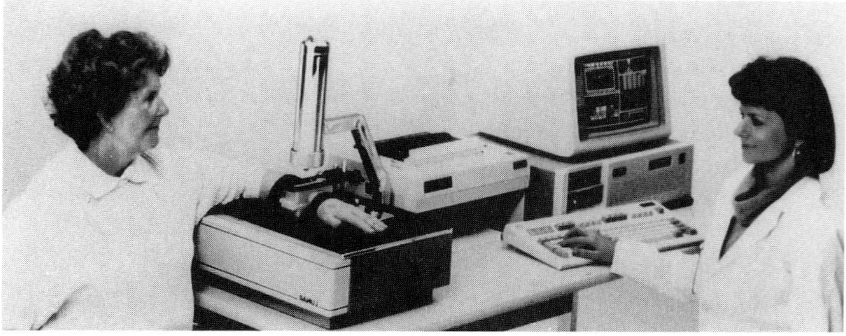

Fig. 1-4. SPA of the radius. Photo courtesy of Lunar Corp.

bone, coupled by a mechanical motor drive system. Iodine-125 at 27.3 keV, or americium-241 at 59.6 keV, were originally used to generate the single-energy photon beam, although most SPA units subsequently developed in the United States employed only ^{125}I.

The physical calculations for SPA determinations of bone mineral are valid only when there is uniform thickness of the bone and soft tissue in the scan path. In order to artificially create this kind of uniform thickness, the limb to be studied had to be submerged in a water bath, or surrounded by a tissue-equivalent material. As a practical matter, this limited SPA to measurements of the distal appendicular skeleton, such as the radius, and, later, the calcaneus. Figure 1-4 illustrates a patient undergoing an SPA study of the midradius. Although difficult to see in the photograph, the area of interest in the forearm is wrapped with a tissue-equivalent gel-filled bag to produce the necessary uniform thickness. After the photon attenuation is quantified, the determination of the amount of bone mineral is based on a comparison to the photon attenuation seen with a calibration standard derived from dried, defatted, human ashed bone of known weight.

SPA is both accurate and precise, although these parameters will vary slightly with the site studied. For SPA measurements of the midradius, accuracy has been reported as ranging from 3 to 5%, and precision as ranging from 1 to 2% *(24,26–28)*. In expert hands, the precision of midradial measurements should approach 1%. Early measurements of the distal and ultradistal radius did not demonstrate the same high degree of precision, primarily because of the marked changes in composition of the bone, with very small changes in location within the distal and ultradistal radius. With newer instruments, which employ computer-enhanced localization routines and rectilinear scanning, SPA measurements of the distal and ultradistal radius should approach a precision of 1% *(29)*. Accuracy and precision of measurements at the os calcis with SPA have been reported to be <3% *(27)*. The skin-radiation dose for both the radius and os calcis is 5–10 mrem *(27,28)*. The biologically important radiation dose is negligible. Results are reported as either bone mineral content (BMC) in grams or as bone mineral content per unit length (BMD/l) in g/cm. The time required to perform such studies is approximately 10 minutes. The cost for SPA studies of the appendicular skeleton ranges from $35 to $125 *(28,30)*.

The ability to predict the risk of appendicular fractures with SPA measurements of the radius is well established *(31–33)*. SPA measurements of the radius also appear to be good predictors of fracture risk of the spine, and good predictors of global fracture risk *(31,34,35)*. The prediction of fracture risk is discussed in detail in Chapter 6.

Dual-Photon Absorptiometry (DPA)

The basic principle involved in dual-photon absorptiometry (DPA) for the measurement of bone density is the same as for SPA: the ability to quantify the degree of attenuation of a photon energy beam after passage through bone and soft tissue. In dual-photon systems, however, an isotope that emits photon energy at two distinct photoelectric peaks, or two isotopes, each emitting photon energy at separate and distinct photoelectric peaks, are used. When the beam is passed through a region of the body containing both bone and soft tissue, attenuation of the photon beam will occur at both energy peaks. If one energy peak is preferentially attenuated by bone, however, the contributions of soft tissue in beam attenuation can be mathematically subtracted *(36)*. As in SPA, the remaining contributions of beam attenuation from bone can be quantified and then compared to standards created from ashed bone. The ability to separate bone from soft tissue in this manner finally allowed quantification of the bone density in those areas of the skeleton that were surrounded by large or irregular soft tissue masses, notably the spine and proximal femur. DPA can also be used to determine total-body bone density. The development of DPA, and its application to the spine, proximal femur, and total body, is attributed to a number of investigators: Dunn, Wahner, and Riggs *(37)*; Reed *(38)*; Roos *(39)*; Mazess *(40)*; Wilson and Madsen *(41)*; and Peppler *(42)*.

The isotope most commonly employed in DPA is gadolinium-153, which naturally emits photon energy at two photoelectric peaks, 44 and 100 keV. It is the photoelectric peak of 44 keV at which bone preferentially attenuates the photon energy. The attenuated photon beams are detected by a NaI scintillation detector, and quantified after passage through pulse-height analyzers set at 44 and 100 keV. The shielded holder for the ^{153}Gd source, which is collimated and equipped with a shutter that is operated by a computer, moves in tandem with the NaI detector in a rectilinear scan

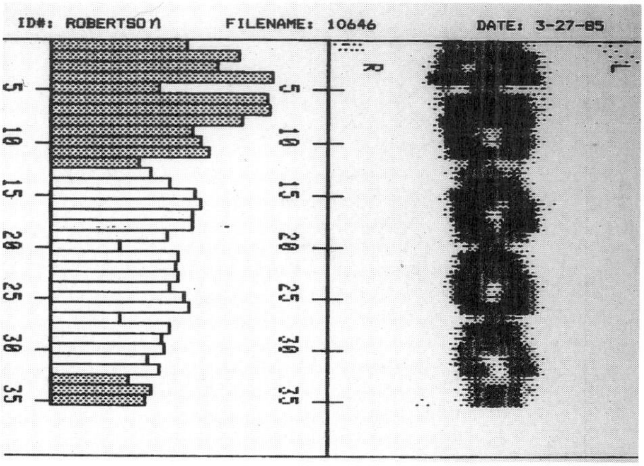

Fig. 1-5. The intensity-modulated image of the spine created with an early DPA device.

path over the region of interest. A point-by-point calculation of bone density in the scan path can be made. Figure 1-5 is the intensity-modulated image of the spine created with an early DPA device. Figure 1-6 demonstrates the intensity-modulated images of the same spine created with a later DPA device, and newer pencil-beam and fan-array dual-energy X-ray absorptiometers.

Bone-density studies of the lumbar spine are performed with the photon energy beam passing in a posterior-to-anterior (PA) direction. Because of the direction of the beam, the vertebral body and the posterior elements are included in the scan path. The transverse processes are eliminated. This results in a combined measurement of cortical and trabecular bone, which includes the more trabecular vertebral body surrounded by its cortical shell and the highly cortical posterior elements. The results are reported as an areal density in grams of mineral per square centimeter of bone (g/cm^2) of mineral. The bone mineral density of the proximal femur is also an areal density that is acquired with the beam passing in a posterior to anterior direction. Figure 1-7 shows an early DPA device, with the patient positioned for a study of the lumbar spine.

DPA studies of the spine require approximately 30 minutes to complete. Studies of the proximal femur take 30–45 minutes to perform. Total-body bone density studies with DPA require 1 hour. Skin radiation dose is low during spine or proximal femur studies, at 15 mrem. Accuracy of DPA measurements of the spine ranges from 3 to 6%, and, for the proximal femur, 3 to 4% *(43)*. Precision for measurements of spine bone density is 2–4%, and around 4% for the femoral neck. The cost of a DPA study of

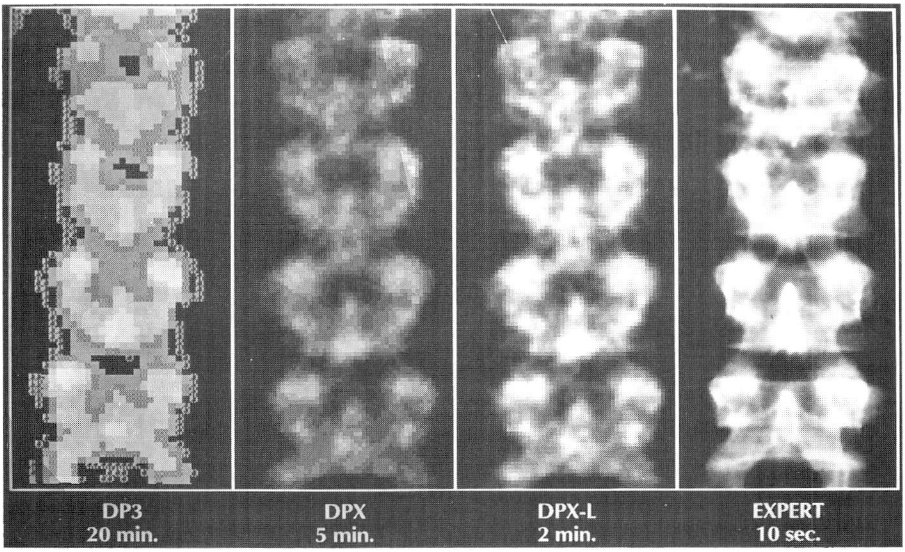

Fig. 1-6. An intensity-modulated image of the spine of the same patient created with four different devices. From left to right, a late DPA device, early DXA pencil-beam device, late DXA pencil-beam device, and a fan-array DXA device. Photo courtesy of Lunar Corp.

the spine or proximal femur ranges from $125 to $200 or $75 to $125, respectively *(27,30)*.

DPA was considered a major advance from SPA, because it allowed the quantification of bone density in the spine and proximal femur. DPA does have several limitations, however. Machine maintenance is expensive. The ^{153}Gd source must be replaced yearly, at a cost of approximately $5000 or more. It has also been noted that, as the radioactive source decays, values obtained with DPA increase by as much as 0.6%/month *(44)*. With replacement of the source, values may fall by as much as 6.2%. Although mathematical formulas have been developed to compensate for this effect of source decay, it remains a cause for concern, potentially affecting both accuracy and reproducibility. The precision of 2–4% for DPA measurements of the spine and proximal femur limited its application for serial measurements of bone density. Two measurements performed with a technique that has a precision of 2% will yield a difference that is accurate at a 95% confidence level within ±5.5%. If the precision is only 4%, the resulting difference is accurate to within ±11.1% *(45)*. Even at an 80% confidence level, these numbers fall to only ±3.6 and ±7.3%, respectively. Using only two measurements creates a margin of error that is too great to

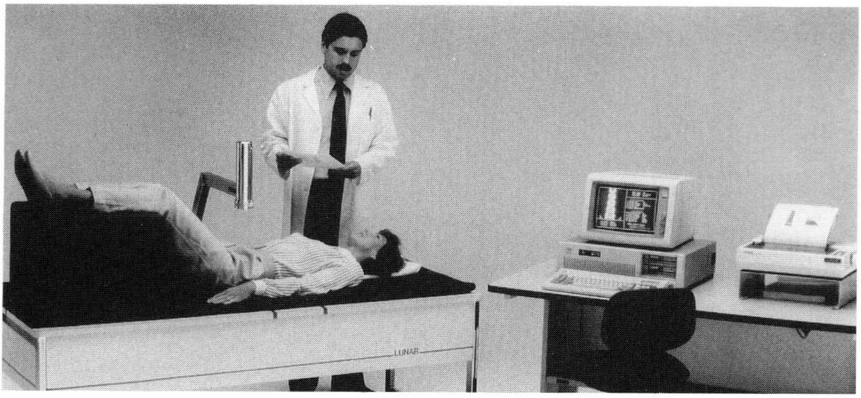

Fig. 1-7. DPA of the spine. Photo courtesy of Lunar Corp.

be clinically useful in following changes in bone density over time. Although these ranges can be narrowed by performing multiple measurements within a given period of time, this increases the costs associated with the testing, which similarly serves to reduce its clinical utility in this regard.

As a practical matter, all spine bone-density studies in which the photon beam passes in an AP or PA direction will be unable to separate the highly trabecular vertebral body from its more cortical posterior elements. Calcifications in the overlying soft tissue or abdominal aorta will attenuate such a beam, falsely elevating the bone-density values. Arthritic changes in the posterior elements of the spine will also affect the measurement *(46)*. This is discussed in greater detail in Chapter 2.

The ability to make site-specific predictions of fracture risk of the spine and proximal femur, or global fracture-risk predictions, with DPA has been established in prospective trials *(15,34)*.

Dual-Energy X-Ray Absorptiometry (DXA)

The underlying principles of dual-energy X-ray absorptiometry (DXA) are the same as those of DPA. With DXA, however, the radioactive isotope source of photon energy has been replaced by an X-ray tube. There are several advantages of X-ray sources over radioactive isotopes. There is no source decay that would otherwise require costly replacement of the radioactive source. Similarly, there is no concern of a drift in patient values caused by source decay. The greater source intensity, or photon flux, produced by the X-ray tube, and the smaller focal spot, allows for better beam collimation, which results in less dose overlap between scan lines and greater image resolution. Scan times are faster, and precision is improved.

Because X-ray tubes produce a beam that spans a wide range of photon energies, the beam must be narrowed in some fashion in order to produce the two distinct photoelectric peaks necessary to separate bone from soft tissue. The major manufacturers of dual-energy X-ray absorptiometers in the United States have chosen to do this in one of two ways. Lunar Corp. of Madison, WI, and Norland Medical Systems, Inc. of Fort Atkinson, WI, use rare earth K-edge filters to produce two distinct photoelectric peaks. Hologic, Inc., of Waltham, MA, uses a pulsed power source to the X-ray tube to create the same effect.

K-edge filters produce an X-ray beam with a high number of photons in a specific energy range, which is just above the K-absorption edge of the tissue in question. The K-edge is the binding energy of the K-shell electron. This energy level varies from tissue to tissue. The importance of the K-edge is that at photon energies just above this level, the transmission of photons through the tissue in question drops dramatically; that is, the photons are maximally attenuated at this energy level *(47)*. Therefore, to separate bone from soft tissue in a quantifiable fashion, the energy of the photon beam should be just above the K-edge of bone or soft tissue for maximum attenuation. Lunar uses a cerium (Ce) filter that has a K-shell absorption edge at 40 keV. A Ce-filtered X-ray spectrum at 80 kV will contain two photoelectric peaks at about 40 and 70 keV. The samarium (Sm) K-edge filter employed by Norland has a K-shell absorption edge of 46.8 keV. The Sm-filtered X-ray beam at 100 kV produces a low-energy peak at 46.8 keV. In the Norland system, the high-energy peak is variable, because the system employs selectable levels of filtration, but the photons are limited to less than 100 keV by the 100 kV employed. The K-edge of both Ce and Sm results in a low-energy peak, which approximates the 44 keV low-energy peak of ^{153}Gd used in most dual-photon systems.

The Hologic dual-energy X-ray absorptiometer utilizes a different system to produce the two photoelectric peaks necessary to separate bone from soft tissue. Instead of employing K-edge filtering of the X-ray beam, Hologic employs alternating pulses to the X-ray source at 70 and 140 kV.

Most regions of the skeleton are accessible with DXA. Studies can be made of the spine in both an anterior–posterior* and lateral direction. Although access to the lumbar spine in the lateral projection is limited by rib overlap of L1, and L2, and pelvic overlap of L4, the lateral projection

*Although spine bone-density studies with DXA are often referred to as AP spine studies, the beam actually passes in a posterior-to-anterior direction. Such studies are correctly characterized as PA spine studies, but it has become an accepted convention to refer to them as AP spine bone-density studies. One of the new fan-array DXA scanners, the Lunar Expert, does perform AP spine studies.

offers the ability to eliminate the confounding effects of dystrophic calcification on densities measured in the AP direction *(48)*. Lateral scans also eliminate the highly cortical posterior elements, which contribute as much as 47% of the mineral content measured in the AP direction *(49)*. The proximal femur, radius, calcaneus, and total body can also be evaluated with DXA.

Scan times are dramatically shorter with DXA compared to DPA. Early DXA units required approximately 4 minutes for studies of the AP spine or proximal femur. Total body studies required 20 minutes in the medium-scan mode and only 10 minutes in the fast-scan mode. Later DXA units scan even faster, with studies of the AP spine or proximal femur requiring only 2 minutes to perform.

The values obtained with dual-energy X-ray studies of the skeleton are highly correlated with values from earlier studies performed with DPA. Consequently, its accuracy is considered comparable to that of DPA *(50–53)*. DXA spine values, and Hologic and Norland DXA proximal femur values, are consistently lower than values obtained with DPA. There are also differences in the values obtained with DXA equipment from the three major manufacturers. Values obtained with either a Hologic or Norland DXA unit are consistently lower than those obtained with a Lunar DXA unit, although all are highly correlated with each other *(54–56)*. Comparison studies using all three manufacturers' equipment have resulted in formulas that allow for conversion of the values between manufacturers, but the margin of error in such conversions is too large to make such comparisons clinically useful. The development of a universal standard to which the machines could be calibrated, or a standardized bone mineral density, should eliminate this problem in the future. The conversion of data from one manufacturer to another, and the standardized BMD, is discussed in Chapter 8.

Radiation exposure with dual-energy X-ray equipment is extremely low for all scan types. Expressed as skin dose, radiation exposure during an AP spine or proximal femur study is only 2–5 mrem. The biologically important effective dose, or whole-body equivalent dose, is only 0.1 mrem *(57)*.

Perhaps the most significant advance seen with DXA is the marked improvement in precision. Expressed as a coefficient of variation, short-term precision in normal subjects has been reported as low as 0.9% for the AP lumbar spine, and 1.4% for the femoral neck *(50)*. Precision studies over the course of 1 year have reported values of 1% for the lumbar spine and 1.7–2.3% for the femoral neck *(53)*.

DXA has been used in prospective studies to predict fracture risk. In one of the largest studies of its kind, DXA studies of the proximal femur were demonstrated to have the greatest predictive ability for hip fracture, compared to measurements at other sites with SPA or DPA *(15)*.

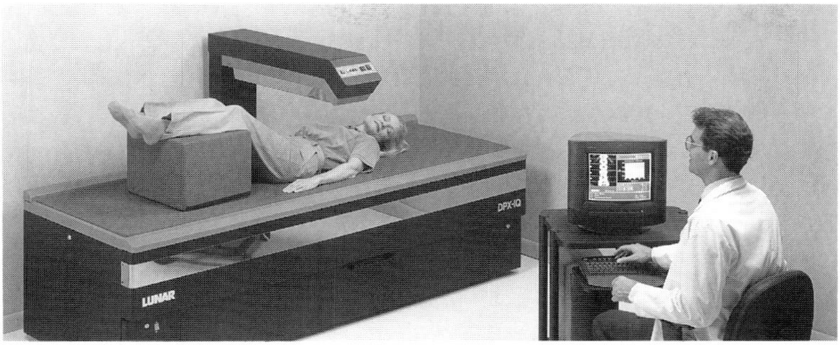

Fig. 1-8. The Lunar IQ, a DXA pencil-beam absorptiometer. Photo courtesy of Lunar.

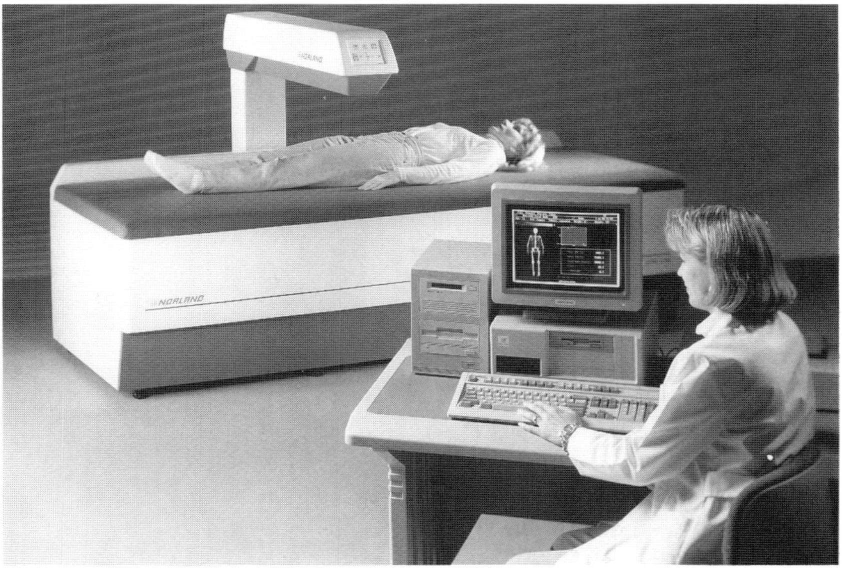

Fig. 1-9. The Norland XR-36, a DXA pencil-beam absorptiometer. Photo courtesy of Norland Corp.

Figures 1-8 to 1-10 are DXA units from the three major manufacturers in the United States. These units are considered first-generation DXA units, or pencil-beam scanners. The next generation of DXA scanners are fan-array scanners. The difference between these two types of scanners is illustrated in Figs. 1-11 and 1-12. Pencil-beam scanners employ a collimated X-ray beam that moves in tandem in a rectilinear pattern with a single detector, or, in the case of the Norland unit, two sequential detectors. Fan-array scanners employ an array of detectors, which obviates the need for a rectilinear scan path. Scan times are reduced to as short as 30 seconds

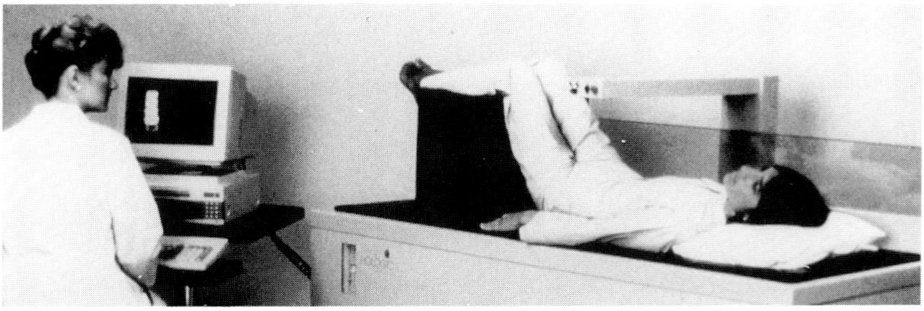

Fig. 1-10. The Hologic QDR 1000, a DXA pencil-beam absorptiometer. Photo courtesy of Hologic, Inc.

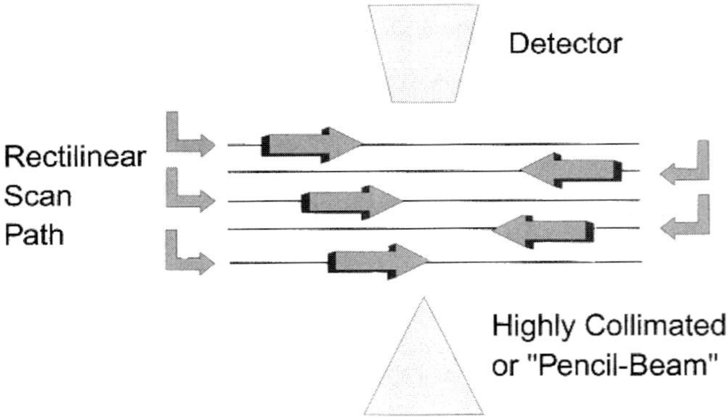

Fig. 1-11. Pencil-beam DXA absorptiometers. The detector and highly collimated X-ray beam move in tandem in a rectilinear scan path.

for a study of the spine in the AP direction. Figure 1-13 is the Lunar fan-array scanner, the Expert; Fig. 1-14 is the Hologic fan-array scanner, the QDR-4500. Image resolution is also enhanced with the fan-array scanners. Images of radiographic, or near-radiographic, quality can be obtained, as shown in Fig. 1-15. This has created a new application for bone densitometry scanning called morphometric X-ray absorptiometry, or MXA. With MXA, images of the spine obtained in the lateral projection can be used for computer analysis of the vertebral dimensions, and for diagnosis of vertebral fracture. It is also conceivable that MXA software will be developed to measure hip-axis length from studies of the proximal femur. Hip-axis length has been shown to be an independent predictor of hip-fracture risk *(58)*.

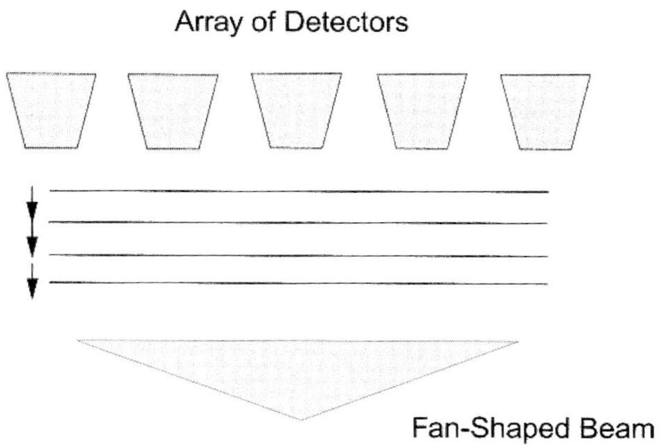

Fig. 1-12. Fan-array DXA absorptiometers. An array of detectors obviates the need for a rectilinear scan path. Data is acquired across an entire scan line simultaneously.

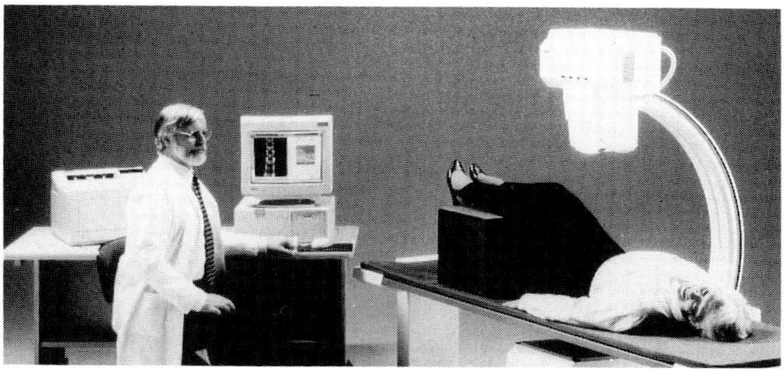

Fig. 1-13. The Lunar Expert, a fan-array DXA device. Photo courtesy of Lunar Corp.

DXA is progressively replacing older DPA units in most clinical sites. The improved scan times, improved image resolution, lower radiation dose, greater precision, greater flexibility in application to a variety of skeletal sites, and lower cost of operation give DXA clear advantages over DPA.

Peripheral DXA Units

Several new devices are now available that utilize dual-energy X-ray technology. These devices are unique, because they are dedicated to the measurement of one or two appendicular sites. As such, these devices are often characterized as peripheral devices. They tend to be small, compact,

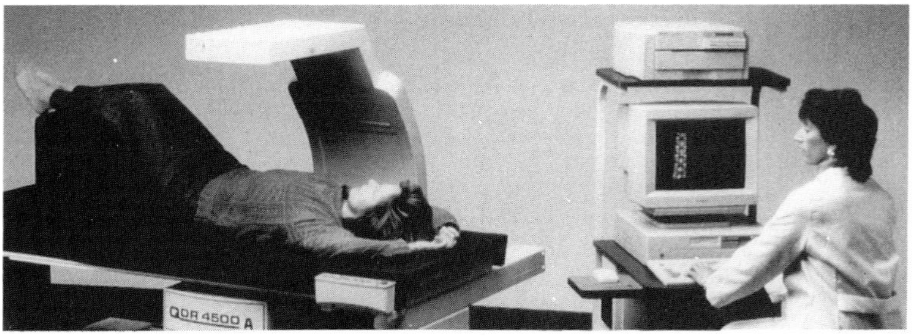

Fig. 1-14. The Hologic QDR 4500, a fan-array DXA device. Photo courtesy of Hologic, Inc.

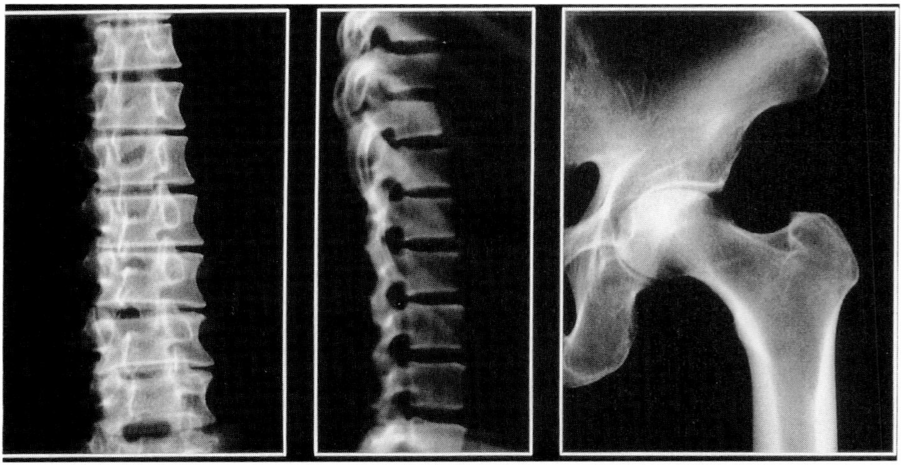

Fig. 1-15. Fan-array DXA Images. Photo courtesy of Lunar Corp.

and portable. Equipment costs are generally much less than the full-size central DXA units.

DTX-200

The DTX-200 (Fig. 1-16) is from Osteometer Meditech A/S, in Roedovre, Denmark. This portable device weighs approximately 79 lb (36 kg). It is a dual-energy, rectilinear scanner that uses a K-edge filter. The dimensions of the machine are 32" height × 24" depth × 12" width (80 × 62 × 30 cm). Measurements can be made of the ultradistal and distal sites on the forearm. Radiation exposure is reported as an effective dose of 0.01 mrem. Precision for the distal site is reported as 0.9%, and for the ultradistal site, 1.1%.

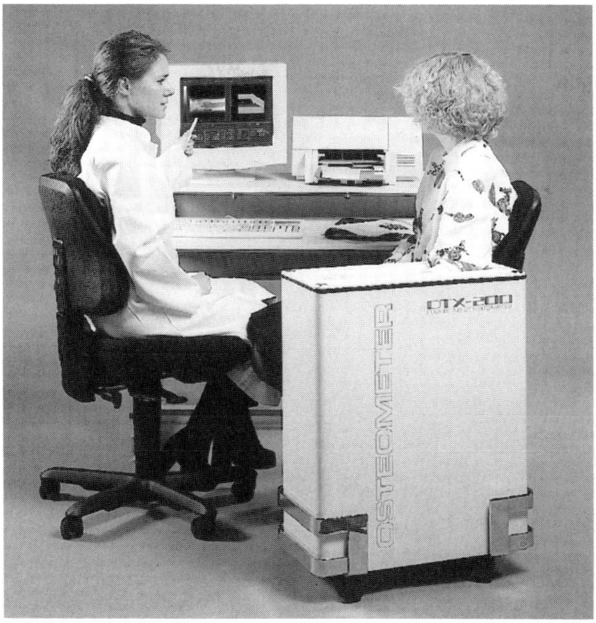

Fig. 1-16. The Osteometer DTX-200, a portable DXA device dedicated for measurements of bone density in the forearm. Photo courtesy of Osteometer MediTech A/S.

pDEXA

The Norland pDEXA® (Fig. 1-17) is a dual-energy X-ray densitometer that uses a tin K-edge filter to produce energy peaks at 28 and 48 keV. Bone density is quantified in the distal radius and ulna, the proximal (33%) radius and ulna, and the proximal radius alone. The device weighs 59 lb (27 kg) and measures 16.7" height × 17" depth × 20.5" width (42.5 × 43 × 52 cm). In vivo precision is reported as 0.88–1.5% for the distal radius and ulna, 1.07–1.4% for the proximal radius and ulna, and 1.10–1.68% for the proximal radius. Radiation exposure is reported as a skin dose of <2 mrem at standard scan speeds.

Peripheral Instantaneous X-Ray Imager (PIXI)

The Peripheral Instantaneous X-ray Imager, or PIXI™ (Fig. 1-18), utilizes a dual-energy high-voltage supply with a fixed anode tube. The device can be used to quantify the bone mass in either the forearm or calcaneus. Short-term precision in vivo is reported as 1.0–1.5%. The device weighs 55 lb (25 kg) and is 25" depth × 12" width × 13" height (63 × 30 × 33 cm) The radiation skin dose is 20 mrem. The PIXI is manufactured by Lunar.

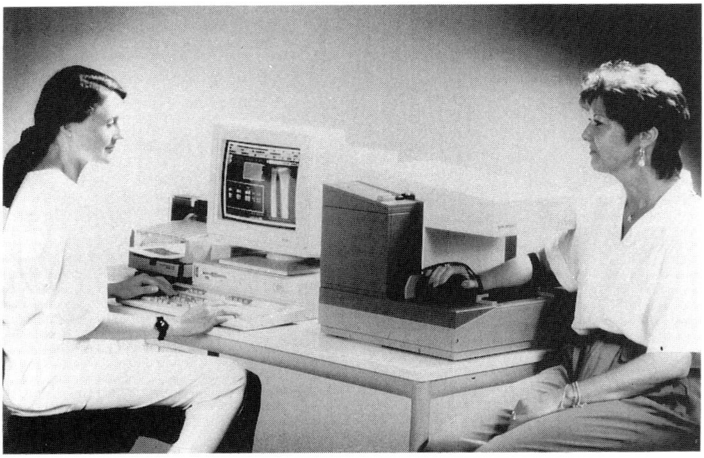

Fig. 1-17. The Norland pDEXA, a portable DXA device dedicated for measurements of bone density in the forearm. Photo courtesy of Norland.

Single-Energy X-Ray Absorptiometry (SXA)

Single-energy X-ray absorptiometry (SXA) is the X-ray-based counterpart of SPA, much as DXA is the X-ray-based counterpart of DPA. SXA units are being used to measure bone density in the distal radius and ulna and os calcis. Like their DXA counterparts, SXA units do not utilize radioactive isotopes, which reduces the cost of operating the equipment, and should result in more reliable long-term performance. The accuracy and precision of SXA appears to be comparable to SPA *(59)*.

Figure 1-19 is a photograph of the SXA 3000™, the OsteoAnalyzer from Norland Medical Systems, Inc., Ft. Atkinson, WI. This is a single-energy X-ray device that utilizes a K-edge tin filter to perform rectilinear scans of the calcaneus in under 4 minutes. This portable machine weighs approximately 45 lb (20.4 kg) and measures 14" height × 19" depth × 18" width (34.5 × 48.5 × 45.5 cm). Radiation exposure is reported to be a skin dose of 1.3 mrem.

Quantitative Computed Tomography (QCT)

Although quantitative computed tomography (QCT) is a photon absorptiometric technique like SPA, SXA, DPA, and DXA, it is unique in that it provides a three-dimensional image, which makes possible a direct measurement of density, and a spatial separation of trabecular from cortical bone. In 1976, Ruegsegger et al. *(60)* developed a dedicated peripheral quantitative CT scanner, using ^{125}I for measurements of the radius. Genant

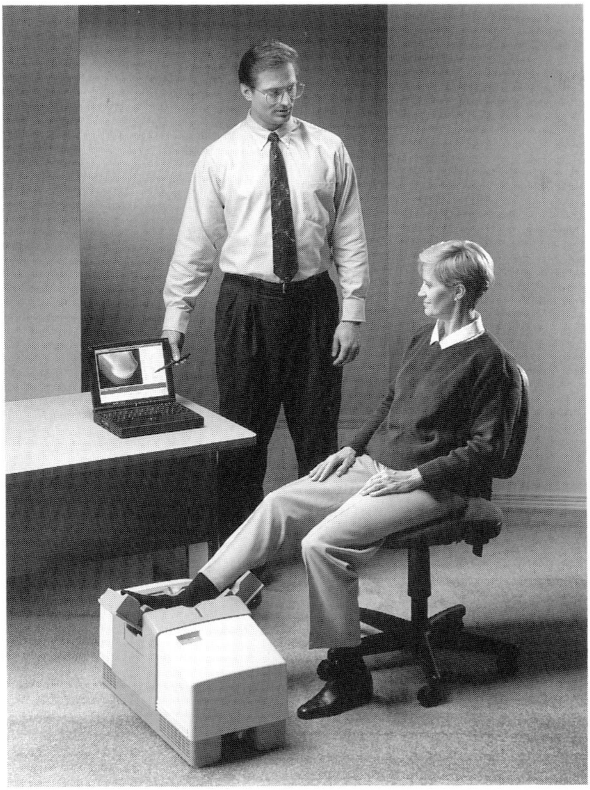

Fig. 1-18. The Lunar PIXI, a portable DXA device for measurements of bone density in the os calcis and forearm. Photo courtesy of Lunar.

and Cann *(61,62)* are credited with adapting commercially available CT scanners for the quantitative assessment of spinal bone density. It is this approach that has received the most widespread use in the United States, although dedicated CT units for the measurement of the peripheral skeleton, or pQCT units, are beginning to appear in clinical centers.

QCT studies of the spine utilize a reference standard or phantom, which is scanned simultaneously with the patient. The phantom, which contains varying concentrations of K_2HPO_4, is placed underneath the patient during the study. A scout view is required for localization, and then an 8–10-mm-thick slice is measured through the center of two or more vertebral bodies, which are generally selected from T12 to L3 *(63)*. A region of interest within the anterior portion of the vertebral body is analyzed for bone density, and is reported as mg/cm^3 K_2HPO_4 equivalents. This region of interest

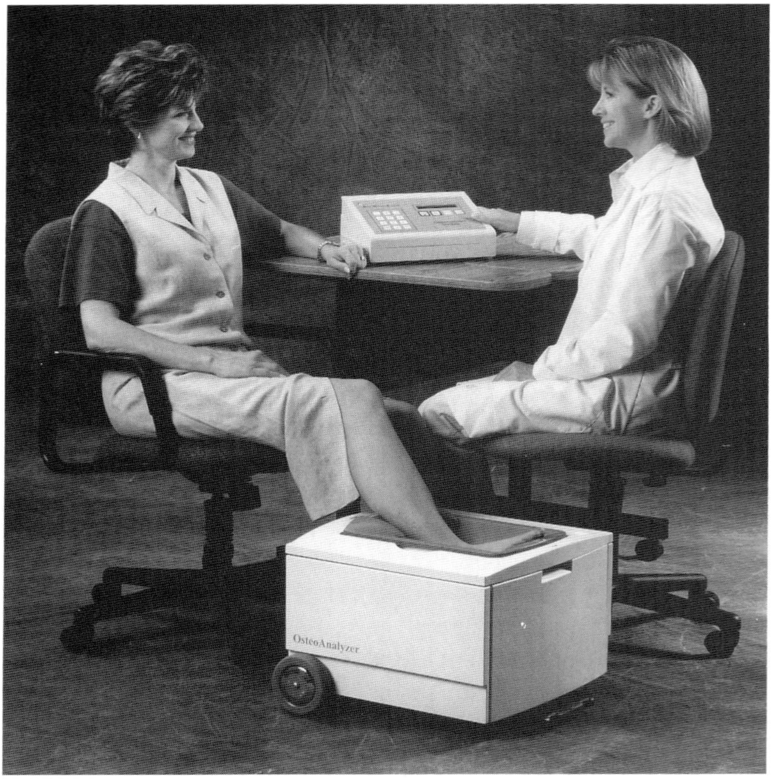

Fig. 1-19. The Norland Analyzer, a portable SXA device for measurement of bone density in the os calcis. Photo courtesy of Norland Medical Systems.

is carefully placed to avoid the cortical shell of the vertebral body. The result is a three-dimensional trabecular density, unlike the two-dimensional areal mixed cortical and trabecular densities reported with AP studies of the spine utilizing DPA or DXA. Figure 1-20 shows a QCT study of the spine.

A study of the spine with QCT requires about 30 minutes *(30)*. The skin-radiation dose is generally 100–300 mrem. This overestimates the biologically important effective radiation dose, because only a small portion of marrow is irradiated during a QCT study of the spine *(57)*. The effective dose, or whole-body equivalent dose, is generally in the range of only 3 mrem. The localizer scan that precedes the actual QCT study will add an additional 3 mrem to the effective dose. Nevertheless, these values are still quite acceptable in the context of natural background radiation of approximately 20 mrem per month. CT units, which, by their design are

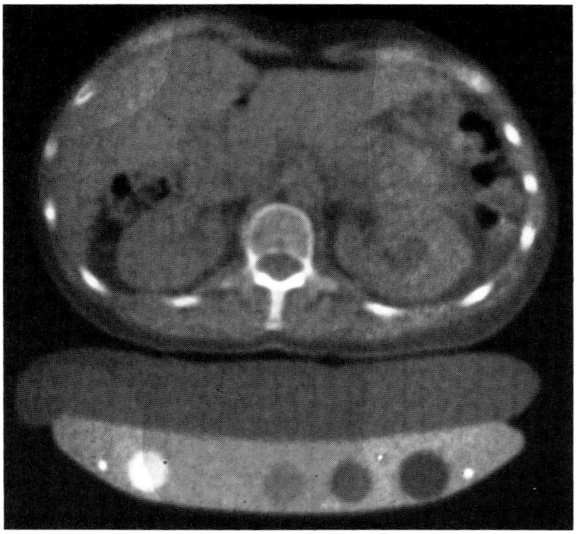

Fig. 1-20. QCT of the spine. The K_2HPO_4 phantom is seen underneath the patient. Photo courtesy of Dr. David Sartoris.

unable to utilize low kVp settings for QCT studies, may deliver skin and absorbed doses 3–10-× higher.

The accuracy of QCT for measurements of spine BMD is affected by the presence of marrow fat *(63–65)*. Marrow fat increases with age, resulting in an increasingly large error in the accuracy of spine QCT measurements in older patients. The accuracy of QCT is reported to range from 5 to 15%, depending on the age of the patient and percentage of marrow fat. The presence of marrow fat results in an underestimation of bone density in the young of about 20 mg/cm^3, and as much as 30 mg/cm^3 in the elderly *(63)*. The error introduced by marrow fat can be partially corrected by applying data on vertebral marrow fat with aging, originally developed by Dunnill et al. *(66)*. In an attempt to eliminate the error introduced by marrow fat, dual-energy QCT, or DEQCT, was developed by Genant and Boyd *(67)*. This method clearly reduced the error introduced by the presence of marrow fat, to as low as 1.4% in cadaveric studies *(64,65)*. In vivo, the accuracy with DEQCT is 3–6% *(30,63)*. Radiation dose with DEQCT is increased approximately 10-fold, compared to regular or single-energy QCT (SEQCT), and precision is not as good. The precision of SEQCT for vertebral measurements, in expert hands, is 1–3%, and for DEQCT, 3–5% *(63,68)*. Expertise in either SEQCT or DEQCT is, in the opinion of most, severely limited. The cost of a QCT spinal bone density measurement is around $150 *(30)*.

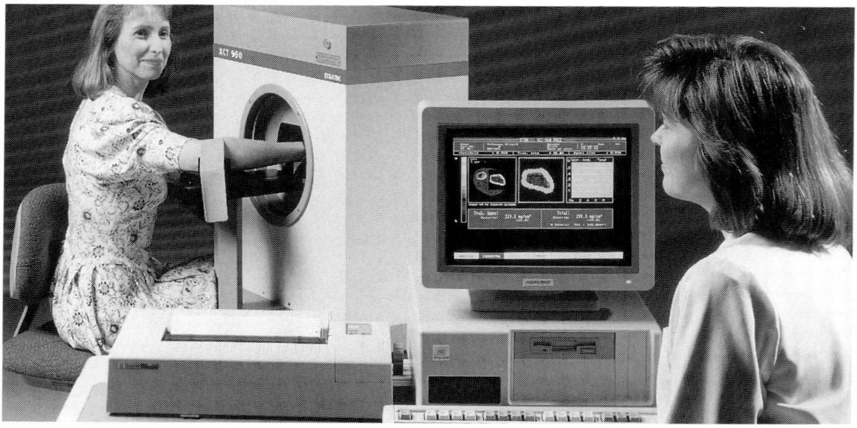

Fig. 1-21. The Norland/Stratec XCT 960, a peripheral QCT device dedicated for measurements of bone density in the forearm. Photo courtesy of Norland.

The ability to measure bone density in the proximal femur with QCT is also limited. Using both dedicated QCT and standard CT units, investigators have attempted to utilize QCT for measurements of the proximal femur *(69,70)*. This capability remains restricted to a few research centers.

QCT of the spine has been used in studies of prevalent osteoporotic fractures, and it is clear that such measurements can distinguish osteoporotic individuals from normal individuals as well as or even better than DPA *(71–74)*. Fractures are rare with values above 110 mg/cm^3 and extremely common below 60 mg/cm^3 *(75)*. Because QCT measures only trabecular bone, which is more metabolically active than cortical bone, rates of change in disease states observed with QCT spine measurements tend to be greater than those observed with AP spine studies performed with DPA or DXA *(61,76)*. This greater magnitude of change partially offsets the effects of the poorer precision seen with QCT, compared to DXA. The correlations between spine bone-density measurements with QCT and skeletal sites measured with other techniques are statistically significant, but too weak to allow accurate prediction of bone density at another site from measurement of the spine with QCT *(22,73,74)*.

Peripheral QCT

Peripheral QCT is becoming more widely available. These are dedicated units that are utilized primarily for the measurement of bone density in the forearm. Figure 1-21 is the Norland/Stratec XCT 960 pQCT™ X-ray Bone Densitometer, which is a peripheral QCT unit, designed to quantify the bone density in the forearm.

REFERENCES

1. Johnston CC, Epstein S (1981) Clinical, biochemical, radiographic, epidemiologic, and economic features of osteoporosis. *Orthop Clin North Am* 12:559–569.
2. Aitken M (1984) Measurement of bone mass and turnover, in *Osteoporosis in Clinical Practice*. Bristol: John Wright, pp. 19,20.
3. Singh J, Nagrath AR, Maini PS (1970) Changes in trabecular pattern of the upper end of the femur as an index of osteoporosis. *J Bone Joint Surg Am* 52-A:457–467.
4. Bohr H, Schadt O (1993) Bone mineral content of femoral bone and lumbar spine measured in women with fracture of the femoral neck by dual photon absorptiometry. *Clin Orthop* 179:240–245.
5. Nordin BEC (1983) Osteoporosis with particular reference to the menopause. In: Avioli LV, ed. *The Osteoporotic Syndrome*, New York: Grune and Stratton, pp. 13–44.
6. Shimmins J, Anderson JB, Smith DA, et al. (1972) The accuracy and reproducibility of bone mineral measurements "in vivo." (a) The measurement of metacarpal mineralisation using an X-ray generator. *Clin Radiol* 23:42–46.
7. Exton-Smith AN, Millard PH, Payne PR, Wheeler EF (1969) Method for measuring quantity of bone. *Lancet* 2:1153,1154.
8. Dequeker J (1982) Precision of the radiogrammetric evaluation of bone mass at the metacarpal bones. In: Dequeker J, Johnston CC, eds. *Non-invasive Bone Measurements: Methodological Problems*, Oxford: IRL Press, pp. 27–32.
9. Aitken JM, Smith CB, Horton PW, et al. (1974) The interrelationships between bone mineral at different skeletal sites in male and female cadavera. *J Bone Joint Surg Br* 56B:370–375.
10. Meema HE, Meindok H (1992) Advantages of peripheral radiogrammetry over dual-photon absorptiometry of the spine in the assessment of prevalence of osteoporotic vertebral fractures in women. *J Bone Miner Res* 7:897–903.
11. Bywaters EGL (1948) The measurement of bone opacity. *Clin Sci* 6:281–287.
12. Barnett E, Nordin BEC (1961) Radiologic assessment of bone density. 1. The clinical and radiological problem of thin bones. *Br J Radiol* 34:683–692.
13. Mack PB, Brown WN, Trapp HD (1949) The quantitative evaluation of bone density. *Am J Roentgenol Rad Ther* 61:808–825.
14. Vose GP, Mack PB (1963) Roentgenologic assessment of femoral neck density as related to fracturing. *Am J Roentgenol Rad Ther Nucl Med* 89:1296–1301.
15. Cummings SR, Black DM, Nevitt MC, et al. (1993) Bone density at various sites for prediction of hip fractures. *Lancet* 341:72–75.
16. Mazess RB (1983) Noninvasive methods for quantitating trabecular bone. In: Avioli LV, ed. *The Osteoporotic Syndrome*, New York: Grune and Stratton, pp. 85–114.
17. Mack PB, O'Brien AT, Smith JM, Bauman AW (1939) A method for estimating degree of mineralization of bones from tracings of roentgenograms. *Science* 89:467.
18. Mack PB, Vogt FB (1971) Roentgenographic bone density changes in astronauts during representative Apollo space flight. *Am J Roentgenol Rad Ther Nucl Med* 113:621–633.
19. Cosman F, Herrington B, Himmelstein S, Lindsay R. (1991) Radiographic absorptiometry: a simple method for determination of bone mass. *Osteoporosis Int* 2:34–38.
20. Yates AJ, Ross PD, Lydick E, Epstein RS (1995) Radiographic absorptiometry in the diagnosis of osteoporosis. *Am J Med* 98:41S–47S.
21. Yang S, Hagiwara S, Engelke K, et al. (1994) Radiographic absorptiometry for bone mineral measurement of the phalanges: precision and accuracy study. *Radiology* 192:857–859.

22. Kleerekoper M, Nelson DA, Flynn MJ, Pawluszka AS, Jacobsen G, Peterson EL (1994) Comparison of radiographic absorptiometry with dual-energy X-ray absorptiometry and quantitative computed tomography in normal older white and black women. *J Bone Miner Res* 9:1745–1749.
23. Mussolino ME, Looker AC, Madans JH, Edelstein D, Walker RE, Lydick E, Epstein RS, Yates AJ (1997) Phalangeal bone density and hip fracture risk. *Arch Intern Med* 157:433–438.
24. Cameron JR, Sorenson G (1963) Measurements of bone mineral in vivo: an improved method. *Science* 142:230–232.
25. Vogel JM (1987) Application principles and technical considerations in SPA. In: Genant HK, ed. *Osteoporosis Update 1987*, San Francisco: University of California Printing Services, pp. 219–231.
26. Johnston CC (1983) Noninvasive methods for quantitating appendicular bone mass. In: Avioli LV, ed. *The Osteoporotic Syndrome*, New York: Grune and Stratton, pp. 73–84.
27. Barden HS, Mazess RB (1989) Bone densitometry of the appendicular and axial skeleton. *Top Geriatric Rehabil* 4:1–12.
28. Kimmel PL (1984) Radiologic methods to evaluate bone mineral content. *Ann Intern Med* 100:908–911.
29. Steiger P, Genant HK (1987) The current implementation of single-photon absorptiometry in commercially available instruments. In: Genant HK, ed. *Osteoporosis Update 1987*, San Francisco: University of California Printing Services, pp. 233–240.
30. Chesnut CH (1993) Noninvasive methods for bone mass measurement. In: Avioli L, ed. *The Osteoporotic Syndrome*, 3rd ed., New York: Wiley-Liss, pp. 77–87.
31. Gardsell P, Johnell O, Nilsson BE (1991) The predictive value of bone loss for fragility fractures in women: a longitudinal study over 15 years. *Calcif Tissue Int* 49:90–94.
32. Hui SL, Slemenda CW, Johnston CC (1989) Baseline measurement of bone mass predicts fracture in white women. *Ann Intern Med* 111:355–361.
33. Ross PD, Davis JW, Vogel JM, Wasnich RD (1990) A critical review of bone mass and the risk of fractures in osteoporosis. *Calcif Tissue Int* 46:149–161.
34. Melton LJ, Atkinson EJ, O'Fallon WM, Wahner HW, Riggs BL (1993) Long-term fracture prediction by bone mineral assessed at different skeletal sites. *J Bone Miner Res* 8:1227–1233.
35. Black DM, Cummings SR, Genant HK, Nevitt MC, Palermo L, Browner W (1992) Axial and appendicular bone density predict fracture in older women. *J Bone Miner Res* 7:633–638.
36. Nord RH (1987) Technical considerations in DPA. In: Genant HK, ed. *Osteoporosis Update 1987*, San Francisco: University of California Printing Services, pp. 203–212.
37. Dunn WL, Wahner HW, Riggs BL (1980) Measurement of bone mineral content in human vertebrae and hip by dual photon absorptiometry. *Radiology* 136:485–487.
38. Reed GW (1966) The assessment of bone mineralization from the relative transmission of ^{241}Am and ^{137}Cs radiations. *Phys Med Biol* 11:174.
39. Roos B, Skoldborn H (1974) Dual photon absorptiometry in lumbar vertebrae. I. Theory and method. *Acta Radiol Ther Phys Biol* 13:266–290.
40. Mazess RB, Ort M, Judy P (1970) Absorptiometric bone mineral determination using ^{153}Gd. In: Cameron JR, ed. *Proceedings of Bone Measurements Conference*, U.S. Atomic Energy Commission, pp. 308–312.
41. Wilson CR, Madsen M (1977) Dichromatic absorptiometry of vertebral bone mineral content. *Invest Radiol* 12:180–184.

42. Madsen M, Peppler W, Mazess RB (1976) Vertebral and total body bone mineral content by dual photon absorptiometry. *Calcif Tissue Res* 2:361–364.
43. Wahner WH, Dunn WL, Mazess RB, et al. (1985) Dual-photon Gd-153 absorptiometry of bone. *Radiology* 156:203–206.
44. Lindsay R, Fey C, Haboubi A (1987) Dual photon absorptiometric measurements of bone mineral density increase with source life. *Calcif Tissue Int* 41:293,294.
45. Cummings SR, Black DB (1986) Should perimenopausal women be screened for osteoporosis? *Ann Intern Med* 104:817–823.
46. Drinka PJ, DeSmet AA, Bauwens SF, Rogot A (1992) The effect of overlying calcification on lumbar bone densitometry. *Calcif Tissue Int* 50:507–510.
47. Curry TS, Dowdey JE, Murry RC (1990) *Christensen's Physics of Diagnostic Radiology*. Philadelphia: Lea and Febiger.
48. Rupich RC, Griffin MG, Pacifici R, Avioli LV, Susman N (1992) Lateral dual-energy radiography: artifact error from rib and pelvic bone. *J Bone Miner Res* 7:97–101.
49. Louis O, Van Den Winkel P, Covens P, Schoutens A, Osteaux M (1992) Dual-energy X-ray absorptiometry of lumbar vertebrae: relative contribution of body and posterior elements and accuracy in relation with neutron activation analysis. *Bone* 13:317–320.
50. Lees B, Stevenson JC (1992) An evaluation of dual-energy X-ray absorptiometry and comparison with dual-photon absorptiometry. *Osteoporosis Int* 2:146–152.
51. Kelly TL, Slovik DM, Schoenfeld DA, Neer RM (1988) Quantitative digital radiography versus dual photon absorptiometry of the lumbar spine. *J Clin Endocrinol Metab* 76:839–844.
52. Holbrook TL, Barrett-Connor E, Klauber M, Sartoris D (1991) A population-based comparison of quantitative dual-energy X-ray absorptiometry with dual-photon absorptiometry of the spine and hip. *Calcif Tissue Int* 49:305–307.
53. Pouilles JM, Tremollieres F, Todorovsky N, Ribot C (1991) Precision and sensitivity of dual-energy X-ray absorptiometry in spinal osteoporosis. *J Bone Miner Res* 6: 997–1002.
54. Laskey MA, Crisp AJ, Cole TJ, Compston JE (1992) Comparison of the effect of different reference data on Lunar DPX and Hologic QDR-1000 dual-energy X-ray absorptiometers. *Br J Radiol* 65:1124–1129.
55. Pocock NA, Sambrook PN, Nguyen T, Kelly P, Freund J, Eisman J (1992) Assessment of spinal and femoral bone density by dual X-ray absorptiometry: comparison of Lunar and Hologic instruments. *J Bone Miner Res* 7:1081–1084.
56. Lai KC, Goodsitt MM, Murano R, Chesnut CC (1992) A comparison of two dual-energy X-ray absorptiometry systems for spinal bone mineral measurement. *Calcif Tissue Int* 50:203–208.
57. Kalender WA (1992) Effective dose values in bone mineral measurements by photon-absorptiometry and computed tomography. *Osteoporosis Int* 2:82–87.
58. Faulkner KG, Cummings SR, Black D, Palermo L, Gluer C, Genant HK (1993) Simple measurement of femoral geometry predicts hip fracture: the study of osteoporotic fractures. *J Bone Miner Res* 8:1211–1217.
59. Kelly TL, Crane G, Baran DT (1994) Single X-ray absorptiometry of the forearm: precision, correlation, and reference data. *Calcif Tissue Int* 54:212–218.
60. Ruegsegger P, Elsasser U, Anliker M, Gnehn H, Kind H, Prader A (1976) Quantification of bone mineralisation using computed tomography. *Radiology* 121:93–97.
61. Genant HK, Cann CE, Ettinger B, Gorday GS (1982) Quantitative computed tomography of vertebral spongiosa: a sensitive method for detecting early bone loss after oophorectomy. *Ann Intern Med* 97:699–705.

62. Cann CE, Genant HK (1980) Precise measurement of vertebral mineral content using computed tomography. *J Comput Assist Tomogr* 4:493–500.
63. Genant HK, Block JE, Steiger P, Gluer C (1987) Quantitative computed tomography in the assessment of osteoporosis. In: Genant HK, ed. *Osteoporosis Update 1987*, San Francisco: University of California Printing Services.
64. Laval-Jeantet AM, Roger B, Bouysse S, Bergot C, Mazess RB (1986) Influence of vertebral fat content on quantitative CT density. *Radiology* 159:463–466.
65. Reinbold W, Adler CP, Kalender WA, Lente R (1991) Accuracy of vertebral mineral determination by dual-energy quantitative computed tomography. *Skeletal Radiol* 20:25–29.
66. Dunnill MS, Anderson JA, Whitehead R (1967) Quantitative histological studies on age changes in bone. *J Pathol Bacteriol* 94:274–291.
67. Genant HK, Boyd D (1977) Quantitative bone mineral analysis using dual energy computed tomography. *Invest Radiol* 12:545–551.
68. Cann CE (1987) Quantitative computed tomography for bone mineral analysis: technical considerations. In: Genant HK, ed. *Osteoporosis Update 1987*, San Francisco: University of California Printing Services, pp. 131–144.
69. Sartoris DJ, Andre M, Resnick C, Resnick D (1986) Trabecular bone density in the proximal femur: quantitative CT assessment. *Radiology* 160:707–712.
70. Reiser UJ, Genant HK (1984) Determination of bone mineral content in the femoral neck by quantitative computed tomography. 70th Scientific Assembly and Annual Meeting of the Radiological Society of North America, Washington, DC.
71. Gallagher C, Golgar D, Mahoney P, McGill J (1985) Measurement of spine density in normal and osteoporotic subjects using computed tomography: relationship of spine density to fracture threshold and fracture index. *J Comput Assist Tomogr* 9:634,635.
72. Raymaker JA, Hoekstra O, Van Putten J, Kerkhoff H, Duursma SA (1986) Osteoporosis fracture prevalence and bone mineral mass measured with CT and DPA. *Skeletal Radiol* 15:191–197.
73. Reinbold WD, Reiser UJ, Harris ST, Ettinger B, Genant HK (1986) Measurement of bone mineral content in early postmenopausal and postmenopausal osteoporotic women. A comparison of methods. *Radiology* 160:469–478.
74. Sambrook PN, Bartlett C, Evans R, Hesp R, Katz D, Reeve J (1985) Measurement of lumbar spine bone mineral: a comparison of dual photon absorptiometry and computed tomography. *Br J Radiol* 58:621–624.
75. Genant HK, Ettinger B, Harris ST, Block JE, Steiger P (1988) Quantitative computed tomography in assessment of osteoporosis. In: Riggs BL, Melton LJ, eds. *Osteoporosis: Etiology, Diagnosis and Management*, New York: Raven, pp. 221–249.
76. Richardson ML, Genant HK, Cann CE, et al. (1985) Assessment of metabolic bone disease by quantitative computed tomography. *Clin Orth Rel Res* 195:224–238.

2 Densitometric Anatomy

Contents

Densitometry was originally developed as a quantitative measurement technique, rather than as an imaging technique. Nevertheless, there are unique aspects to skeletal anatomy in the context of densitometric analysis that should be appreciated in order to properly utilize the technology and interpret the results.

THE SKELETON IN DENSITOMETRY

Axial and Appendicular Skeleton

The skeleton has traditionally been divided into two components: the appendicular skeleton and the axial skeleton. The appendicular skeleton includes the extremities, scapula, and pelvis *(1)*. The axial skeleton consists of the skull, ribs, sternum, and the spine. In the context of densitometry, however, the term "axial skeleton" generally refers only to the spine. Similarly, the term "appendicular" generally refers only to the extremities. These more limited definitions of the terms axial and appendicular are the result of the historic lack of applications of densitometry to the other skeletal regions normally included in such divisions.

Weight-Bearing and Nonweight-Bearing Skeleton

Regions of the skeleton are also characterized as weight-bearing or nonweight-bearing. This division is intuitively obvious and not without clinical significance. The spine and lower extremities are considered weight-bearing regions; the remainder of the skeleton is nonweight-bearing.

Central and Peripheral Skeleton

Skeletal sites that are quantified with bone densitometry may also be classified as central or peripheral sites. Although it is obvious that the spine would be considered a central site, the proximal femur is also considered a central site, even though it is part of the appendicular skeleton. The calcaneus and the various sites on the forearm are considered peripheral sites, although the calcaneus is obviously a weight-bearing site, but the sites on the forearm are not. By extension, bone densitometers that can measure the spine, hip, or both are often referred to as central machines, even though the machines may also have the capability of being used to measure a peripheral site like the forearm. The designation of these machines as central machines is intended to differentiate them from smaller machines that are dedicated to measurements of the distal appendicular skeleton, such as the forearm or calcaneus. These machines are called peripheral machines.

SKELETAL SITE COMPOSITION

The skeleton is composed of two types of bone: cortical bone and trabecular bone. Cortical bone is also called compact or haversian bone. Trabecular bone may also be described as cancellous or spongious bone. Eighty percent of the skeleton is cortical bone. The remaining 20% is trabecular bone, which is found primarily in the distal ends of the long bones and in the axial skeleton. Trabecular bone may be described as consisting of plates, arches, and struts, with marrow occupying the spaces between these structures; cortical bone is a more solid structure, forming the outer casing of the bones *(1)*.

Trabecular bone has a higher metabolic rate than cortical bone *(2)*. As a consequence, rates of change may be greater at sites that are predominantly trabecular in composition, compared to sites that are predominantly cortical. If a patient is being followed over time to look for changes in the bone mineral density from a disease process or therapeutic intervention, the greatest magnitude of change will generally be seen at a site that is predominantly trabecular bone. There are certain disease processes, however, that seem to have a predilection for sites that are predominantly cortical in composition. Hyperparathyroidism, for example, may cause demineralization at predominantly cortical sites, such as the femoral neck or 33% radial site.

The exact composition of many of the sites used in densitometry remains controversial. In a classic study, Schlenker and VonSeggen *(3)* quantified the average percentage of cortical and trabecular bone along the length of the radius and ulna in four cadaveric female forearms. The forearms were taken from women aged 21, 43, 63, and 85 years. The distribution and percentage of trabecular bone in the radius and ulna were similar. The maximum percentage of trabecular bone was seen in the first 2 cm proximal to the radial and ulnar styloids. The percentage of trabecular bone then dropped precipitously in both bones in a transitional region that lay between 2 and 3 cm proximal to either styloid, and remained very small throughout the remainder of the proximal radius and ulna. The percentage of trabecular bone in the four subjects in the most distal 10% of the radius ranged from 50 to 67%; in the region that represented 30–40% of the total length measured from the styloid tip, the percentage of trabecular bone ranged from only 0.6 to 6.8%. In the region called the ultradistal radius, the percentage of trabecular bone is approximately 66% *(4)*.

The composition of either whole vertebra or the isolated vertebral body remains in dispute. The traditional view is that in whole vertebra, 55–75% of the calcium content is found in trabecular bone. These figures are largely derived from early anatomic studies, in which the methods used to arrive at such conclusions were poorly described *(5,6)*. The traditional view was challenged in 1987 by Nottestad et al. *(7)* who performed anatomic dissections of 24 vertebrae taken from 14 normal individuals: 10 women whose average age was 72 years, and 4 men whose average age was 63 years. The vertebrae were ashed and the calcium content assayed using atomic absorption spectrophotometry. Nottestad et al. *(7)* found that trabecular bone accounted for only 24.4% of the calcium content of whole female vertebrae. Trabecular calcium accounted for 41.8% of the calcium content in the vertebral body. The percentages were less in men, averaging 18.8 and 33.5%, respectively. Eastell et al. *(8)* refuted this finding, based on anatomic dissections of L2 from 13 individuals: 6 men whose average age was 38.5 years, and 7 women whose average age was 40.9 years. In this study, cortical and trabecular contributions to calcium content were determined by microdensitometry, and by dissection and ashing. They reported that the whole vertebra was 72% trabecular bone in women and 80% trabecular bone in men. Adjusting these figures to compensate for the expected difference between the two-dimensional measurements that were actually performed and the three-dimensional structure of whole vertebrae, the percentages dropped slightly, to 69% in women and 77% in men.

The composition of the commonly measured sites in the proximal femur was briefly studied again by Baumel, using anatomic dissection of the upper end of the femur in six cadavers (age at death 49–79 years) *(9)*. In this small study, the percentage of trabecular bone in the femoral neck was 36.45% (±3.85%), and in the trochanter, 39.06% (±3.79%).

Despite these controversies, clinically useful characterizations of the composition of the scan sites can be made. Table 2-1 lists the most com-

Table 2-1
The Relative Percentages of Cortical and Trabecular Bone at Various Skeletal Sites[a]

Region of interest	*% of Trabecular bone*	*% of Cortical bone*
AP spine (DPA/DXA)	66	34
AP spine (QCT)	100	
Lateral spine (DXA)[b]	++++	
Femoral neck	25	75
Ward's area[b]	++++	
Trochanteric region	50	50
Os calcis	95	5
Midradius	1	99
Distal radius	20	80
8-mm radius	25	75
5-mm radius	40	60
Ultradistal radius	66	34
Phalanges	40	60
Total body	20	80

[a]The exact composition of some of these skeletal sites is controversial. These are considered clinically useful characterizations of the percentages of cortical and trabecular bone.

[b]This site is highly trabecular, but the exact composition is not defined in the literature.

Reproduced with permission of the publisher from ref. *10*.

monly assessed skeletal sites and their relative percentages of trabecular and cortical bone *(10)*. Note that the spine, when measured with quantitative computed tomography (QCT), is described as 100% trabecular bone. This is because the three-dimensional, volumetric measure that is obtained with QCT allows the center of the vertebral body to be isolated from its cortical shell and the highly cortical posterior elements. The two-dimensional areal measurement employed in dual-photon absorptiometry (DPA) and dual-energy X-ray absorptiometry (DXA) measurements of the spine cannot do this. Although the posterior elements are eliminated from the scan path on a lateral spine study performed with DXA, elements of the cortical shell remain. Therefore, although the measurement of the spine in the lateral projection with DXA is a highly trabecular measurement of bone density, the measurement is not a measurement of 100% trabecular bone.

THE SPINE IN DENSITOMETRY

Studies of the lumbar spine performed with DPA or DXA are generally acquired by the passage of photon energy from the posterior-to-anterior

Spine Artifacts

Compression Fx
Osteophytes
Osteochondrosis
facet scerosis
A rotic Calcification

cterized as PA spine studies; nevertheless, spine studies. Some of the newer fan-array uire lumbar spine bone-density images in o plain radiography, however, the beam spine has less influence on the appearance n the measured BMC or BMD. Studies of uired in the lateral projection, using DXA. with the patient supine, or in the left lateral on the type of DXA unit being employed.

bral Anatomy

ided into two major components: the body posterior elements consist of the pedicles, the transverse processes, and the inferior and superior articulating surfaces. The appearance of the image of the spine on an AP or PA study is predominantly determined by the relative density of the various elements that make up the entire vertebra. Figure 2-1A is a photograph of a posterior view of the lumbar spine with the intervertebral disks removed. Figure 2-1B,C demonstrates the appearance of the spine as the transverse processes are removed, and then as the vertebral bodies are removed from the photograph. What remains in Fig. 2-1C is characteristic of the appearance of the lumbar spine on a DXA lumbar-spine study. The transverse processes are eliminated from the scan field and the vertebral bodies are not well seen, because they are behind and equally or less dense than the posterior elements. In a study of 34 lumbar vertebrae taken from three men and seven women ranging in age from 61 to 88 years, the mineral content of the posterior elements averaged 47% of the mineral content of the entire vertebrae *(11)*.

The posterior elements that remain in Fig. 2-1C form the basis of the DXA lumbar-spine image as seen in Fig. 2-2. The unique shapes of the posterior elements of the various lumbar vertebrae have led to the use of these shapes as an aid in the identification of the lumbar vertebrae. L1, L2, and L3 are often characterized as having a U- or Y-shaped appearance. L4 is described as looking like a block H or X. L5 has the appearance of a block I on its side. Figure 2-3 is a graphic illustration of these shapes. Compare these shapes to the actual posterior elements seen in Fig. 2-1C and the DXA lumbar-spine study shown in Fig. 2-2. Although the transverse processes are generally not seen on a spine bone-density study, the processes at L3 will sometimes be partially visible, since this vertebra tends to have the largest transverse processes. Figure 2-4A,B is the spine image only from the study shown in Fig. 2-2. In Fig. 2-4B, the shapes of the posterior elements have been outlined for emphasis.

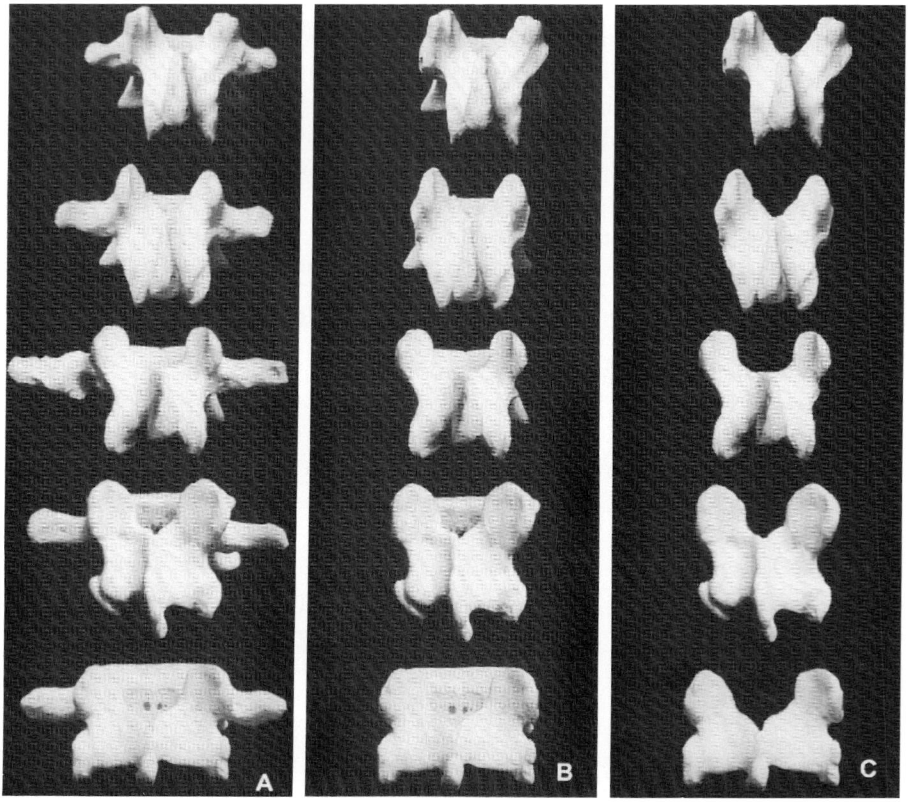

Fig. 2-1. The lumbar spine viewed from behind. **(A)** Intact vertebrae. **(B)** The transverse processes have been removed. **(C)** The vertebral bodies have been removed, leaving only the posterior elements. (Photo from McMinn RMH, Hutchings RT, Pegington J, and Abrahams PH. [1993] *Color Atlas of Human Anatomy*, 3rd ed. By permission of Mosby International) (*see* color plate 1 appearing after p. 78)

The bone mineral densities (BMDs) and bone mineral contents (BMCs) for the individual lumbar vertebrae are highly correlated with each other, and with the average BMD for L2–L4 as shown in Table 2-2 *(12)*. The correlation between individual vertebrae is approx 0.83 for BMD and 0.79 for BMC. A higher correlation is seen between individual vertebrae and the average for L2–L4 for both BMD and BMC: 0.95 and 0.90, respectively. The correlation between L1 and the L2–L4 average BMD or BMC is poorer, at 0.83 and 0.78, respectively. L1 frequently has the lowest BMC and BMD of the four lumbar vertebrae measured *(13)*. In a study of 148 normal

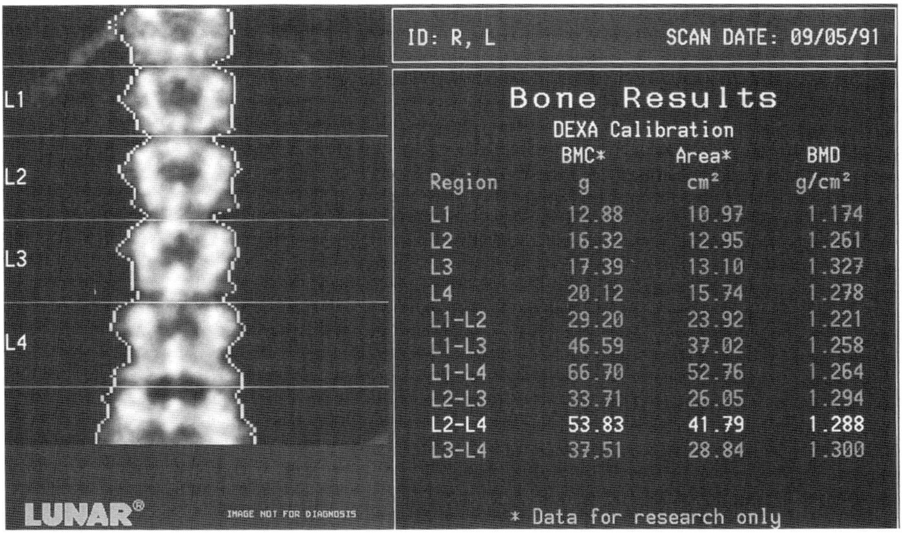
L1
L2
L3
L4
LUNAR®
IMAGE NOT FOR DIAGNOSIS
ID: R, L
SCAN DATE: 09/05/91
Bone Results
DEXA Calibration
BMC* Area* BMD
Region g cm² g/cm²
L1 12.88 10.97 1.174
L2 16.32 12.95 1.261
L3 17.39 13.10 1.327
L4 20.12 15.74 1.278
L1-L2 29.20 23.92 1.221
L1-L3 46.59 37.02 1.258
L1-L4 66.70 52.76 1.264
L2-L3 33.71 26.05 1.294
L2-L4 53.83 41.79 1.288
L3-L4 37.51 28.84 1.300
* Data for research only

Fig. 2-2. A DXA AP spine study acquired on the Lunar DPX. The shapes of the vertebrae in this image are primarily created by the posterior elements. The shapes in this study are classic. The expected increase in BMC and area is also seen from L1 to L4. The increase in BMD from L1 to L3, with a decline from L3 to L4, is also typical. (*see* color plate 2 appearing after p. 78)

women ages 50–60, Peel et al. *(13)* found that the BMC increased between L1–L2, L2–L3, and L3–L4 although the increase between L3 and L4 was roughly half that seen at the other levels, as shown in Table 2-3. BMD increased between L1–L2 and L2–L3, but showed no significant change between L3 and L4. The average change between L3 and L4 was actually a decline of 0.004 g/cm^2. The larges increase in BMD occurred between L1 and L2. The apparent discrepancies in the magnitude of the change in BMC and BMD between the vertebrae are the result of the progressive increase in area of the vertebrae from L1 to L4. The DXA AP lumbar spine study shown in Fig. 2-2 illustrates the progressive increase in BMC and area from L1 to L4, and the expected pattern of change in BMD between the vertebral levels.

Studies from Peel et al. *(13)* and Bornstein and Peterson *(14)* suggest that the majority of individuals have five lumbar vertebrae, with the lowest set of ribs on T12. Bornstein and Peterson found that only 17% of 1239 skeletons demonstrated a pattern of vertebral segmentation and rib placement other than five lumbar vertebrae, with the lowest ribs on T12. Similarly, Peel et al. *(13)* found something other than the expected pattern of five lumbar vertebrae, with the lowest ribs on T12, in 16.5% of 375 women.

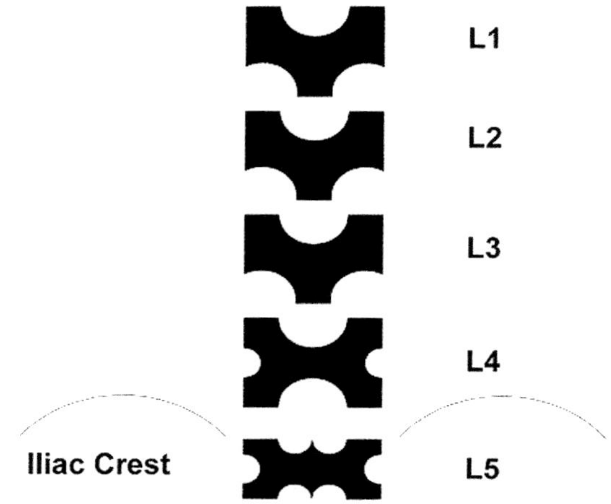

Fig. 2-3. The characteristic shapes of the lumbar vertebrae as seen on a DXA AP spine study.

An additional 7.2% had five lumbar vertebrae, but had the lowest level of ribs on T11. Therefore, 90.7% of the women studied by Peel et al. had five lumbar vertebrae. Only 1.9%, or 7, women had six lumbar vertebrae. In three of these women, ribs were seen on L1. This was the only circumstance in which ribs were seen on L1. Of the entire group, 7.5% had only four lumbar vertebrae. In the majority of cases here, the lowest ribs were seen on T11. Table 2-4 summarizes these findings.

A knowledge of the frequency of anomalous vertebral segmentation, the characteristic shapes created by the posterior elements on an AP spine bone density study, and the expected incremental change in BMC and BMD are used to ensure that the vertebrae are labeled correctly. If the vertebrae are mislabeled, comparisons to the normative databases will be misleading. The expected effect of mislabeling T12 as L1 would be to lower the BMC or BMD at L1, which would compare unfavorably to the reference value for L1. The BMC and BMD averages for L1–L4 or L2–L4 would also be lowered. The degree to which BMC is lowered by mislabeling is substantially greater than BMD, as shown in Table 2-5 *(13)*. The assumption that the lowest set of ribs is found at the level of T12 is often used as the basis for labeling the lumbar vertebrae. As can be seen from Table 2-4, this assumption would result in the vertebrae being labeled incorrectly in 13.3% of the population. As a consequence, all of the criteria noted above should be employed in determining the correct labeling of the lumbar vertebrae. This should obviate the need for plain films for the sole purpose of labeling the vertebrae in the vast majority of instances. Figure 2-5 is an

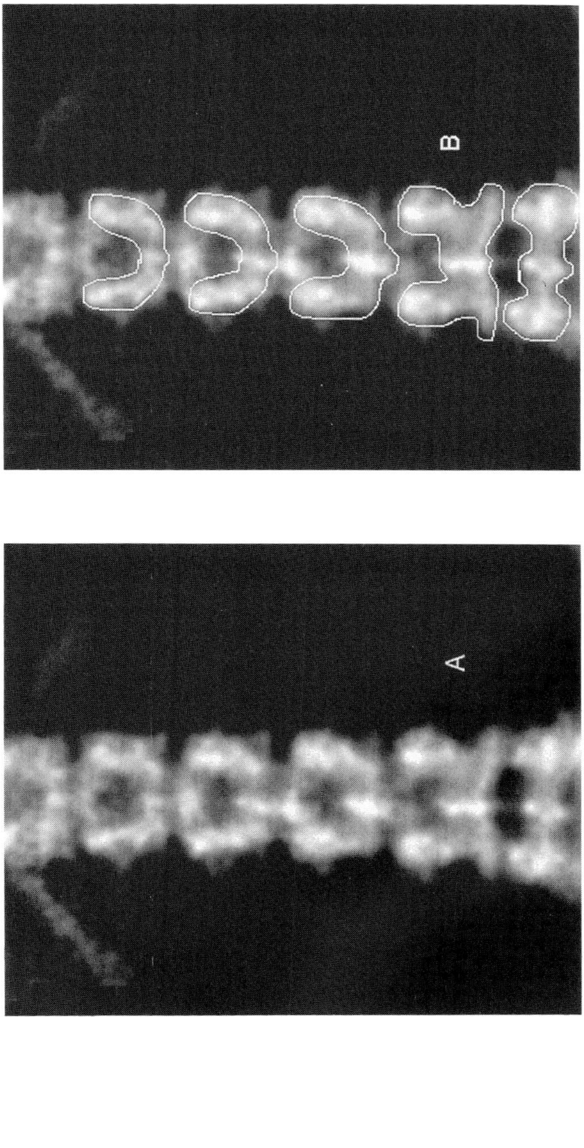

Fig. 2-4. (A) An DXA AP spine image acquired on the Lunar DPX. This is the spine image seen in the study shown in Fig. 2-2, with the intervertebral disk markers and bone-edge markers removed for clarity. **(B)** The shapes have been outlined for emphasis.

Table 2-2
Correlation of BMD Between Individual Lumbar Vertebrae and L2–4 Average BMD

	L1	*L2*	*L3*	*L4*
L1		0.80	0.78	0.75
L2	0.85		0.84	0.76
L3	0.79	0.90		0.79
L4	0.75	0.83	0.85	
L2–4	0.83	0.94	0.96	0.95

All correlations were significant at $P < 0.001$.

Adapted from Mazess RB, Barden HS. (1990) Interrelationships among bone densitometry sites in normal young women. *Bone and Mineral* 11:347–356, with kind permission from Elsevier Science Ireland, Ltd., Bay 15K, Shannon Industrial Estate, Co. Clare, Ireland.

Table 2-3
Incremental Change in BMC and BMD Between Adjacent Vertebrae in 148 Normal Women Age 50–60 as Measured by DXA

Vertebrae	*Increase in BMC (g)*	*% Increase in BMC*	*Increase in BMD (g/cm²)*	*% Increase in BMD*
L1–2	2.07	13.7	0.090	7.9
L2–3	2.43	14.8	0.050	4.3
L3–4	1.13	5.0	–0.004[a]	–0.8[a]

[a]Not statistically significant.

Reprinted from the *Journal of Bone and Mineral Research* (1993) 8:719–723 with permission from the American Society for Bone and Mineral Research.

AP spine study in which the labeling of the lumbar vertebrae was not straightforward. The characteristic shapes of the vertebrae are easily seen, but ribs appear to be projecting from what should be L1. The labeling shown in Fig. 2-5 is correct.

As will be seen in Chapters 6 and 7, AP spine bone density measurements are extremely useful in predicting fracture risk and following the effects of a variety of disease processes and therapeutic interventions. Unfortunately, the AP spine is also the site most commonly affected by structural changes or artifacts that may affect either the accuracy or precision of the measurement, or both.

Artifacts in AP Spine Densitometry

Vertebral Fractures

Any type of vertebral fracture is expected to cause an increase in the BMD at the site of the fracture. Because DXA measurements of the AP

Table 2-4
Percentage of Women with Various Combinations of Numbers of Lumbar Vertebrae and Position of Lowest Ribs

No. of lumbar vertebrae	*Position of lowest ribs*	*% of Women*
5	T12	83.5
5	T11	7.2
4	T12	2.1
4	T11	5.3
6	T12	1.1
6	L1	0.8

Reprinted from the *Journal of Bone and Mineral Research* (1993) 8:719–723 with permission from the American Society for Bone and Mineral Research.

Table 2-5
Effect of Mislabeling T12 as L1 on BMC and BMD in AP-DXA Spine Measurements

Measurement	*Difference*	*Mean %*
BMC		
L1	1.61 g	11.5
L2–L4	3.47 g	8.4
L1–L4	4.8 g	8.4
BMD		
L2–L4	0.035 g/cm^2	3.6
L1–L4	0.039 g/cm^2	3.5

Reprinted from the *Journal of Bone and Mineral Research* (1993) 8:719–723 with permission from the American Society for Bone and Mineral Research.

spine are often employed in patients with osteoporosis, osteoporotic fractures in the lumbar spine are a common problem, rendering the measurement of BMD inaccurate if the fractured vertebra is included. An increased precision error would also be expected if the fractured vertebra is included in BMD measurements performed as part of a serial evaluation of BMD. Although a fractured lumbar vertebra can be excluded from consideration in the analysis of the data, this reduces the maximum number of contiguous vertebrae in the lumbar spine that are available for analysis. For reasons of statistical accuracy and precision, the average BMD for 3–4 contiguous vertebrae is preferred over two-vertebrae averages or the BMD of a single vertebra. Figure 2-6 illustrates an AP spine study in which a fracture was apparent at L3. Although the BMD at L3 is expected to be higher than at

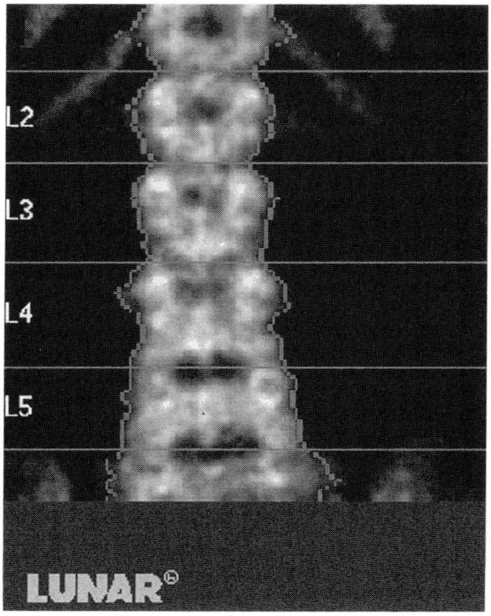

Fig. 2-5. A DXA AP spine image acquired on the Lunar DPX. The characteristic shapes of the vertebrae are easily seen, but ribs appear to be projecting from L1, making vertebral identification unclear. The labeling shown is correct. Case courtesy of Dr. David Nichols, Texas Woman's University. (*see* color plate 3 appearing after p. 78).

either L2 or L4, it is disproportionately higher. The L2–L4 BMD average will be increased, because of the effect of the fracture on the BMD at L3. In the DXA AP lumbar-spine study shown in Fig. 2-7, the image does not as readily suggest a fracture. The BMD at L1, however, is higher than the BMD at L2, which is unusual. A plain lateral film of the lumbar spine of this patient, shown in Fig. 2-8, confirmed a fracture at L1.

Other structural changes within the spine can affect the BMD measurements. Osteophytes, osteochondrosis, and facet sclerosis can increase the BMD when measured in the AP direction. Aortic calcification will also potentially affect the BMD when measured in the AP spine, because the X-ray beam will detect the calcium in the aorta as it passes through the body on a PA path. It is therefore useful to note how often these types of changes are expected in the general population, and the potential magnitude of the effect these changes may have on the BMD.

Effect of Osteophytes on BMD

In 1982, Krolner et al. *(15)* observed that osteophytes caused a statistically significant increase in the BMD in the AP spine, when compared to

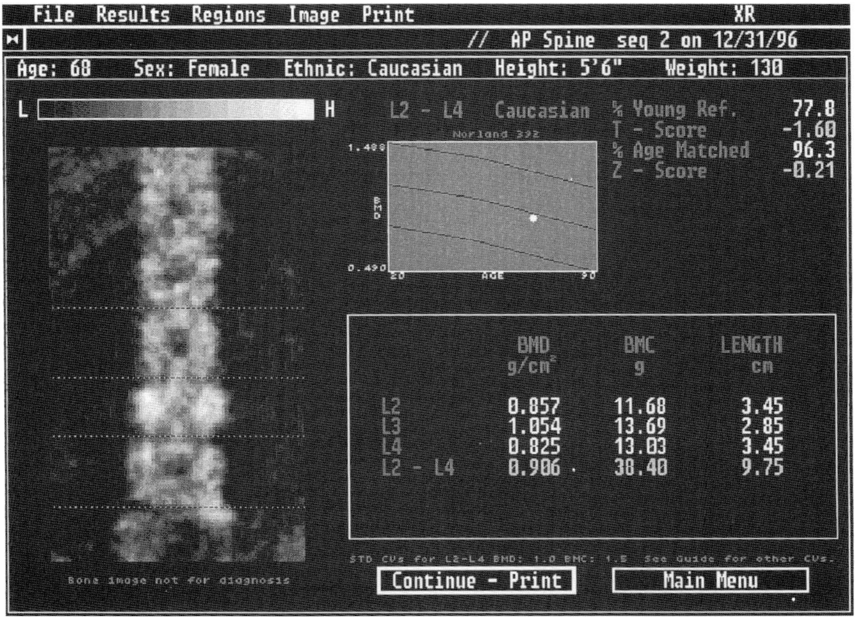

Fig. 2-6. A DXA AP spine study acquired on the Norland XR-36. A compression fracture is apparent at L3 on the image. The BMD at L3 is also clearly increased. Case courtesy of Norland Medical Systems, Inc., Ft. Atkinson, WI. (*see* color plate 4 appearing after p. 78)

controls without osteophytes. More recently, Rand et al. *(16)* evaluated a population of 144 postmenopausal women aged 40–84 years, with a mean age of 63.3 years, for the presence of osteophytes, osteochondrosis, scoliosis, and aortic calcification. These women, although generally healthy, were referred for the evaluation of BMD because of suspected postmenopausal osteoporosis. Table 2-6 lists the percentages of these women found to have these types of degenerative changes. Based on these findings, Rand et al. estimated the probability of degenerative changes in the spine as being <10% in women under the age of 50. In 55-year-old women, however, the probability jumped to 40%, and, in 70-year-old women, to 85%. Of these four types of degenerative changes, however, only the presence of osteophytes or osteochondrosis significantly increased the BMD. The magnitude of the increase caused by the osteophytes ranged from 9.5% at L4 to 13.9% at L1. The effect on BMD from osteochondrosis ranged from 3.9% at L3 to 11.9% at L1. Cann et al. *(17)* also estimated the effect of osteophytes on BMD in the spine at 11%. In Fig. 2-9, osteophytes are clearly visible at L2 on the lateral lumbar radiograph. The appearance of

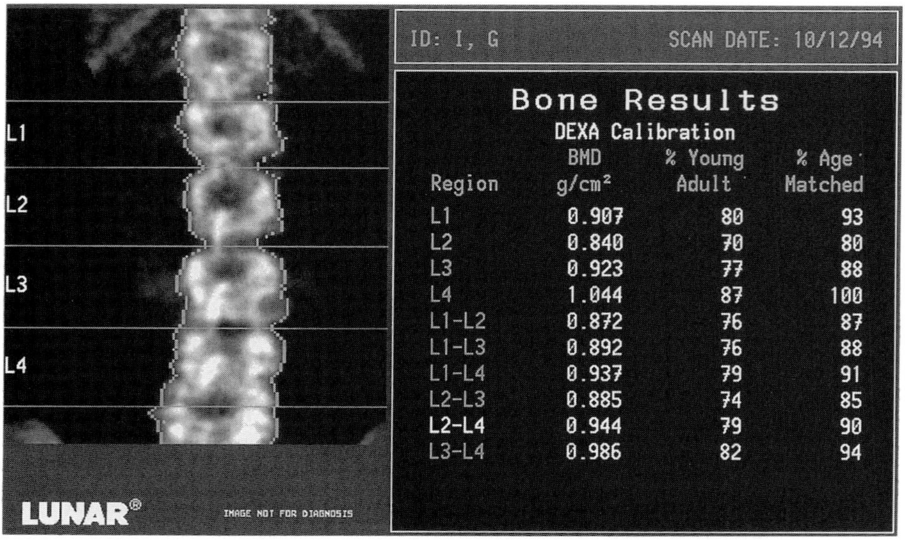
L1
L2
L3
L4
LUNAR®
IMAGE NOT FOR DIAGNOSIS
ID: I, G
SCAN DATE: 10/12/94
Bone Results
DEXA Calibration
Region | BMD g/cm² | % Young Adult | % Age Matched
L1 | 0.907 | 80 | 93
L2 | 0.840 | 70 | 80
L3 | 0.923 | 77 | 88
L4 | 1.044 | 87 | 100
L1-L2 | 0.872 | 76 | 87
L1-L3 | 0.892 | 76 | 88
L1-L4 | 0.937 | 79 | 91
L2-L3 | 0.885 | 74 | 85
L2-L4 | 0.944 | 79 | 90
L3-L4 | 0.986 | 82 | 94

Fig. 2-7. A DXA spine study acquired on the Lunar DPX. The image is not particularly remarkable, but the individual BMD values are. The BMD at L1 is higher than L2, which is unusual. A lateral lumbar X-ray of this patient shown in Fig. 2-8 confirms a fracture at L1.

this region on the DXA AP lumbar-spine study in Fig. 2-10 suggests a sclerotic process at this level. Osteophytes and endplate sclerosis are also seen on the plain film in Fig. 2-11. The effect on the DXA image of the lumbar spine, shown in Fig. 2-12, is dramatic. There is also an obvious increase in the BMD at L2 and L3.

Effect of Aortic Calcification on BMD

Although it did not significantly increase BMD, vascular calcification was seen in 24.3% of the population studied by Rand et al. *(16)*. In an extensive study of aortic calcification in 200 women, age 50 or older, by Frye et al. *(18)*, the overall prevalence of aortic calcification was noted, in addition to the relative severity and corresponding quantitative effect on BMD measured in the AP spine. A grading system for both linear calcifications and calcified plaques was applied to lateral spine films, with a grade of 0 indicating neither type of calcification, and a grade of 2 indicating the most severe degree. The prevalence of any degree of aortic calcification and severe (grade 2) calcification is shown in Fig. 2-13. The prevalence of any degree of aortic calcification is extremely low in women under age 60, but does increase dramatically in women age 60 and older. The prevalence of severe aortic calcification, however, remains low

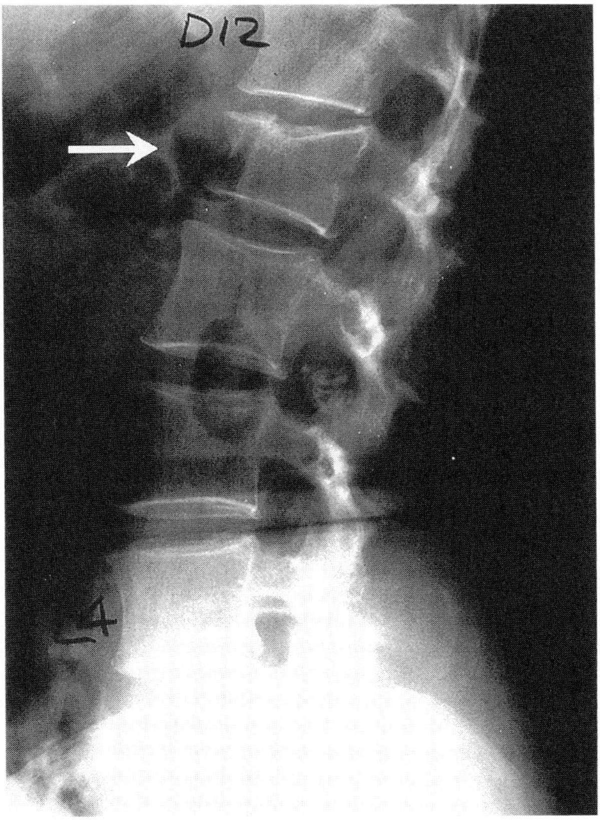

Fig. 2-8. A lateral lumbar X ray of the patient whose DXA study is shown in Fig. 2-7. A fracture at L1 is indicated by the arrow.

throughout the fifties, sixties, and seventies. Even in women aged 80 and older, the prevalence did not exceed 30%. Table 2-7 summarizes the effect on BMD in women with any degree of aortic calcification and severe aortic calcification. Neither effect was statistically significant. These findings are similar to those of Frohn et al. *(19)*, Orwoll et al. *(20)*, Reid et al. *(21)*, Banks et al. *(22)*, and Drinka et al. *(23)*, in which no significant effect of aortic calcification was seen on the BMD measured in the AP spine. The studies from Orwoll et al. and Drinka et al. were performed in men.

Aortic calcification is not easily seen on most DXA AP lumbar-spine studies. In Fig. 2-14A, however, the faint outline of the calcified aorta is visible. The aorta is easily seen on the lateral DXA image in Fig. 2-14B. Figure 2-15

Table 2-6
Frequency of Specific Types of Degenerative Changes in the Spines of 144 Women Aged 40–84

Type of degenerative change	*% with change (n)*
Osteophytes	45.8 (66)
Osteochondrosis	21.5 (31)
Vascular calcification	24.3 (35)
Scoliosis	22.2 (32)
Any type	59.0 (72)

From ref. *16*.

shows both studies. In this case, the DXA lateral-spine study can be used to eliminate the effects of the calcified aorta on the BMD measurement.

The Effect of Facet Sclerosis on BMD

Unlike aortic calcification, facet sclerosis can have a profound effect on the measured BMD in the AP projection. In the study by Drinka et al. *(23)* noted earlier, 113 elderly men were evaluated with standard AP and lateral lumbar-spine films and DPA of the lumbar spine. A grading system for facet sclerosis was developed, with a grade of 0 indicating no sclerosis, and a grade of 3 indicating marked sclerosis. As shown in Table 2-8, grade 1 sclerosis had no significant effect on the BMD. Grades 2 and 3, however, markedly elevated the BMD at the vertebral levels at which the facet sclerosis was found. Figure 2-16 is an AP spine BMD study, in which facet sclerosis is suggested at L3 by the appearance of the image. The BMD values at L3 and L4 are also markedly higher than expected, based on the values at L1 and L2. The plain film of this patient, shown in Fig. 2-17, confirms facet sclerosis at the lower lumbar levels.

Other Causes of Artifacts in AP Spine Studies

There are other potential causes of elevations in the BMD in the AP spine. Stutzman et al. *(24)* identified pancreatic calcifications, renal stones, gall stones, contrast agents, and ingested calcium tablets, in addition to osteophytes, aortic calcification, and fractures, as possible causes of error. Figures 2-18 to 2-20 illustrate other structural changes in the spine that will affect the BMD measured in the AP projection.

The Spine in the Lateral Projection

The effect on BMD measured in the spine in the AP projection from aortic calcification, facet sclerosis, osteophytes, and other degenerative changes can be overcome by quantifying the bone density of the spine in

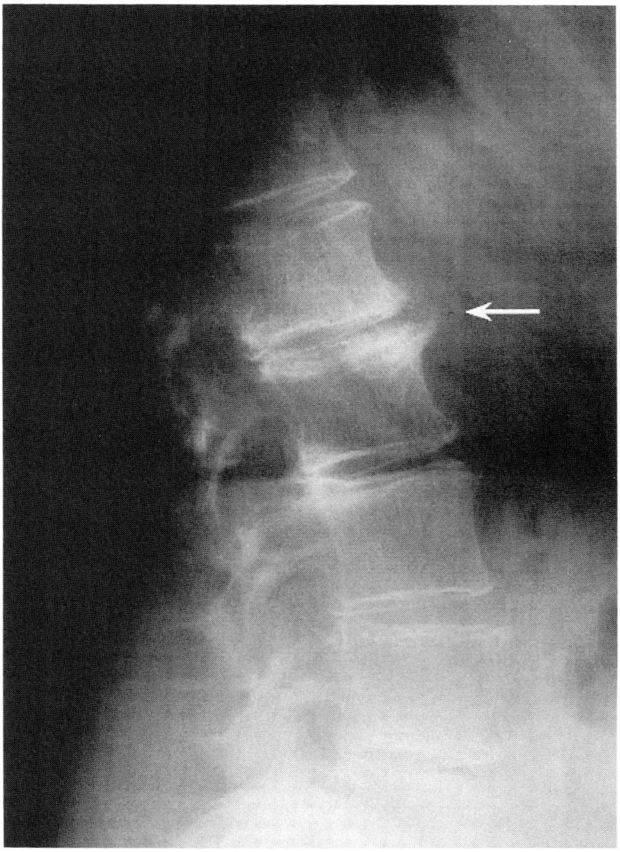

Fig. 2-9. A lateral lumbar X ray of the patient whose DXA study is shown in Fig. 2-10. The arrow indicates a region of endplate sclerosis and osteophyte formation.

the lateral projection, as was shown in Fig. 2-15. In addition, the highly cortical posterior elements and a portion of the cortical shell of the vertebral body can be eliminated from the measurement, resulting in a more trabecular measure of bone density in the spine. This is desirable in those circumstances in which a trabecular measure of bone density is indicated, and particularly in circumstances in which changes in bone density are being followed over time. The higher metabolic rate of trabecular bone, compared to cortical bone, should result in a much larger magnitude of change in this more trabecular measure of bone density, compared to the mixed cortical–trabecular measure of bone density in the AP spine. The measurement of bone density by DXA in the lateral projection is not a

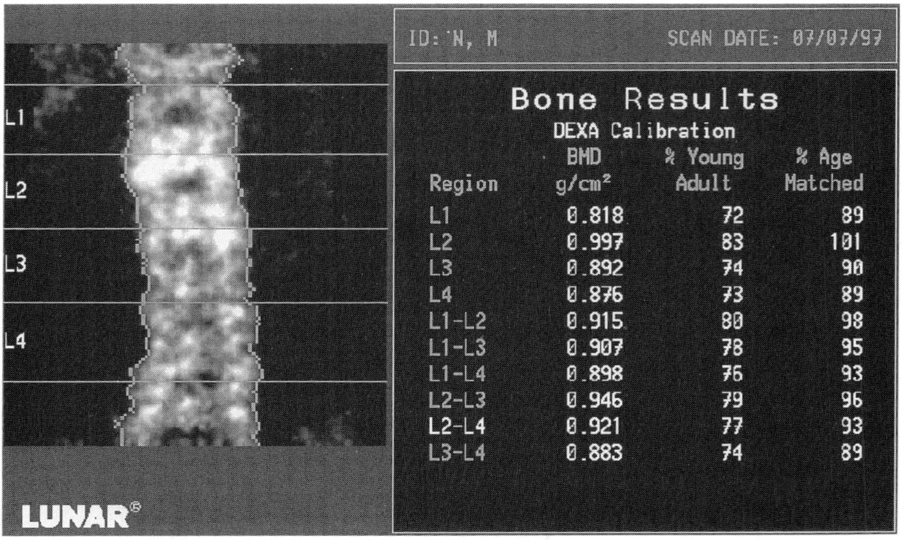

Region	BMD g/cm²	% Young Adult	% Age Matched
L1	0.818	72	89
L2	0.997	83	101
L3	0.892	74	90
L4	0.876	73	89
L1-L2	0.915	80	98
L1-L3	0.907	78	95
L1-L4	0.898	76	93
L2-L3	0.946	79	96
L2-L4	0.921	77	93
L3-L4	0.883	74	89

Fig. 2-10. A DXA AP spine study acquired on the Lunar DPX. A sclerotic reaction should be suspected at L2 from the appearance of the image and the marked increase in BMD at L2, compared to the BMDs at L1 and L3.

measurement of 100% trabecular bone, since all of the cortical vertebral shell is not eliminated from analysis.

Vertebral identification in the lateral projection can be difficult. The lumbar vertebrae are generally identified by the relative position of the overlapping pelvis and the position of the lowest set of ribs. The position of the pelvis tends to differ, however, when the study is performed in the left lateral decubitus position, compared to the supine position. Rupich et al. *(25)* found that the pelvis overlapped L4 in only 15% of individuals, when studied in the supine position. Jergas et al. *(26)* reported a figure of 19.7% for L4 overlap for individuals studied in the supine position. In DXA studies performed in the left lateral decubitus position, pelvic overlap of L4 occurred in 88% of individuals *(13)*. In the other 12%, the pelvis overlapped L5 in 5%, and the L3–L4 disk space or L3 itself in 7%. As a consequence, although the position of the pelvis tends to identify L4 in most individuals scanned in the left lateral decubitus position, it also eliminates the ability to accurately measure the BMD at L4 in those individuals. The ribs are less useful than the pelvis in identifying the lumbar vertebrae. Rib overlap of L1 can be expected in the majority of individuals, whether they are studied in the supine or left lateral decubitus position *(13)*. This may not be seen, however, in the 12.5% of individuals whose lowest set of ribs is on T11.

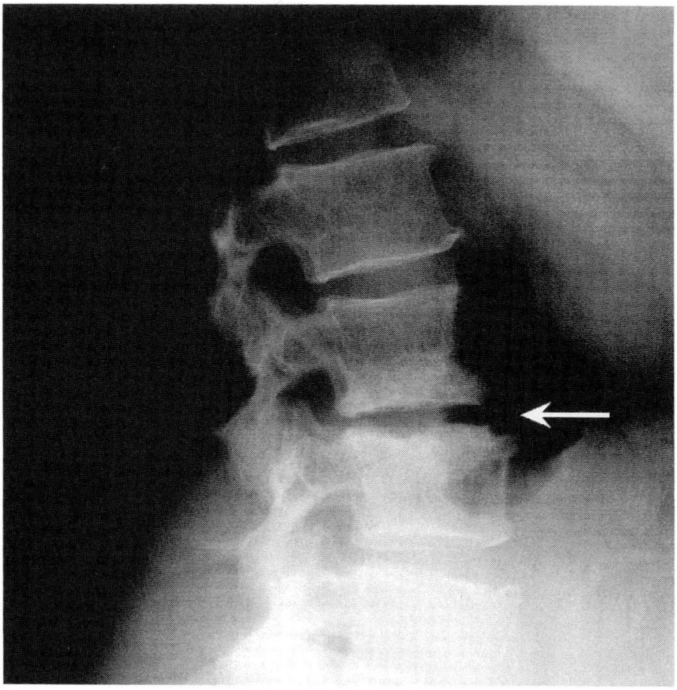

Fig. 2-11. A lateral lumbar X ray of the patient whose DXA study is shown in Fig. 2-12. The arrow indicates a region of marked endplate sclerosis.

The location of the pelvis and the presence of rib overlap may aid in identification of the vertebrae, but they also limit the available vertebrae for analysis. When a lateral spine DXA study is performed in the left lateral decubitus position, L4 cannot be analyzed in the majority of individuals, because of pelvic overlap. L1 is generally not analyzed because of rib overlap, regardless of whether the study is performed supine or in the left lateral decubitus position. Rupich et al. *(25)* also found that rib overlay L2 in 90% of individuals studied in the supine position. It was estimated that rib BMC added 10.4% to the L2 BMC. As a consequence, when lateral DXA studies are performed in the left lateral decubitus position, L3 may be the only vertebra that is not affected by either pelvic overlap or rib overlap. In the supine position, L3 and L4 are generally unaffected. This means that, depending on the positioning required by the technique, the value from a single vertebra, or from only a two-vertebrae average, may have to be used. This is undesirable, although sometimes unavoidable, from the standpoint of statistical accuracy and precision.

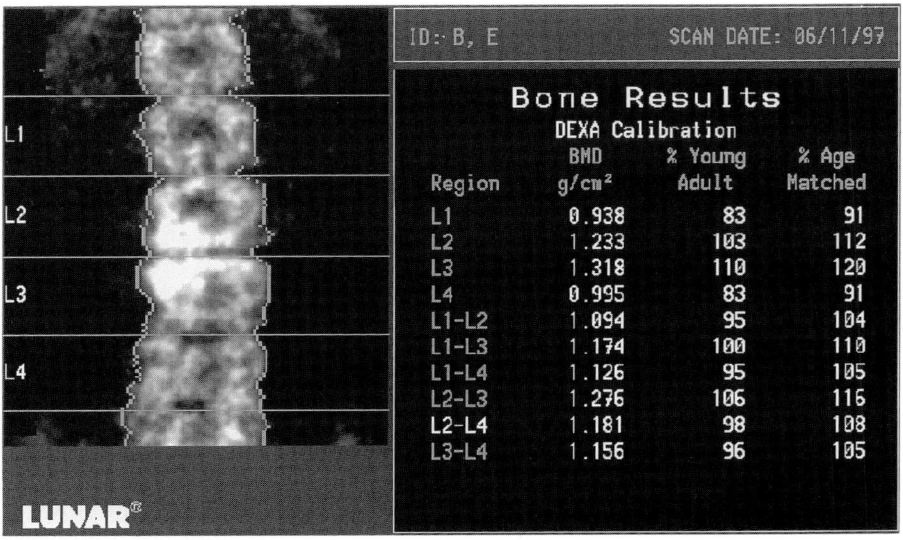
L1
L2
L3
L4
LUNAR®
ID: B, E
SCAN DATE: 06/11/97
Bone Results
DEXA Calibration
Region
BMD g/cm²
% Young Adult
% Age Matched
L1 0.938 83 91
L2 1.233 103 112
L3 1.318 110 120
L4 0.995 83 91
L1-L2 1.094 95 104
L1-L3 1.174 100 110
L1-L4 1.126 95 105
L2-L3 1.276 106 116
L2-L4 1.181 98 108
L3-L4 1.156 96 105

Fig. 2-12. A DXA AP spine study acquired on the Lunar DPX. The image dramatically suggests the sclerotic process seen on the X ray in Fig. 2-11. There is a marked increase in the BMD at L2 and L3.

If the vertebrae are misidentified in the lateral projection, the effect on BMD can be significant. In the study by Peel et al. *(13)*, misidentification of the vertebral levels would have resulted in 12% of individuals in which the pelvis did not overlap L4 in the left lateral decubitus position. If L2 was misidentified as L3, the BMD of L3 was underestimated by an average of 5.7%. When L4 was misidentified as L3, the BMD at L3 was overestimated by an average of 3.1%. Although spine X rays are rarely justified for the sole purpose of vertebral identification on a DXA study performed in the AP projection, this may be required for DXA lumbar spine studies performed in the lateral projection, particularly when performed in the left lateral decubitus position. Because analysis may be restricted to only one or two vertebrae, reducing statistical accuracy, consideration should be given to combining lateral DXA spine studies with bone density assessments of other sites, for diagnostic purposes.

THE PROXIMAL FEMUR IN DENSITOMETRY

Proximal Femur Anatomy

The gross anatomy of the proximal femur is shown in Fig. 2-21A,B. In densitometry, the proximal femur has been divided into specific regions of interest. The proximal femur study shown in Fig. 2-22 illustrates these

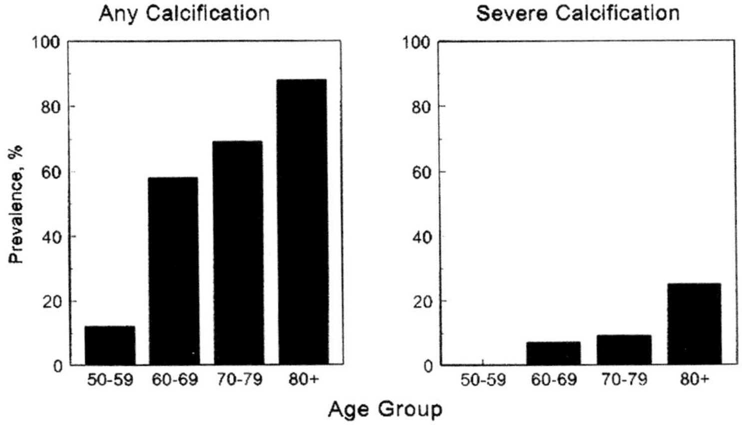

Fig. 2-13. The prevalence of aortic calcification in women aged 50 and over. (Reprinted from Frye MA, et al. [1992] Osteoporosis and calcification of the aorta. Bone and Mineral 19:185–194, with kind permission from Elsevier Science Ireland Ltd., Bay 15K, Shannon Industrial Estate, Co. Clare, Ireland.)

Table 2-7
Effect of Aortic Calcification on BMD in the Spine

	BMD			
Site	*Observed*	*Expected*	*Difference*	*% of Expected*
BMD spine				
Any grade 1 or 2	0.93	0.92	0.01	101.4%
Any grade 2	0.94	0.89	0.05	106.7%

Values are in g/cm^2.

Adapted from Frye MA, et al. (1992) Osteoporosis and calcification of the aorta. *Bone Min* 19:185–194, with kind permission from Elsevier Science Ireland Ltd., Bay 15K, Shannon Industrial Estate, Co. Clare, Ireland.

regions, which are based upon the anatomy shown in Fig. 2-21A,B. Ward's area is a region with which most physicians are not familiar. Ward's triangle, as it was originally called, is an anatomic region in the neck of the femur that is formed by the intersection of three trabecular bundles, as shown in Fig. 2-23. In densitometry, Ward's triangle is a calculated region of low density in the femoral neck, rather than a specific anatomic region. Because the region in densitometry is identified as a square, the region is generally now called Ward's area, instead of Ward's triangle. The total femur region of interest encompasses all of the individual regions: the

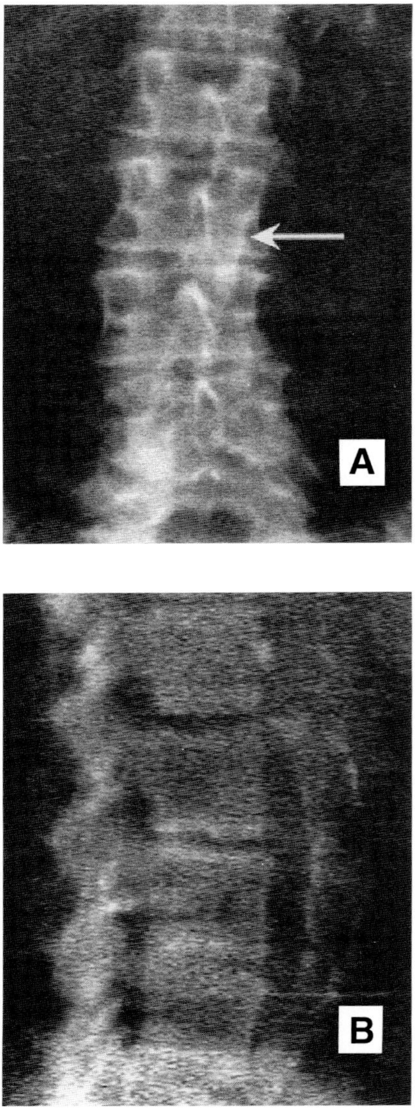

Fig. 2-14. AP and lateral DXA lumbar spine images acquired on the Hologic QDR-4500. The arrow seen in **(A)** indicates the faint outline of the calcified aorta that is easily seen on the lateral study in **(B)**. Case courtesy of Hologic, Inc., Waltham, MA.

femoral neck, Ward's area, the trochanteric region, and the shaft. Each of these regions within this one bone contains a different percentage of trabecular and cortical bone, as noted in Table 2-1.

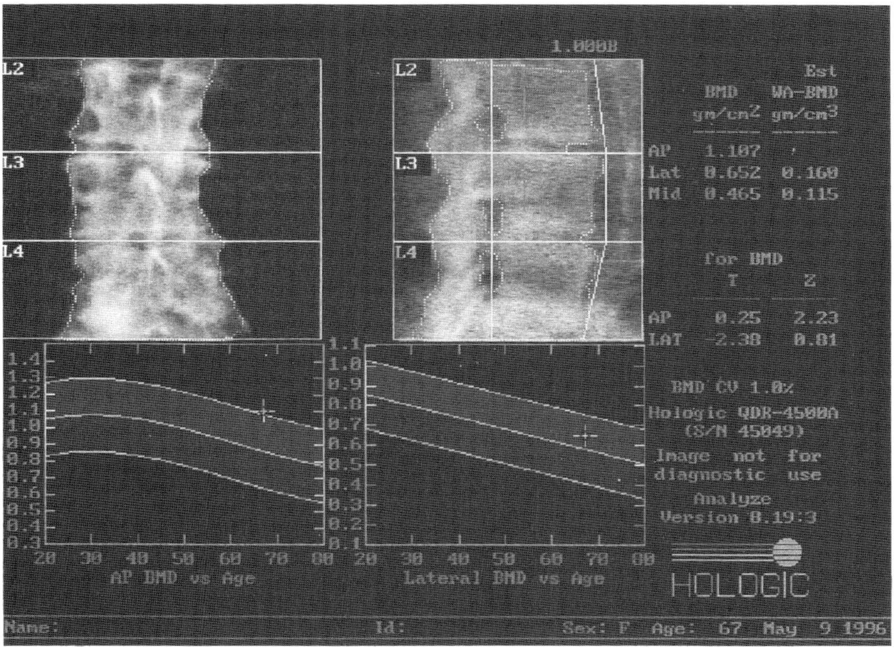

Fig. 2-15. A DXA AP and lateral lumbar spine study acquired on the Hologic QDR-4500. These are the analyzed studies for the images shown in Fig. 2-14. Case courtesy of Hologic, Inc., Waltham, MA. (*see* color plate 5 appearing after p. 78)

Effect of Rotation on BMD in the Proximal Femur

The lesser trochanter is an important anatomic structure from the perspective of recognizing the degree to which the femur has been rotated during positioning for a proximal femur bone-density study. Precision in proximal femur bone density testing is highly dependent on reproducing the degree of rotation of the proximal femur from study to study. Internally rotating the femur approximately 15° will result in the femoral neck being parallel to the plane of the scan table. BMD values in the femoral neck are the lowest in this position. As femoral rotation is either increased or decreased from this position, the femoral neck BMD value will increase. Table 2-9 illustrates the magnitude of the increase in BMD in a cadaver study from Goh et al. *(27)*. The apparent length of the neck of the femur will decrease as rotation is increased or decreased from the basic position. When the neck of the femur is parallel to the plane of the scan table, the X-ray beam passes through the neck at a 90° angle to the neck. With changes in rotation, the neck is no longer parallel to the scan table, and the

Table 2-8
Increase in BMD from Facet Sclerosis

	Grade 2	*Grade 3*
L1	0.275	0.465
L2	0.312	0.472
L3	0.184	0.343
L4	0.034	0.247
Average	0.201	0.382

Values are in g/cm^2.

Adapted with permission of the publisher from Drinka PJ et al. (1992) The effect of overlying calcification on lumbar bone densitometry. *Calcified Tissue International* 50:507–510.

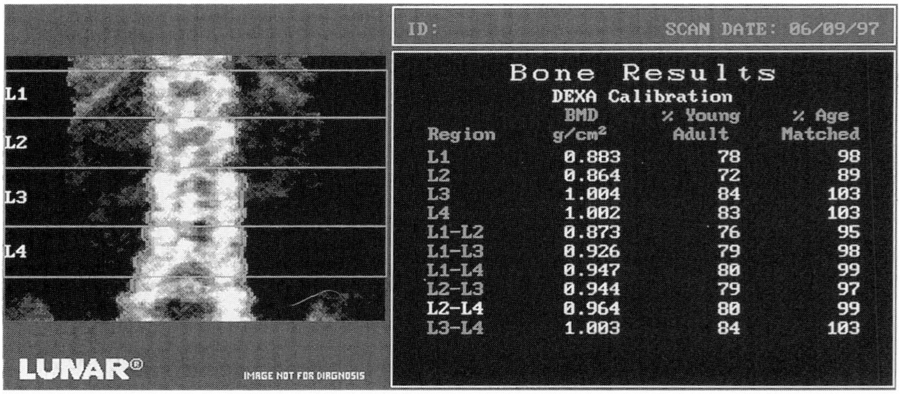

Fig. 2-16. A DXA AP lumbar-spine study acquired on the Lunar DPX. There is a marked increase in the BMD between L2 and L3, which is maintained at L4. The image faintly suggests sclerosis in the region of the facet joints at L3 and L4. This is more dramatically seen in the plain film of this patient shown in Fig. 2-17.

beam enters the neck at an angle that is greater or less than 90°. The result is an apparent shortening of the length of the neck and an increase in the mineral content in the path of the beam. The combination results in an apparent increase in BMD. The only visual clue to consistent rotation is the reproduction of the size and shape of the lesser trochanter. Because the trochanter is a posterior structure, leg positioning in which the femur has not been rotated sufficiently internally tends to produce a very large and pointed lesser trochanter. Excessive internal rotation of the proximal femur will result in a total disappearance of the lesser trochanter. The size of the lesser trochanter in the DXA proximal femur image in Fig. 2-24A indicates

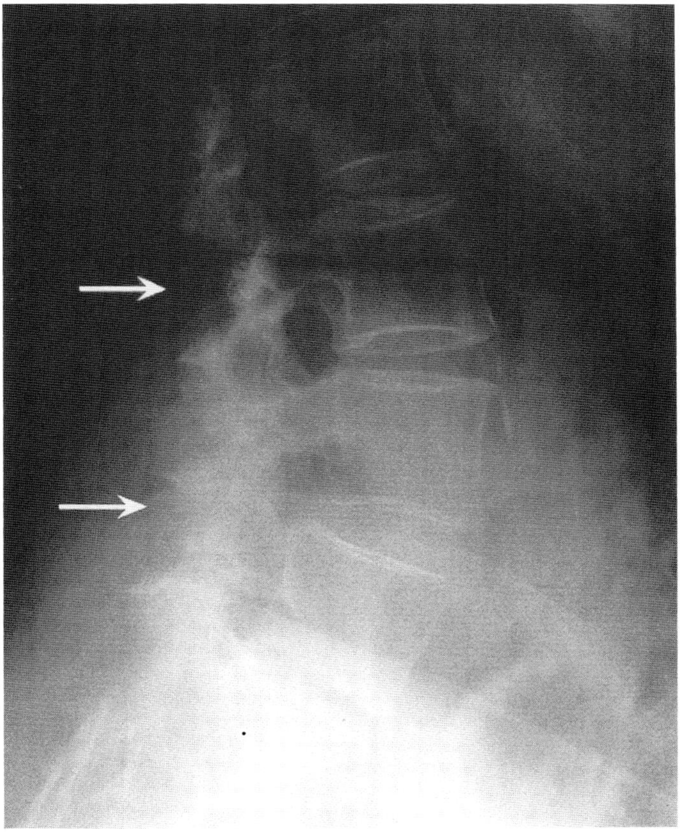

Fig. 2-17. A lateral lumbar spine X ray of the patient whose bone-density study is shown in Fig. 2-16. The arrows indicate regions of sclerosis in the posterior elements.

correct internal rotation. This can be compared to the size of the lesser trochanter seen in the DXA proximal femur study in Fig. 2-24B, in which the lesser trochanter is very large and pointed, indicating insufficient internal rotation. Although this would be undesirable in a baseline study of the proximal femur, follow-up studies using the proximal femur in this patient should be done with this same degree of rotation. Any change in rotation from the baseline study would be expected to affect the magnitude of change in the BMD, decreasing the precision of the study.

Effect of Leg Dominance on BMD in the Proximal Femur

In general, there does not seem to be a significant difference in the BMD in the regions of the proximal femur between the right and left legs of

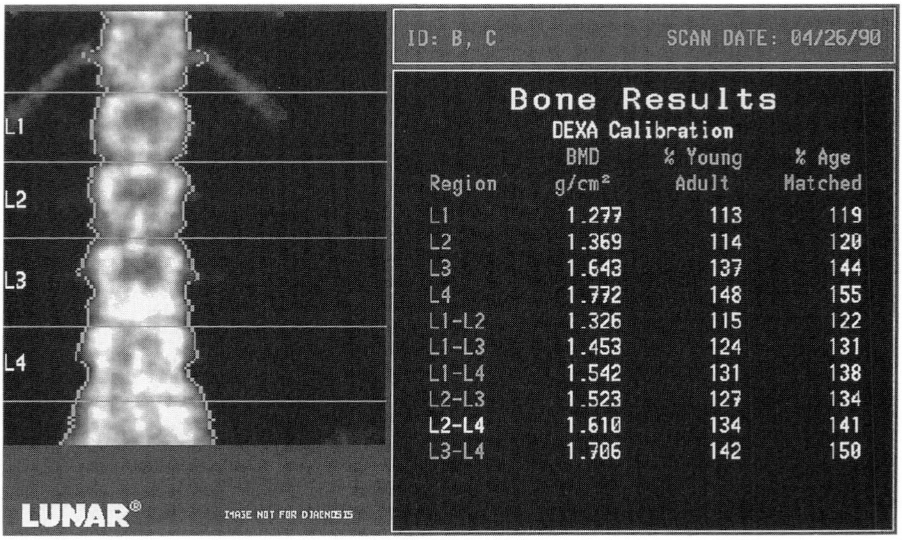
ID: B, C
SCAN DATE: 04/26/90
Bone Results
DEXA Calibration
Region | BMD g/cm² | % Young Adult | % Age Matched
L1 1.277 113 119
L2 1.369 114 120
L3 1.643 137 144
L4 1.772 148 155
L1-L2 1.326 115 122
L1-L3 1.453 124 131
L1-L4 1.542 131 138
L2-L3 1.523 127 134
L2-L4 1.610 134 141
L3-L4 1.706 142 150
L1
L2
L3
L4
LUNAR®
IMAGE NOT FOR DIAGNOSIS

Fig. 2-18. A DXA AP spine study acquired on the Lunar DPX. The image suggests increased density at L3 and L4, but there is also a linear vertical lucency over L4. The BMD values are markedly increased at L3 and L4. This patient had previously undergone an L3–4, L4–5 interbody fusion and laminectomy at L4.

normal individuals *(28,29)*. Leg dominance, unlike arm dominance, does not appear to exert a significant effect on the bone densities in the proximal femur, and is not used to determine which femur should be studied. In patients with scoliosis, however, lower bone densities have been reported on the side of the convexity *(30)*.

Effect of Artifacts on BMD in the Proximal Femur

Structural change and artifact interfering with DXA proximal femoral BMD measurements seem to occur less often than in the spine. Osteoarthritic change in the hip joint may cause thickening of the medial cortex and hypertrophy of the trabeculae in the femoral neck, which would be expected to increase the BMD in the neck and Ward's area *(31)*. The trochanteric region is not apparently affected by such change, and has been recommended as the preferred site to evaluate in patients with osteoarthritis of the hip *(32)*. The effects of osteoarthritis of the hip on BMD in other regions of the skeleton are discussed in Chapter 7. Proximal femur fracture and surgically implanted prostheses will render measurements of bone density in the proximal femur inaccurate.

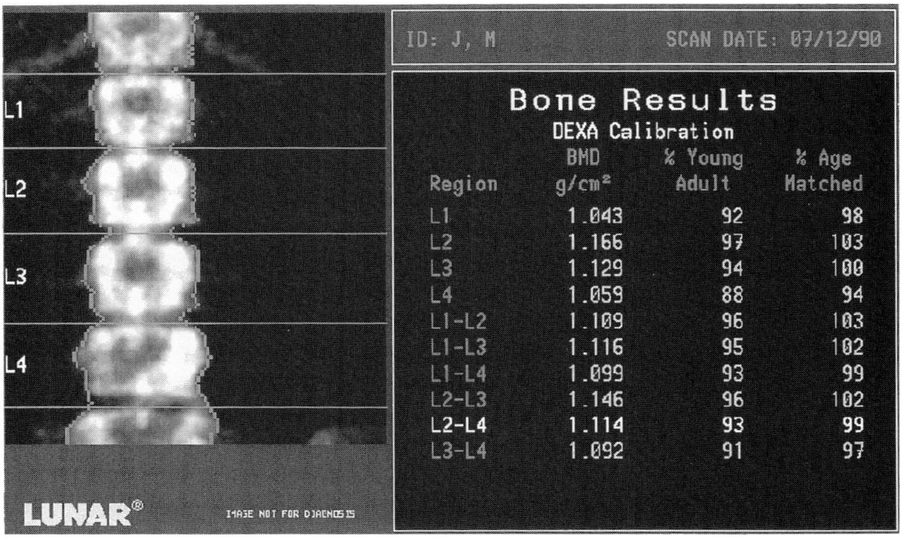

Fig. 2-19. A DXA AP spine study acquired on the Lunar DPX. The image is unusual at L4, with what appears to be an absence of part of the posterior elements. This was confirmed with plain films. This would be expected to decrease the BMD at L4. (*see* color plate 6 appearing after p. 78)

THE FOREARM IN DENSITOMETRY

Nomenclature

The nomenclature used to describe the various sites in the forearm that are assessed with densitometry can be confusing. Commonly used sites are the 33% or one-third site,* the 50% and 10% sites, the 5 and 8 mm sites, and the ultradistal site. The sites designated by a percentage are named based on the location of the site in relationship to the overall length of the ulna. This is true regardless of whether the site is on the ulna or the radius. In other words, the 50% site on the radius is located directly across from the site on the ulna that marks 50% of the overall ulnar length, not 50% of the overall radial length. The 5 and 8 mm sites are located on either bone at the point where the separation distance between the radius and ulna is 5 or 8 mm, respectively. The 33% and 50% sites are often referred to as

*Although a mathematical conversion of one-third to a percentage would result in a value of 33.3%, the site, when named as a percentage, is called the 33% site, and is located on the radius or ulna at a location that represents 33%, not 33.3%, of the length of the ulna.

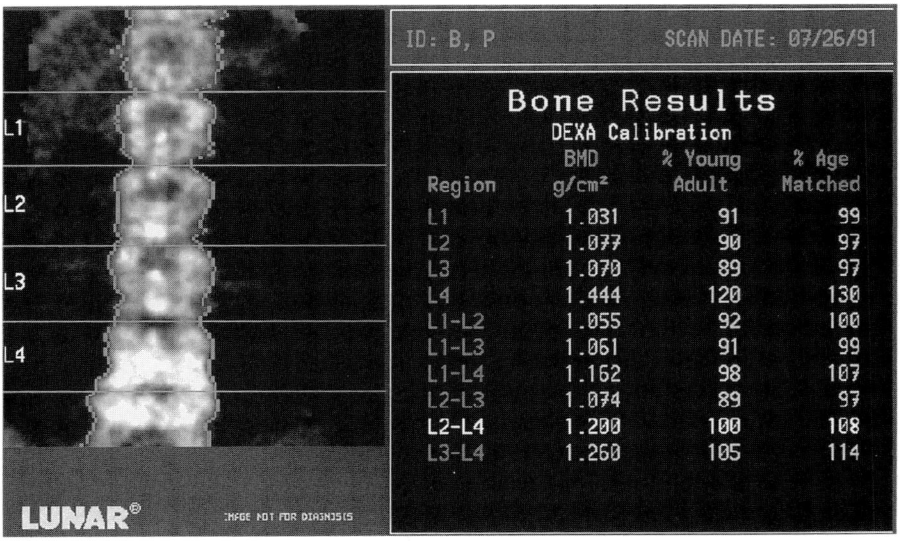

Fig. 2-20. A DXA AP spine study acquired on the Lunar DPX. The image suggests a marked sclerotic reaction at L4 and L5. There is also a marked increase in the BMD at L4, compared to L3. This sclerotic process was thought to be the result of an episode of childhood disciitis. (*see* color plate 7 appearing after p. 78)

midradial sites, but the 10% site is considered a distal site. The ultradistal site is variously located at a distance of either 4 or 5% of the ulnar length. The difference between these sites is the relative percentage of cortical and trabecular bone found at the site. Table 2-1 summarizes the percentages of cortical and trabecular bone in the various sites on the radius.

Effect of Arm Dominance on Forearm BMD

Unlike the proximal femur, arm dominance has a pronounced effect on the bone density of the arm. In healthy individuals, the BMC at the 33% radial site differs by 6–9% between the dominant and nondominant arms *(33)*. A difference of 3% has been reported at the 8 mm site *(34)*. If the individual is involved in any type of repetitive activity that involves unilateral arm activity, the difference between the dominant and nondominant arm densities will be magnified to an even greater extent. Two studies of individuals who play tennis, an activity in which the dominant arm is subjected to repeated loading and impact, illustrate the effect of unilateral activity. In a study by Huddleston et al. *(35)*, the BMC in the dominant arm at the 50% radial site, measured by SPA, was 13% greater than in the nondominant arm. In a more recent study from Kannus et al. using DXA

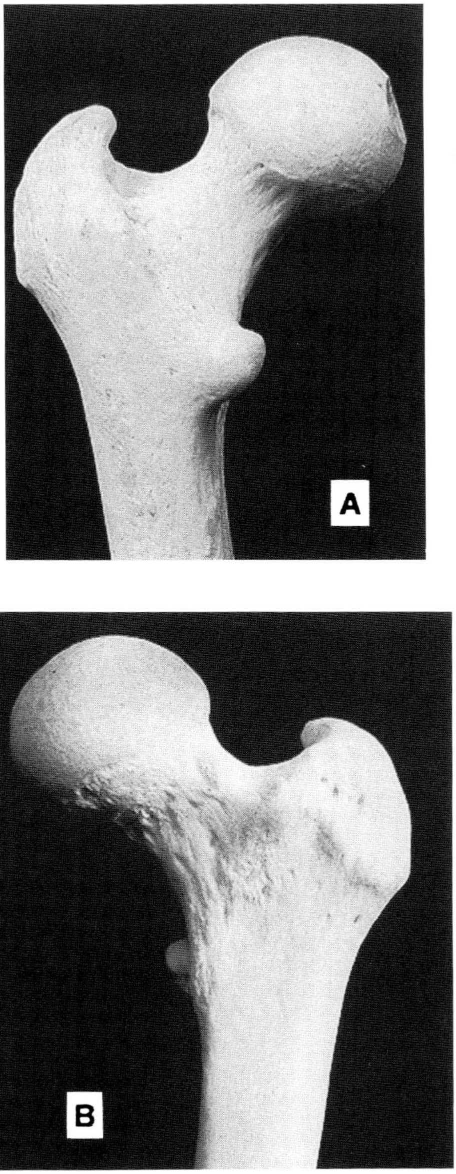

Fig. 2-21. (A) The proximal femur as viewed from behind. The lesser trochanter is clearly seen to be a posterior structure. **(B)** The proximal femur as seen from the front. The lesser trochanter is now behind the shaft of the femur. (Photos from McMinn RMH, Hutchings RT, Pegington J, and Abrahams PH. [1993] *Color Atlas of Human Anatomy*, 3rd ed. By permission of Mosby International) (*see* color plates 8 and 9 appearing after p. 78)

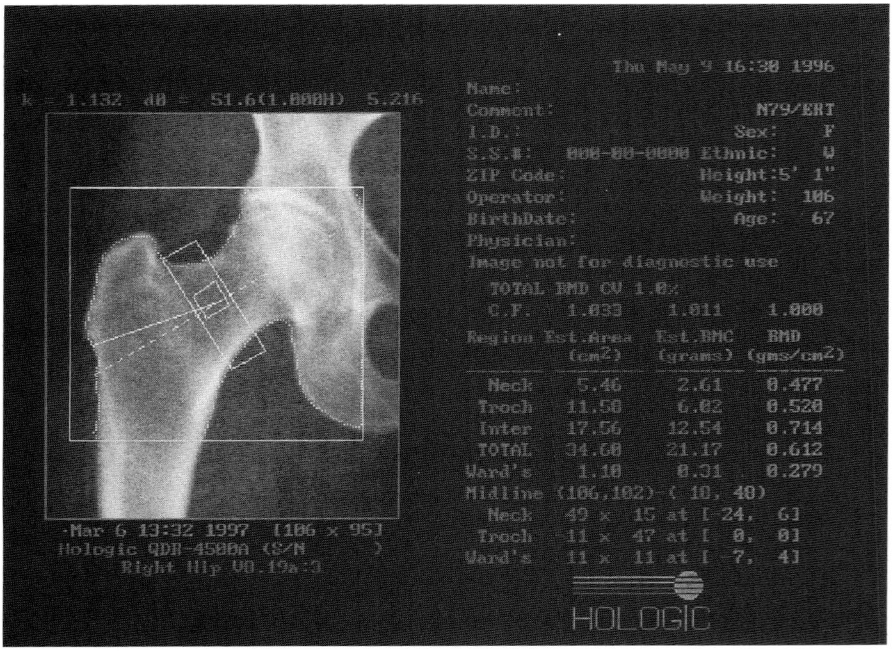

Fig. 2-22. A DXA proximal femur study acquired on the Hologic QDR-4500. Five regions of the interest are defined in this study. Case courtesy of Hologic, Inc., Waltham, MA. (*see* color plate 10 appearing after p. 78)

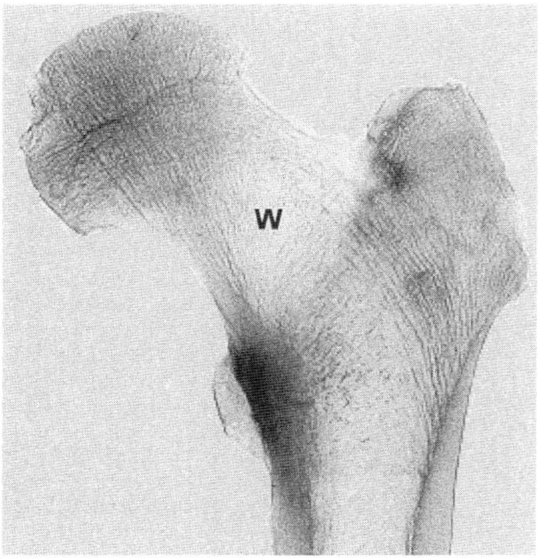

Fig. 2-23. Ward's triangle, indicated by the letter W, is formed by the intersection of bundles of trabeculae in the femoral neck. (Photo from McMinn RMH, Hutchings RT, Pegington J, and Abrahams PH. [1993] *Color Atlas of Human Anatomy*, 3rd ed. By permission of Mosby International) (*see* color plate 11 appearing after p. 78)

Table 2-9
Effect of Increasing Internal or External Rotation from the Neutral Position on the Femoral Neck BMD (g/cm^2) of Cadaveric Femurs

	Neutral	*External rotation from neutral of*			*Internal rotation from neutral of*		
Cadaver no.	0°	15°	30°	45°	15°	30°	45°
1	0.490	0.524	0.549	0.628	0.510	0.714	0.845
2	0.574	0.567	0.632	0.711	0.581	0.619	0.753
3	0.835	0.872	0.902	1.071	0.874	1.037	1.222
4	0.946	0.977	1.005	1.036	1.102	1.283	1.492

Reproduced with permission of the publisher from Goh JCH et al. (1995) Effect of femoral rotation on bone mineral density measurements with dual energy X-ray absorptiometry. *Calcified Tissue International* 57:340–343.

(36), the side-to-side difference in BMD in tennis players averaged 10.8% at the distal radius and 9.9% at the midradius. The corresponding values in the controls were only 3.4 and 2.5%, respectively. Because of these recognized differences, the nondominant arm has traditionally been studied when the bone content or density is being quantified for the purposes of diagnosis or fracture-risk assessment. Most reference databases for the machines in current use have been created using the nondominant arm. Comparisons of the dominant arm to these reference databases would not be valid.

The Effect of Artifacts on BMD in the Forearm

The forearm sites are relatively free from the confounding effects of most of the types of artifacts that are often seen in the lumbar spine. The presence of a prior fracture in the forearm will affect the accuracy of the BMC or BMD measurements in the forearm, close to the prior fracture site. Akesson et al. *(37)*, suggested that, in women with a prior fracture of the distal radius, the BMC was increased by 20% at the distal radius of the fractured arm, in comparison to the nonfractured arm, irrespective of arm dominance.

OTHER SKELETAL SITES

Many other skeletal sites can be studied using the techniques available today. Total-body bone density, phalangeal bone density, and calcaneal bone density are commonly performed studies. The bone density in regions in the humerus, tibia, and distal femur can also be quantified. The anatomic considerations for these sites are not unique to densitometry, however. Thus, these sites are not discussed in detail here. The relative percentages

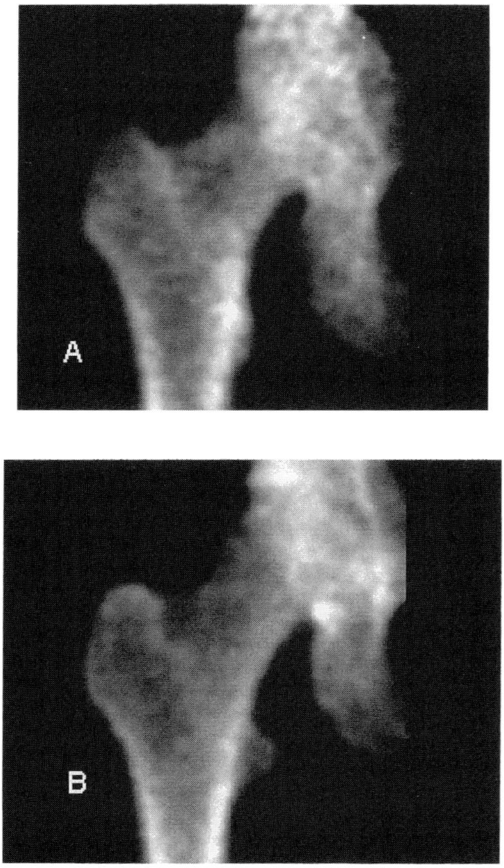

Fig. 2-24. (A) DXA proximal femur study acquired on the Lunar DPX. The lesser trochanter is clearly seen, but small in size, indicating proper rotation of the proximal femur during positioning. Compare this lesser trochanter to the lesser trochanter seen in **(B)** DXA proximal femur study acquired on the Lunar DPX. The lesser trochanter is very large and pointed, indicating insufficient internal rotation during positioning.

of trabecular and cortical bone for the phalanges, calcaneus, and total body are noted in Table 2-1.

REFERENCES

1. Recker RR (1992) Embryology, anatomy, and microstructure of bone. In Coe FL, Favus MJ, eds. *Disorders of Bone and Mineral Metabolism*, New York: Raven, pp. 219–240.
2. Dempster DW (1992) Bone remodeling. In Coe FL, Favus MJ, eds. *Disorders of Bone and Mineral Metabolism*, New York: Raven, pp. 355–380.

3. Schlenker RA, VonSeggen WW (1976) The distribution of cortical and trabecular bone mass along the lengths of the radius and ulna and the implications for in vivo bone mass measurements. *Calcif Tissue Res* 20:41–52.
4. Eastell R, Wahner HW, O'Fallon WM, Amadio PC, Melton LJ III, Riggs BL (1989) Unequal decrease in bone density of lumbar spine and ultradistal radius in Colles' and vertebral fracture syndromes. *J Clin Invest* 83:168–174.
5. Johnson LC (1964) Morphologic analysis in pathology: the kinetics of disease and general biology of bone. In: Frost HM, ed. *Bone Biodynamics*, Boston: Little, pp. 543–564.
6. Rockoff SD, Sweet E, Bleustein J (1969) The relative contribution of trabecular and cortical bone to the strength of human lumbar vertebrae. *Calcif Tissue Res* 3:163–175.
7. Nottestad SY, Baumel JJ, Kimmel DB, Recker RR, Heaney RP (1987) The proportion of trabecular bone in human vertebrae. *J Bone Miner Res* 2:221–229.
8. Eastell R, Mosekilde L, Hodgson SF, Riggs BL (1990) Proportion of human vertebral body bone that is cancellous. *J Bone Miner Res* 5:1237–1241.
9. Heaney RP. Personal communication.
10. Bonnick SL (1996) Bone densitometry techniques in modern medicine. In: Rosen C, ed. *Osteoporosis: Diagnostic and Therapeutic Principles*, Totowa, NJ, Humana, pp. 89–112.
11. Louis O, Van Den Winkel P, Covens P, Schoutens A, Osteaux M (1992) Dual-energy X-ray absorptiometry of lumbar vertebrae: relative contribution of body and posterior elements and accuracy in relation with neutron activation analysis. *Bone* 13:317–320.
12. Mazess RB, Barden HS (1990) Interrelationships among bone densitometry sites in normal young women. *Bone Miner* 11:347–356.
13. Peel NFA, Johnson A, Barrington NA, Smith TWD, Eastell R (1993) Impact of anomalous vertebral segmentation of measurements of bone mineral density. *J Bone Miner Res* 8:719–723.
14. Bornstein PE, Peterson RR (1996) Numerical variation of the presacral vertebral column in three population groups in North America. *Am J Phys Anthropol* 25: 139–146.
15. Krolner B, Berthelsen B, Nielsen SP (1982) Assessment of vertebral osteopenia—comparison of spinal radiography and dual-photon absorptiometry. *Acta Radiol Diagn* 23:517–521.
16. Rand T, Seidl G, Kainberger F, Resch A, Hittmair K, Schneider B, Gluer CC, Imhof H (1997) Impact of spinal degenerative changes on the evaluation of bone mineral density with dual energy X-ray absorptiometry (DXA). *Calcif Tissue Int* 60:430–433.
17. Cann CE, Rutt BK, Genant HK (1983) Effect of extraosseous calcification on vertebral mineral measurement. *Calcif Tissue Int* 35:667.
18. Frye MA, Melton LJ, Bryant SC, Fitzpatrick LA, Wahner HW, Schwartz RS, Riggs BL (1992) Osteoporosis and calcification of the aorta. *Bone Miner* 19:185–194.
19. Frohn J, Wilken T, Falk S, Stutte HJ, Kollath J, Hor G (1990) Effect of aortic sclerosis on bone mineral measurements by dual-photon absorptiometry. *J Nucl Med* 32: 259–262.
20. Orwoll ES, Oviatt SK, Mann T (1990) The impact of osteophytic and vascular calcifications on vertebral mineral density measurements in men. *J Clin Endocrinol Metab* 70:1202–1207.
21. Reid IR, Evans MC, Ames R, Wattie DJ (1991) The influence of osteophytes and aortic calcification on spinal mineral density in post-menopausal women. *J Clin Endocrinol Metab* 72:1372–1374.
22. Banks LM, Lees B, MacSweeney JE, Stevenson JC. (1991) Do degenerative changes and aortic calcification influence long-term bone density measurements? Abstract. 8th International Workshop on Bone Densitometry, Bad Reichenhall, Germany.

23. Drinka PJ, DeSmet AA, Bauwens SF, Rogot A (1992) The effect of overlying calcification on lumbar bone densitometry. *Calcif Tissue Int* 50:507–510.
24. Stutzman ME, Yester MV, Dubovsky EV (1987) Technical aspects of dual-photon absorptiometry of the spine. *Technique* 15:177–181.
25. Rupich RC, Griffin MG, Pacifici R, Avioli LV, Susman N (1992) Lateral dual-energy radiography: artifact error from rib and pelvic bone. *J Bone Miner Res* 7:97–101.
26. Jergas M, Breitenseher M, Gluer CC, Black D, Lang P, Grampp S, Engelke K, Genant HK (1995) Which vertebrae should be assessed using lateral dual-energy X-ray absorptiometry of the lumbar spine? *Osteoporosis Int* 5:196–204.
27. Goh JCH, Low SL, Bose K (1995) Effect of femoral rotation on bone mineral density measurements with dual energy X-ray absorptiometry. *Calcif Tissue Int* 57:340–343.
28. Bonnick SL, Nichols DL, Sanborn CF, Payne SG, Moen SM, Heiss CJ (1996) Right and left proximal femur analyses: is there a need to do both? *Calcif Tissue Int* 58: 307–310.
29. Faulkner KG, Genant HK, McClung M (1995) Bilateral comparison of femoral bone density and hip axis length from single and fan beam DXA scans. *Calcif Tissue Int* 56:26–31.
30. Hans D, Biot B, Schott AM, Meunier PJ (1996) No diffuse osteoporosis in lumbar scoliosis but lower femoral bone density on the convexity. *Bone* 18:15–17.
31. Nevitt MC, Lane NE, Scott JC, Hochberg MC, Pressman AR, Genant HK, Cummings SR (1995) Radiographic osteoarthritis of the hip and bone mineral density. *Arthritis Rheum* 38:907–916.
32. Preidler KW, White LS, Tashkin J, McDaniel CO, Brossman J, Andresen R, Sartoris D (1997) Dual-energy X-ray absorptiometric densitometry in osteoarthritis of the hip. Influence of secondary bone remodeling of the femoral neck. *Acta Radiol* 38: 539–542.
33. Karjalainen P, Alhava EM (1976) Bone mineral content of the forearm in a healthy population. *Acta Radiol Oncol Radiat Phys Biol* 16:199–208.
34. Borg J, Mollgaard A, Riis BJ (1995) Single X-ray absorptiometry: performance characteristics and comparison with single photon absorptiometry. *Osteoporosis Int* 5:377–381.
35. Huddleston AL, Rockwell D, Kulund DN, Harrison B (1980) Bone mass in lifetime tennis athletes. *JAMA* 244:1107–1109.
36. Kannus P, Haapasalo H, Sievanen H, Oja P, Vuori I (1994) The site-specific effects of long-term unilateral activity on bone mineral density and content. *Bone* 15:279–284.
37. Akesson K, Gardsell P, Sernbo I, Johnell O, Obrant KJ (1992) Earlier wrist fracture: a confounding factor in distal forearm bone screening. *Osteoporosis Int* 2:201–204.

3 Statistics in Densitometry

CONTENTS

Many physicians in clinical practice have not had formal training in statistics, but a basic knowledge of certain aspects of statistics is essential for the physician densitometrist. Quality control procedures for the various machines require some statistical analyses. The computer-generated reports of bone density data include statistical devices, such as *T*- and *z*-scores and confidence intervals. In order to interpret serial studies, the physician must understand the concept of precision, and be able to calculate the precision of repeat measurements in his or her facility. These concepts and others are discussed in this chapter.

MEAN, VARIANCE, AND STANDARD DEVIATION

Most statistical textbooks begin with a discussion of the mean, variance, and standard deviation. This is appropriate here as well, because many of the statistical devices used in densitometry begin with a calculation of the mean and standard deviation of a set of bone-density measurements.

Table 3-1
Individual and Mean Spine BMD Values for Patient, Mrs. J.

Patient	*Scan 1*	*Scan 2*	*Scan 3*	*Mean or $\bar{X}$*
Mrs. J.	1.010	1.019	1.100	1.043

Values are in g/cm^2.

The Mean

The mean is the average value for a set of measurements. For example, Mrs. J. underwent three spine bone-density studies on the same day. Between each study, she stood up and then resumed her position on the scan table. The results of her three studies are shown in Table 3-1. The average of the three spine bone-density studies is simply the sum of the three studies divided by the number of studies. In statistical terminology, the average is called the mean. Statistical shorthand for the formula for calculating the average, or mean, is as follows:

$$\bar{X} = \frac{\Sigma X}{n}$$

The mean or $\bar{X}$ (pronounced X-bar) is equal to the sum, Σ, of all X measurements, divided by the number of measurements, n. In this case, the mean of the three spine bone-density measurements on Mrs. J. is 1.043 g/cm^2.

Variance and Standard Deviation

Although the average, or mean, value for the set of three measurements on Mrs. J. is 1.043 g/cm^2, it is reasonable to ask how much the individual measurements vary from the average measurement. This question can be answered by calculating the variance and standard deviation for this set of data.

The variance, abbreviated s^2, is the average of the squares of the differences between each individual measurement and the mean. The formula is as follows:

$$s^2 = \frac{\Sigma(X - \bar{X})^2}{n - 1}$$

Each measurement, X, is subtracted from the mean, $\bar{X}$, in order to find the difference between the measurement and the mean. Because some of the differences will be negative, the differences are squared in order to remove the negative sign. Each of the squared differences is added, and then divided by $n - 1$, or the number of measurements minus 1, to find the average squared difference between the individual measurements and the mean. The rationale behind the use of $n - 1$, instead of n, to find the average is beyond the scope of this discussion.

Remember that the variance is the average of the squared differences between the individual values and the mean. The square root of the variance is called the standard deviation, written as s in statistical formulas, and often abbreviated as SD in medical literature. It is apparent now why the variance is abbreviated as s^2. Both the standard deviation and the variance are measures of variability in a set of data around a central value.

If we were to calculate the variance for the set of three measurements on Mrs. J., the calculations would proceed as follows:

1. The difference between each of the three measurements and the mean is calculated.

$$1.010 - 1.043 = -0.033$$

$$1.019 - 1.043 = -0.024$$

$$1.100 - 1.043 = 0.057$$

2. Each of the three differences is squared.

$$(-0.033)^2 = 0.001089$$

$$(-0.024)^2 = 0.000576$$

$$(0.057)^2 = 0.003249$$

3. The three squared differences are added.

$$0.001089 + 0.000576 + 0.003249 = 0.004914$$

4. This sum is divided by the number of measurements $(n) - 1$. This number is the variance.

$$s^2 = 0.004914 \div 2 = 0.002457$$

The square root of the variance is the standard deviation. Therefore,

$$s = \sqrt{0.002457} = 0.0496$$

The mean or average BMD, based on the three spine bone density measurements on Mrs. J., is 1.043 g/cm^2. The variance and standard deviation from this set of data on Mrs. J. are 0.003 and 0.05 g/cm^2, respectively (with rounding). Since the standard deviation represents a measure of variability of the individual measurements about the mean, it is reasonable to ask what proportion or percentage the standard deviation is of the mean. This brings us to a discussion of the coefficient of variation.

COEFFICIENT OF VARIATION

The coefficient of variation is an important concept in bone densitometry, because it is frequently used to describe the accuracy and precision of the various technologies in use today. The coefficient of variation, abbreviated CV, is calculated by dividing the standard deviation, *s*, by the mean, $\bar{X}$, for a set of data. The formula is as follows:

$$CV = s \div \bar{X}$$

This can be expressed as a percentage by multiplying by 100.

To calculate the CV for the three measurements on Mrs. J., the standard deviation of 0.05 g/cm^2 is divided by the mean of 1.043 g/cm^2. This value is 0.048. To express this as a percentage, 0.048 is multiplied by 100, yielding 4.8%. The percent coefficient of variation, or %CV, is therefore 4.8%.

STANDARD SCORES

Standard scores allow you to compare values on different scales to a common or standard scale *(1)*. Standard scores, such as the *T*-score and *z*-score, are used extensively, but not exclusively, in bone densitometry.

For example, imagine that a group of physicians, group A, was tested on their knowledge of bone densitometry. Arbitrarily, the highest score that could be made on the test was 75, and the lowest score that could be made was 25. A second group of physicians, group B, was also tested on their knowledge of bone densitometry. On this test, however, the highest score that could be made was 100, and the lowest score that could be made was 50. Sometime later, a physician from group A confided to a physician from group B that his score on the test was 70 and that he thought this score was generally above average for the test. The physician from Group B, whose score was 75, was initially relieved that he had outperformed his colleague on the test. Unfortunately, the physician from group B failed to recognize that very different scales were used to grade the two tests, making it impossible to directly compare the raw scores of 70 and 75. The only way to compare how well the two physicians actually did, is to convert their test scores to a third, or standard, scale.

Z-Scores

The *z*-score scale relies on an understanding of the concepts of the mean and SD. Arbitrarily, the mean value for a set of data is assigned a *z*-score of 0. For each SD increase above or below the mean, the *z*-score increases by a value of 1. If the value lies above the mean, the *z*-score value is preceded by a plus sign. If it lies below the mean, a minus sign precedes it. In essence, the *z*-score tells you how many SDs above or below the mean the value in question lies. For example, if the *z*-score is –3.2, the value in question lies 3.2 SDs below the mean. If the *z*-score is +1.5, the value in question lies 1.5 SDs above the mean. *Z*-Scores are not unique to bone densitometry. Any type of numerical data can be converted to a *z*-score, as long as the mean and SD are known. Psychologists have used this type of scale extensively in psychological and IQ testing.

In order to compare the test scores of the two physicians from group A and group B, it becomes clear that it is necessary to calculate the mean and SD for the test scores for group A, and also for group B. When this is done, it is found that the average score for group A was a raw score of 60, with an SD of 5. The average for group B was 80, with an SD of 5. Since the physician from group A had a raw score of 70, his score is 10 points above the average. Because the SD for this group was 5, the group A physician's raw score is 2 SDs above the mean. His *z*-score, therefore, is +2. Although the raw score of the physician from group B appears to be higher, since the average from group B was 80 and the SD was 5, the *z*-score for the physician from group B is actually –1. The physician from group A has the better score in comparison to his peers than does the physician from group B.

T-Scores

The *T*-score is another type of standard score that relies upon the mean value and the SD for a set of numerical data. In this case, however, the mean value is arbitrarily assigned a *T*-score value of 50. For each SD change, the *T*-score increases or decreases by a value of 10, depending on whether the value is above or below the mean. For example, if the value in question is 3 SDs above the mean, the corresponding *T*-score would be 80. If the value were 1.5 SDs below the mean, the *T*-score would be 35. For the two physicians from group A and group B discussed previously, the *T*-scores would be 70 and 40, respectively.

T-scores and *z*-scores are found on the computer-generated bone densitometry printouts from virtually every manufacturer of bone density equipment. Criteria proposed by the World Health Organization for the diagnosis of osteoporosis utilize a *T*-score, and some calculations of fracture risk are based on a *T*-score and *z*-score. In these contexts, however, the *T*-score has undergone some modification, and both the *T*-score and z-score have acquired specific characteristics that are quite distinct from their use in general statistics.

Figure 3-1 is the printout from a spine bone density study performed on a Lunar (Madison, WI) DPX device. The individual BMD values for each vertebra are listed, as well as the average BMD values for each possible combination of contiguous vertebrae. Two of the four columns adjacent to the BMD values reflect *z*-scores. One column is entitled "young-adult *z*" and the other, "age-matched *z*." Based on an understanding of the *z*-score,

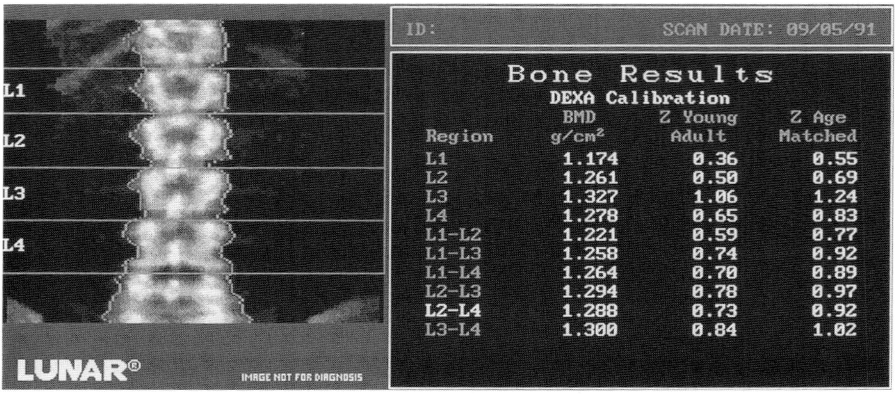
L1
L2
L3
L4
LUNAR®
IMAGE NOT FOR DIAGNOSIS
ID:
SCAN DATE: 09/05/91
Bone Results
DEXA Calibration
Region | BMD g/cm² | Z Young Adult | Z Age Matched
L1 | 1.174 | 0.36 | 0.55
L2 | 1.261 | 0.50 | 0.69
L3 | 1.327 | 1.06 | 1.24
L4 | 1.278 | 0.65 | 0.83
L1-L2 | 1.221 | 0.59 | 0.77
L1-L3 | 1.258 | 0.74 | 0.92
L1-L4 | 1.264 | 0.70 | 0.89
L2-L3 | 1.294 | 0.78 | 0.97
L2-L4 | 1.288 | 0.73 | 0.92
L3-L4 | 1.300 | 0.84 | 1.02

Fig. 3-1. A DXA AP spine study acquired on the Lunar DPX. In addition to the BMD values, young-adult *z*-scores and age-matched *z*-scores are presented for each individual vertebra, and for the average of each combination of contiguous vertebrae.

it is clear that these *z*-scores indicate how many SDs above or below the mean value the particular BMD value lies. But what mean value and SD were used to calculate these *z*-scores? The young-adult *z*-score is calculated using the average peak bone density and SD for the young adult. The column entitled age-matched *z* reflects the use of the average bone density that would have been predicted on the basis of the patient's age. In this case, the L2–L4 BMD average of 0.747 g/cm^2 has a young-adult *z*-score of –3.78 and an age-matched *z*-score of –1.73. This means that the L2–L4 BMD average is 3.78 SDs below the average peak bone density of the young adult, and 1.73 SDs below the BMD value that would have been predicted on the basis of the patient's age.

Figure 3-2 is a bone-density printout from a spine study performed on a Hologic (Waltham, MA) QDR-4500. The BMD values for each individual vertebra and the average BMD value for L1–L4 are evident. Adjacent to these values, two of the four columns are now entitled simply "*T*-score" and "*z*-score." There is nothing in the title of these columns to indicate which average value is being used to calculate these standard scores.

Figure 3-3 is a Norland (Fort Atkinson, WI) DXA AP spine study. A *T*-score of –0.51 and *z*-score of 0.01 are noted for the L2–L4 average BMD. When this format is employed, the average value used to calculate the *T*-score is always the average peak BMD of the young adult. The average value used to calculate the *z*-score is always the average age-matched BMD. The values in the *T*-score column, however, do not look like *T*-scores. *T*-scores, after all, should be scores like 30 or 75. The use of either a plus or minus sign to indicate the position relative to the mean value is not required.

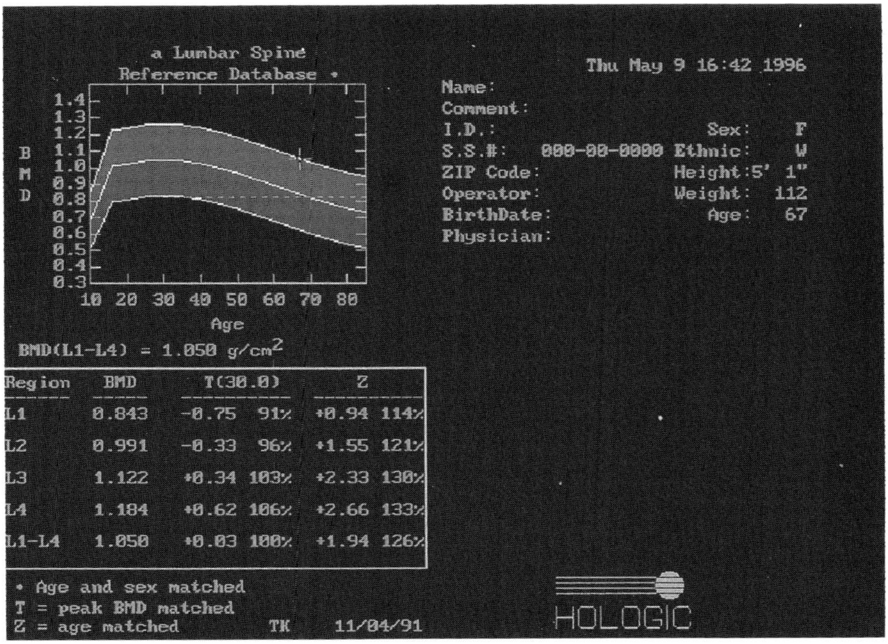

Fig. 3-2. BMD data acquired on the Hologic QDR-4500. In addition to the BMD values, *T*-scores and *z*-scores are presented for each vertebra, and for the L1–L4 average BMD. Case courtesy of Hologic, Inc., Waltham, MA.

These values in the *T*-score column actually look more like *z*-scores. And in fact, that is exactly what they are. These are *z*-scores, which, in bone densitometry only, are renamed *T*-scores. This allows one to understand without so stating that the reference average in use here is the young-adult peak BMD, and that the reference average in use for the calculation of the *z*-score is the age-matched BMD. Therefore, the *T*-score of –1.11 for the L1–L4 average BMD means that the L1–L4 average BMD is 1.11 SDs below the average peak BMD of the young adult. This convention of renaming the young-adult *z*-score the *T*-score has been increasingly adopted by manufacturers of bone density equipment, and has also found its way into much of the bone density literature. It is important to remember that the young-adult *z*-score is identical to the *T*-score in this context. The age-matched *z*-score is identical to what is simply called the *z*-score.

MEASURES OF RISK

Many of the applications of densitometry involve the assessment of risk for fragility fracture. There are several different measures of risk that are

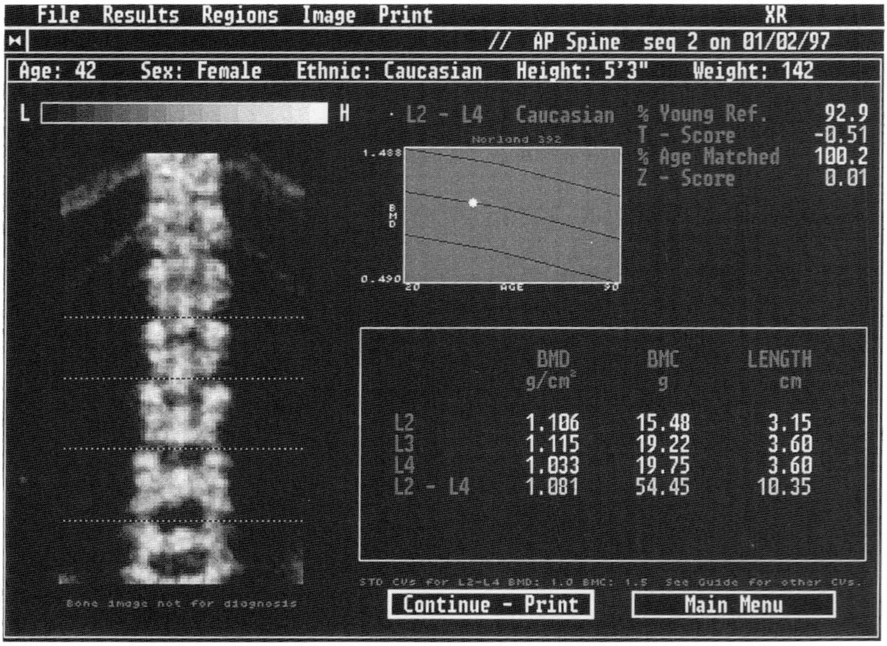

Fig. 3-3. A DXA AP spine study acquired on the Norland XR-36. The *T*-score and *z*-score are presented for the L2–L4 average BMD. Case courtesy of Norland Medical Systems, Inc., Ft. Atkinson, WI. (*see* color plate 12 appearing after p. 78).

commonly used in bone densitometry: prevalence, incidence rate, incidence or absolute risk, relative risk, attributable risk, and odds ratios.

Prevalence and Incidence

Both prevalence and the incidence rate can be considered as measures of a disease experience within a population. They differ principally in that prevalence is derived from observations of a population made at a single point in time, and the incidence rate is derived from observations that are made only after observing a population over a period of time.

Prevalence

There are two ways of expressing prevalence: point prevalence and period prevalence. In this context, it is not terribly important to distinguish between the two, but the information is presented here for the sake of completeness.

Point prevalence is the number of persons with a disease at the time of the observation, divided by the total number of individuals in the population at risk for the disease. This is often expressed as a percentage. If the point prevalence is very small, it may be expressed as the number of cases per 1000 individuals in the population at risk, in order to utilize whole numbers instead of fractions.

The period prevalence is the ratio of the number of individuals with a particular disease at a specific point in time within a specified time interval, divided by the number of individuals in the population at risk for the disease at the midpoint of that time interval.

Both types of measures of prevalence are considered rates. The point prevalence is the more commonly used measure of the two. If the term "prevalence" is used without a modifier, it is reasonable to assume that point prevalence is being discussed. For example, Melton et al. *(2)* reported that the prevalence of a bone density more than 2 SDs below the young-adult mean in the spine in Caucasian women aged 50 and over was 31.8%. This figure is based on a one-time measurement of BMD at the spine in a group of women from Rochester, MN, with extrapolation of the figures to the entire population of Caucasian women over age 50 in the United States in 1990. This is a point prevalence rate.

Incidence

Like prevalence, there are two types of measures of incidence: One is a rate, the other is a risk. Incidence risk, however, is also called absolute risk. To clarify matters, incidence risk will be discussed under the subheading of Absolute Risk.

The incidence rate, or, simply, incidence, is the number of new cases of any disease that have occurred within a specified period of time, divided by the average number of individuals at risk for the disease, multiplied by the length of the time interval. This value may be multiplied by 1000 and expressed as the incidence per 1000 person-years at risk. Other multiples may be used as well. For example, Cooper et al. *(3)* reported that the vertebral fracture incidence rate in women in Rochester, MN, was 145 per 100,000 person-years. The number of individuals at risk for the disease in the population is not the same as the number of individuals in the population at the beginning of the time interval, because, once having developed the disease, the individual is no longer considered at risk. This is important in distinguishing the incidence rate from absolute risk.

Absolute, Relative, and Attributable Risk

Absolute Risk

As noted previously, incidence risk is also known as absolute risk. The term "absolute risk" will be used here. This is the number of individuals developing a disease within a specified period of time, divided by the number of individuals at risk for the disease at the beginning of the time

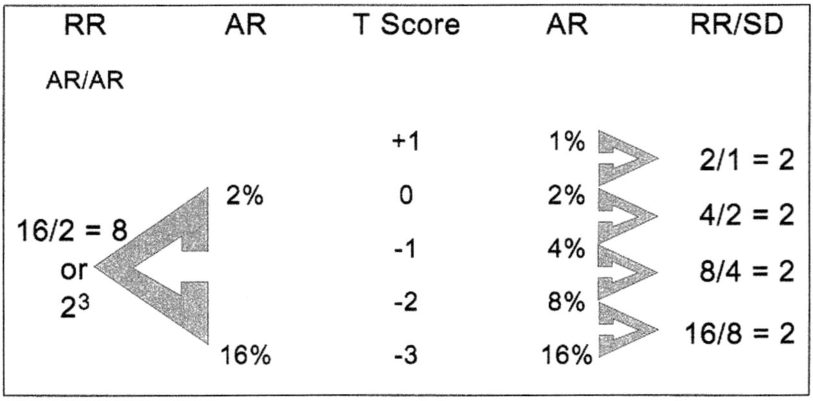

Fig. 3-4. The relationship between absolute risk, relative risk, and the *T*-score. Relative risk is the ratio of two absolute risks.

interval. In the context of this discussion, a certain level of bone density determines risk. The disease is fracture. For example, assume that 1000 women with the same level of bone density in the femoral neck are followed over a period of time. During the observation period, 160 of the women develop a hip fracture. The absolute risk for hip fracture in women with this level of bone density in the femoral neck is 0.16 (160 women with fractures ÷ 1000 women at risk at the beginning of the observation period). Expressed as a percentage, the absolute risk becomes 16%. These values used in the calculation of absolute risk were not taken from the literature. The numbers are for the purpose of illustration only.

Relative Risk

Relative risk is the ratio of two absolute risks. In Fig. 3-4, the relationship between absolute risk and relative risk is illustrated. The values for absolute risk in Fig. 3-4 were not taken from the literature. They are used only for purposes of this exercise. For example, what is the relative risk for fracture for individuals who have a BMD *T*-score of 0, compared to the group with a BMD *T*-score of –1? This simply asks the question, what is the second group's risk (the group with the *T*-score of –1) compared to the first group's (the group with the *T*-score of 0). Another way of putting this would be to say, what is the second group's risk *relative* to the first group's risk?

As shown in Fig. 3-4, the group with the *T*-score of –1 has an absolute risk for fracture of 4%. The group with the *T*-score of 0 has an absolute risk for fracture of 2%. The relative risk is, therefore, 4% ÷ 2%, or 2. An appropriate interpretation of this finding would be that there is a doubling of risk, or a twofold increase in risk, conferred by the decline in BMD of 1 SD, which is, of course, the decline represented by a change in the *T*-score from 0 to –1.

In the medical literature, data from the majority of the prospective fracture trials evaluating the ability of bone-mass measurements to predict fracture risk are presented as the increase in relative risk per SD decline in bone density. For example, based on the prospective fracture trial from Melton et al. *(4)*, the increase in relative risk for spine fracture when measured at the spine was 1.9 for each SD decline in bone density. In other words, when the absolute risk for fracture for any group was divided by the absolute risk for the group whose BMD was 1 SD higher, the ratio, or relative risk, was 1.9.

Using this data from Melton et al. *(4)*, how would the relative risk for spine fracture for an individual with a *T*-score of –3 at the spine be calculated? The relative risk for such an individual would be equal to 1.9^3, or 6.86. It would not be 1.9 × 3. Figure 3-4 illustrates this exponential relationship.

One of the limitations of relative risk is that the relative-risk value alone does not convey information about the absolute risk for any particular group. After all, it would not matter if the absolute risks for two groups used to calculate the relative risk were 2% ÷ 1%, 4% ÷ 2%, or 50% ÷ 25%. The relative risk would be 2 in each case. Nevertheless, relative risk is the strongest indicator of the strength of the relationship between a risk factor, such as low bone mass, and the disease outcome, such as fracture.

Attributable Risk

Attributable risk does not appear frequently in bone density or osteoporosis literature, but it is a useful concept to understand. Attributable risk is the difference between two absolute risks. It is the strongest indicator of the benefits of preventing the risk factor in reducing the occurrence of disease. For example, if the absolute risk for fracture was 10% in a group with a low BMD at the spine, and 2% in a group with a higher BMD at the spine, the attributable risk would be 10% – 2%, or 8%. In other words, 8% of the risk of fracture in the group with the lower BMD can be attributed to the difference in BMD between the two groups. If we could eliminate the difference in BMD between the two groups by increasing the BMD in the group with the lower BMD, we could theoretically eliminate 8% of the fracture risk.

Odds Ratios

Odds ratios are similar to relative risk. The calculation of relative risk, however, requires a knowledge of the absolute risk for the groups being compared, and therefore requires that a prospective study be performed.

When groups are evaluated retrospectively, another measure of risk must be employed. In this circumstance, the odds ratio can be calculated. This is done by calculating the odds of disease for each of the two groups, and then dividing in order to obtain the odds ratio.

For example, 1000 individuals are selected based on the individuals having a low spine bone density. The observation is made that 100 of these individuals have a spine fracture. In another group of 1000 individuals, the controls, who are picked on the basis of having good spine bone densities, only five are observed to have a fracture. What are the odds of having a fracture for an individual in either group, and what is the odds ratio of the low BMD group, compared to the high BMD group?

The odds for fracture in either group are found by dividing the number of individuals with fracture in the group by the number in that group who have not experienced a fracture. Therefore, for the low BMD group, the odds are:

$$100 \div (1000 - 100) = 100 \div 900 = 0.111$$

The odds for the high BMD group are:

$$5 \div (1000 - 5) = 5 \div 995 = 0.005$$

The odds ratio for the low BMD group, compared to the high BMD group, then, is:

$$0.111 \div 0.005 = 22.2$$

The interpretation of this odds ratio is that fracture is 22.2 times more likely in the low BMD group, compared to the high BMD group. These values were not taken from the medical literature, and are used for the purposes of illustration only.

For uncommon diseases, the relative risk and odds ratio will be very similar. For common diseases, however, the odds ratio will be greater than the relative risk.

CONFIDENCE INTERVALS

Remember Mrs. J., who had the three spine bone-density tests for which the mean, SD, and the CV were previously calculated? What if three more measurements were performed on Mrs. J. the next day? After each measurement, Mrs. J. was asked to get up from the scan table and then resume her position, just as she did for the first set of three measurements the day before. The values for the second set of measurements on Mrs. J. are shown in Table 3-2.

Although these values in Table 3-2 are very similar to the values seen in Table 3-1, they are not identical. The fact that the three scans do not produce identical results is not surprising. The ability of the machine to reproduce the results is not perfect. There is a small amount of error that is inherent in

Table 3-2
Individual and Mean Spine BMD Values for Patient, Mrs. J., on Day 2

Patient	*Scan 1*	*Scan 2*	*Scan 3*	*Mean or* $\bar{X}$
Mrs. J.	1.024	1.066	1.070	1.053

Values are in g/cm^2.

the testing, regardless of how well the technician performs the test. This is true for any type of quantitative measurement used in clinical medicine today. The average value for the set of three measurements on the first day and on the second day is different, because the three measurements used to calculate each average were slightly different. The same thing would be true if three measurements were performed on Mrs. J. on a third or fourth day. The average BMD value for each set of three measurements may be different, because the individual measurements used to calculate the average may be slightly different. It is useful, therefore, to know what the range of average values would be if repeated sets of three measurements each were performed on Mrs. J. an infinite number of times. This range is called the confidence interval, and is calculated by finding the standard error of the sample mean. The standard error is different from, but related to, the standard deviation. The formula for the standard error, abbreviated SE, is as follows:

$$\text{SE} = s \div \sqrt{n}$$

where s is the standard deviation, and n is the number of measurements. The SD for the first set of three measurements on Mrs. J. was previously calculated as being 0.05 g/cm^2. The SE, therefore, for that first set of three measurements is:

$$\text{SE} = 0.05 \div \sqrt{3} = 0.03$$

The value of 0.03 g/cm^2 is the SE of the sample mean. The sample refers to the set of three measurements. The mean (or average) for this sample has already been calculated, and was found to be 1.043 g/cm^2. The SE and sample mean are used to calculate the 95% confidence interval (CI) for the sample. The 95% CI is bounded by the mean ± 2× SE.* The formula is written as follows:

$$95\% CI = \bar{X} \pm 2 \times \text{SE}$$

*The actual value by which the SE is multiplied depends on the sample size. For samples in which $n > 20$, the value is very close to 2. For smaller samples, the value will be slightly larger. The formula shown here is a practical characterization of the calculation of the 95% CI.

The 95% CI based on the first set of three measurements on Mrs. J. is:

$$95\%CI = 1.043 \pm 2 \times 0.03$$

$$95\%CI = 0.983 \text{ to } 1.103$$

The interpretation of the 95% CI is that 95% of the means that would be obtained by repeat testing will fall within the range of 0.983 to 1.103 g/cm^2.

There are two characteristics of the SE that become apparent on reviewing the formula for its calculation. First, the SE will always be smaller than the SD. Second, the greater the number of measurements, or *n*, that make up the sample, the smaller the SE will be. The smaller the SE, the more narrow the CI. The more narrow the CI, the greater the likelihood that the average value from the limited sample of scans is representative of the average that would be obtained if Mrs. J. was tested an infinite number of times.

Another example of a CI comes from Cummings et al. *(5)*, who estimated a woman's lifetime risk of having a hip fracture. Using population-based data, it was calculated that the lifetime risk of hip fracture for a 50-year-old white woman was 15.6%. The 95% CI for this risk was 14.8 to 16.4%. This very narrow CI gives increasing credibility to the risk estimate of 15.6%.

CIs and statistical significance are closely related, but CIs tend to provide more useful clinical information. Many medical journals now require that CIs be presented, in addition to assessments of statistical significance for reported data. In densitometry, an understanding of CIs is imperative in interpreting the significance of changes in the BMD over time. This is discussed in the following section on precision, and in greater detail in Chapter 4.

ACCURACY AND PRECISION

Quantitative measurement techniques should be both accurate and precise. In Fig. 3-5, the concepts of accuracy and precision are presented using the analogy of an archer's target. Five arrows have hit target B. One arrow is in the bull's eye and the other four arrows are close. But, of these four arrows, one arrow is off to the right, one is off to the left, one is below the bull's eye, and one is above it. The archer has, at least, hit the target, and could be described as being reasonably accurate, since he has placed one arrow in the bull's eye and the other four around it. But he certainly did not reproduce his shot each time. He is not, therefore, precise. Target A illustrates the abilities of an archer who is precise, but not very accurate. This archer has grouped all five arrows tightly in the upper right quadrant of the target. He has reproduced his shot each time, even though none of the shots

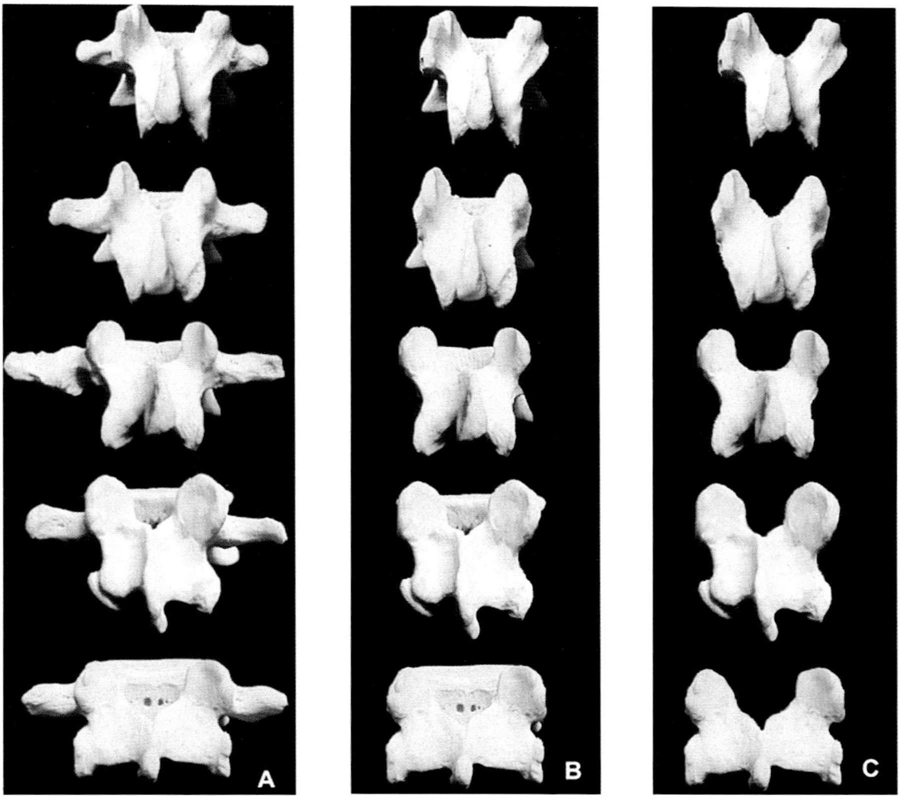

Plate 1 (Fig. 2-1A–C; *see* full caption on p. 36 and discussion in Chapter 2).

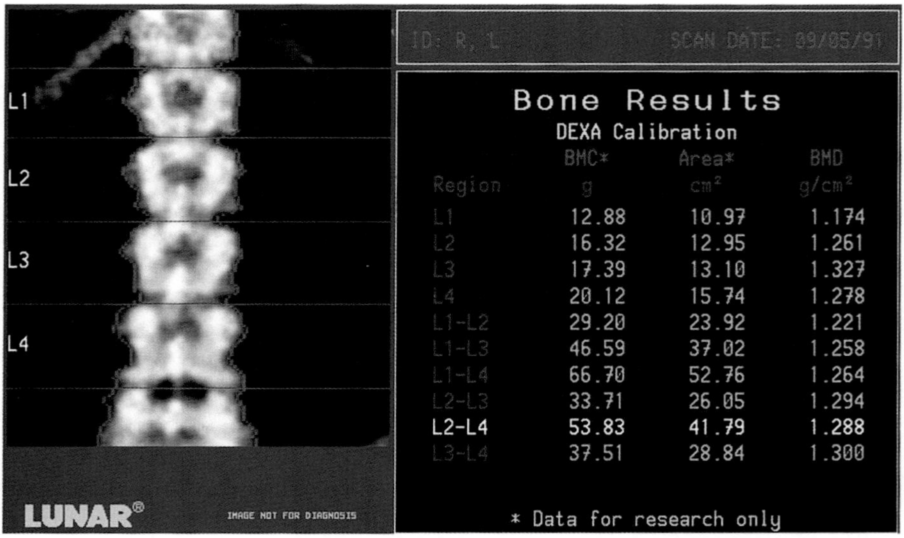

Plate 2 (Fig. 2-2; *see* full caption on p. 37 and discussion in Chapter 2).

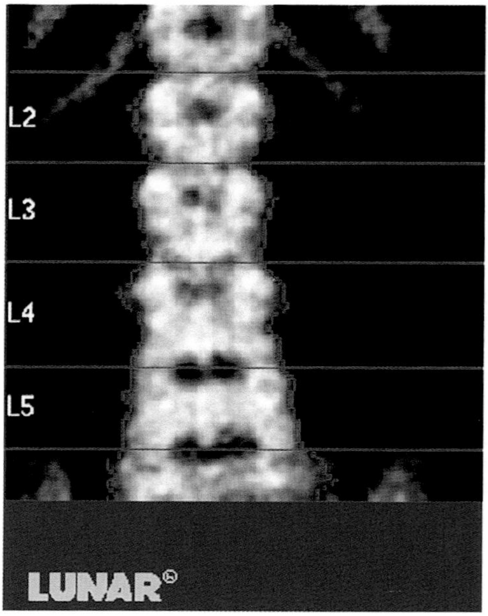

Plate 3 (Fig. 2-5; *see* full caption on p. 42 and discussion in Chapter 2).

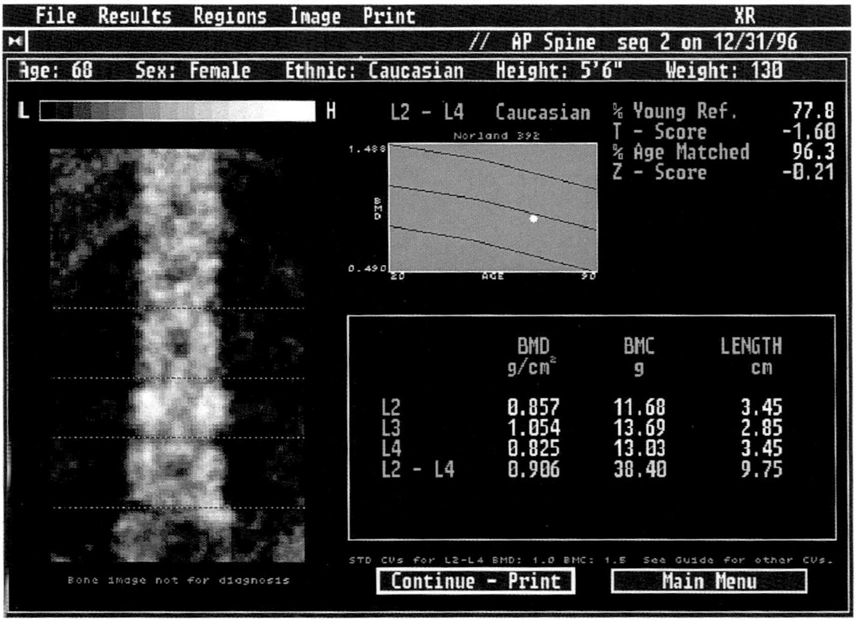

Plate 4 (Fig. 2-6; *see* full caption on p. 43 and discussion in Chapter 2).

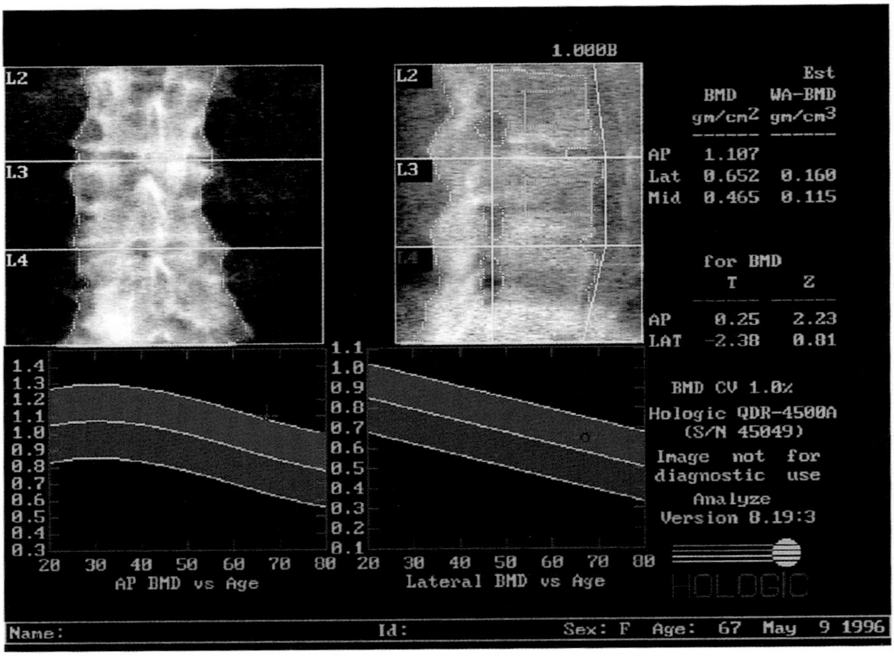

Plate 5 (Fig. 2-15; *see* full caption on p. 53 and discussion in Chapter 2).

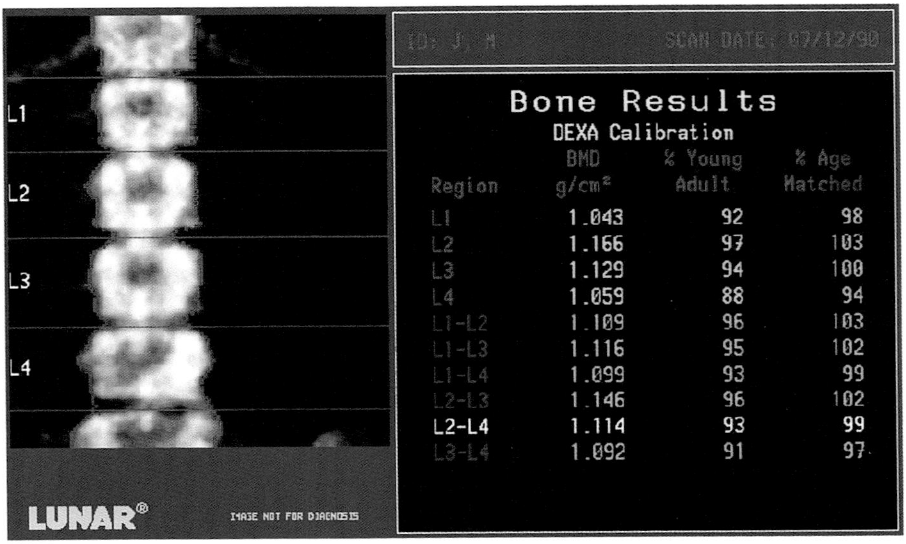
ID: J. M
SCAN DATE: 07/12/90
Bone Results
DEXA Calibration
Region BMD g/cm² % Young Adult % Age Matched
L1 1.043 92 98
L2 1.166 97 103
L3 1.129 94 100
L4 1.059 88 94
L1-L2 1.109 96 103
L1-L3 1.116 95 102
L1-L4 1.099 93 99
L2-L3 1.146 96 102
L2-L4 1.114 93 99
L3-L4 1.092 91 97
L1
L2
L3
L4
LUNAR®
IMAGE NOT FOR DIAGNOSIS

Plate 6 (Fig. 2-19; *see* full caption on p. 57 and discussion in Chapter 2).

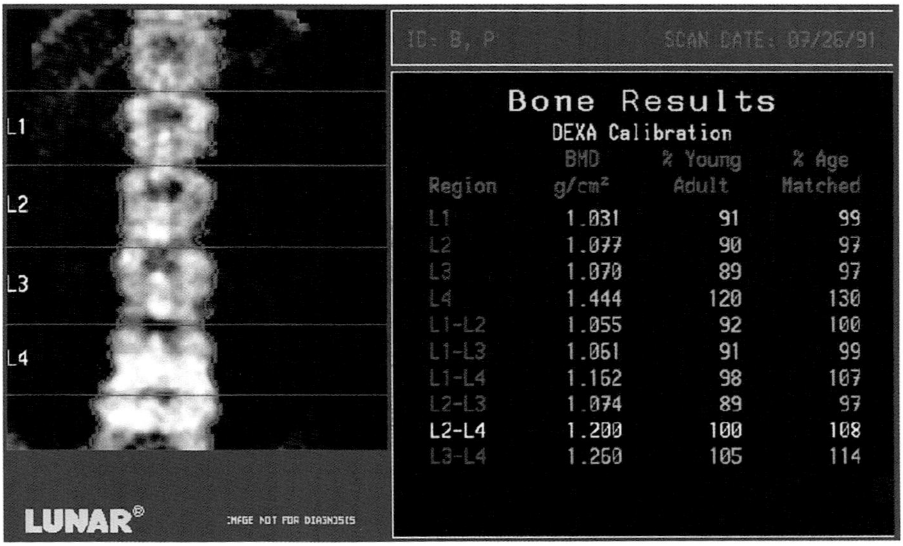
ID: B, P
SCAN DATE: 07/26/91
Bone Results
DEXA Calibration
Region BMD g/cm² % Young Adult % Age Matched
L1 1.031 91 99
L2 1.077 90 97
L3 1.070 89 97
L4 1.444 120 130
L1-L2 1.055 92 100
L1-L3 1.061 91 99
L1-L4 1.162 98 107
L2-L3 1.074 89 97
L2-L4 1.200 100 108
L3-L4 1.260 105 114
L1
L2
L3
L4
LUNAR®
IMAGE NOT FOR DIAGNOSIS

Plate 7 (Fig. 2-20; *see* full caption on p. 58 and discussion in Chapter 2).

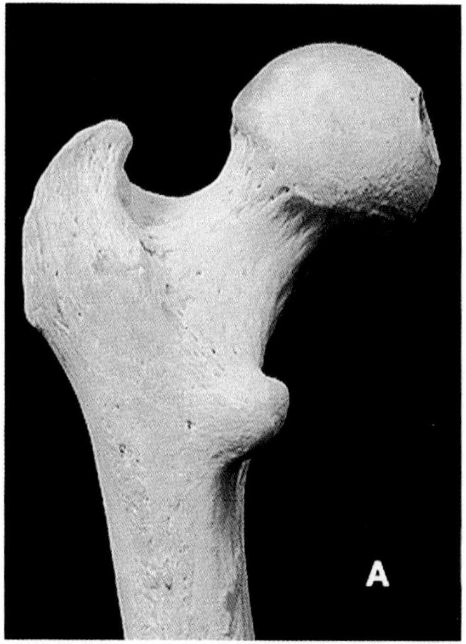

Plate 8 (Fig. 2-21A; *see* full caption on p. 59 and discussion in Chapter 2).

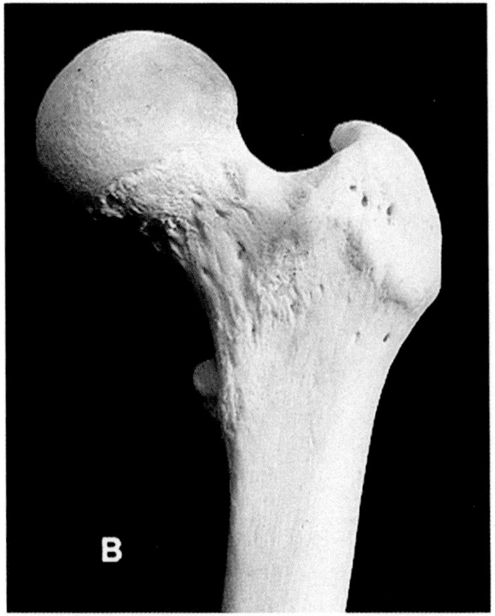

Plate 9 (Fig. 2-21B; *see* full caption on p. 59 and discussion in Chapter 2).

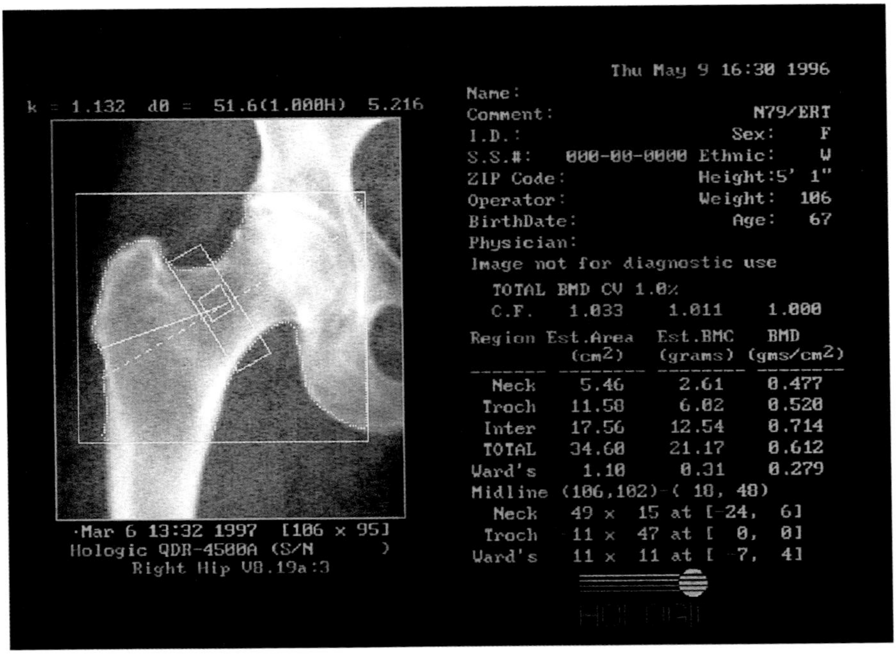

Plate 10 (Fig. 2-22; *see* full caption on p. 60 and discussion in Chapter 2).

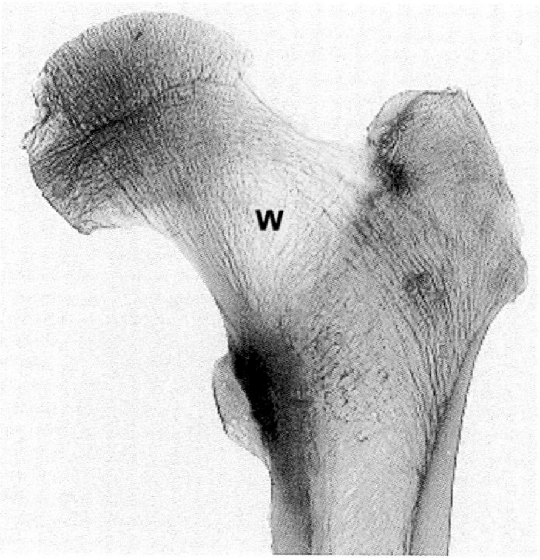

Plate 11 (Fig. 2-23; *see* full caption on p. 60 and discussion in Chapter 2).

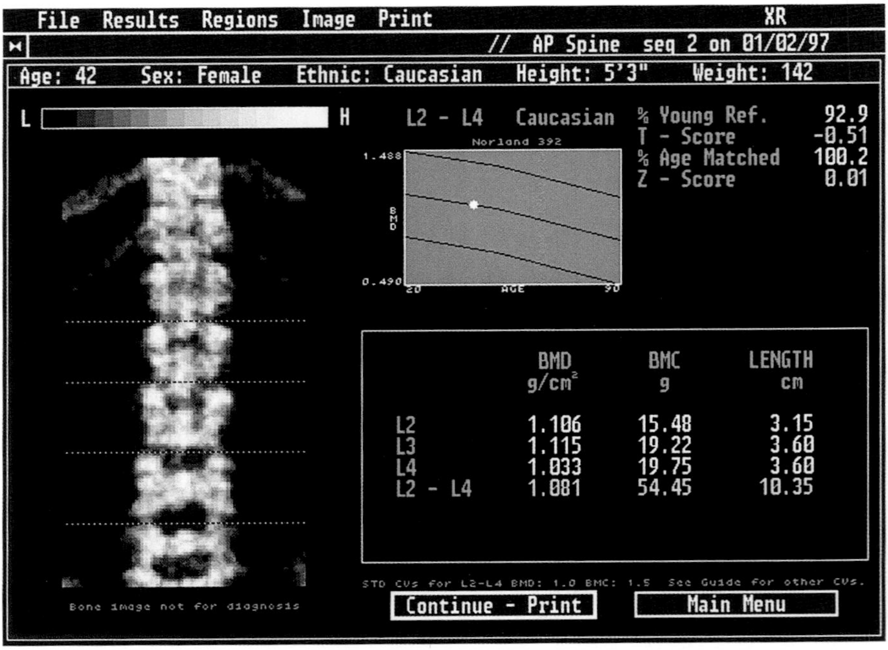

Plate 12 (Fig. 3-3; *see* full caption on p. 72 and discussion in Chapter 3).

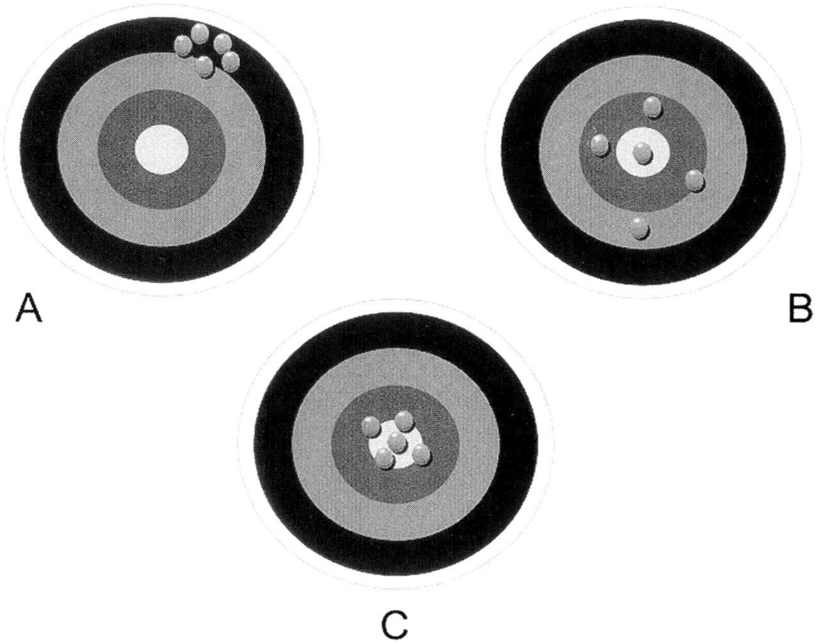

Fig. 3-5. Accuracy and precision. The tightly grouped arrows in target A indicate good precision, but poor accuracy. In target B, the arrows are more accurately placed, but scattered around the bull's eye, indicating good accuracy but poor precision. In target C, the arrows, which are concentrated in the bull's eye and tightly grouped, indicate both good accuracy and good precision.

was accurate. The skill of an archer who is both accurate and precise is illustrated in Fig. 3-5 by the five arrows grouped tightly around the bull's eye on target C.

Accuracy

In bone densitometry, accuracy describes the degree to which the measurement of bone density reflects the true bone density. In other words, if the bone in question was removed from the body, measured, and then ashed and assayed, the true bone density could be determined. How close does a bone density measurement by any technique come to reproducing this true, or real, BMD? Accuracy can be described quantitatively by the percent coefficient of variation (%CV). Remember that the %CV describes the proportion by which the individual measurements vary from the mean value as a percentage. In the context of a discussion of accuracy, the mean value is synonymous with the true BMD. The SD used to calculate the CV represents the variability of the actual individual BMD measurements about this true BMD value. Therefore, if the accuracy of a DXA AP spine bone-density measurement is said to have a %CV of 3–6%, this means that the measurements of BMD tend to vary about the true value by 3–6% of the true value, or real BMD. Even though such a statement describing the accuracy of DXA may at first glance seem to be critical of the technology, remember that the %CV is describing the variability of the measurement about the true value. Therefore, the smaller the %CV, the better.

Precision

Precision is the ability to reproduce the measurement when it is performed under identical conditions, when there has been no real biologic change in the patient. The three spine bone-density measurements on Mrs. J. on the same day, in fact, within a few minutes of each other, did not produce exactly the same result. This was true because there was a certain amount of error introduced by repositioning the patient on the table between measurements. There may also have been a small amount of error introduced during the analysis of the data by the technician. And finally, the technique itself is not perfect, even when the technician exactly reproduces the positioning of the patient and the procedures used to analyze the data.

Like accuracy, precision is often characterized by the %CV. The CV for the first set of three measurements on Mrs. J. was calculated in the discussion of the CV earlier in this chapter, and was found to be 0.048. Expressed as a percentage, the CV becomes 4.8%. In the context of precision, this means that the individual measurements tend to vary from the average of the measurements by 4.8% of the average BMD. Again, the smaller the %CV, the better the precision of the technique.

When a bone-density measurement is being performed for the purposes of diagnosing osteoporosis based on bone-density criteria, the assessment of fracture risk, or to document the effects of any disease process on the bone density, accuracy is a vitally important attribute. Clearly, it is desirable for the measured bone density to be as close to the true or real bone density as possible. When the bone-density measurement is one of a series of measurements being done to detect changes in the bone density over time, accuracy is far less important that precision. This is because it is the magnitude of the difference between measurements that is of interest. It becomes relatively unimportant whether the first measurement was accurate. In order to interpret serial changes in BMD, the densitometrist must have some idea of the precision of the type of testing being employed. If this is not known, there is no way to know if the changes being observed are real, or are simply a result of the error inherent in the test. The calculation of precision for bone-density measurements and the determination of significant change in BMD are discussed in detail in Chapter 4.

CORRELATION

Correlation is a measure of the strength of an association between two variables. It is generally expressed as a dimensionless number known as the correlation coefficient, or Pearson's product-moment correlation coefficient. The correlation coefficient is denoted by the letter *r*. Values for *r* can range from –1 to +1. The greater the numerical value of *r*, the stronger is the association between two variables. Therefore, the strongest associations would be indicated by an *r*-value of either +1 or –1. If the relationship between the two variables is a direct one, the sign in front of the *r*-value will be positive. If the relationship is an inverse one, the sign will be negative. For example, in a study reported by Takada et al. *(6)*, an *r*-value of 0.56 was reported for bone density in the phalanges as measured by radiographic absorptiometry (RA), and bone density in the spine as measured by DXA. The correlation coefficient describes a direct relationship; that is, the BMD as measured by RA increased as the BMD measured by DXA increased. The association between the two variables was not a perfect one. Therefore, the bone density in the phalanges as measured by RA could not be perfectly predicted from the spine bone-density measurement performed with DXA. Nevertheless, there was a direct association or relationship between the BMDs measured at both sites. In another study from Hansen *(7)*, the strength of the association between body weight and BMD at a variety of skeletal sites was reported. The BMDs at the spine, forearm, femoral neck, and trochanter were all noted to be positively related to weight. That is, the BMD increased as weight increased. This association, therefore, will be expressed as a positive *r*-value. The *r*-values ranged from 0.20 to 0.35 between weight and the BMDs at the various skeletal sites. Although these *r*-values were low, and would tend to suggest that the strength of the association between weight and BMD was far from perfect, all of the *r*-values were statistically significant. One could conclude that the association between weight and BMD was positive or direct, but weak. Nevertheless, the *r*-values were statistically significant, implying that the association was unlikely to be a result of chance. An example of an inverse correlation is the finding from Mazess et al. *(8)* of an *r*-value of –0.16 for the association between age and femoral neck BMD, in a cross-sectional study of 218 women, ages 20–39. This means that, as age increased, the BMD in the femoral neck was observed to decrease. Although this value of *r* is again very small, it was statistically significant. Note that correlation does not prove cause and effect. It quantifies the strength of a relationship or association.

STATISTICAL SIGNIFICANCE AND THE *P*-VALUE

Statistical significance is virtually always discussed in the context of the likelihood of coming to an incorrect conclusion based on the acquired data. There are many ways to test for statistical significance. The choice of technique is determined by the nature of the study being performed. The various techniques for significance testing are not relevant to the discussion here. However, the results of significance testing are usually presented in the form of a *P*-value. Traditionally, two levels of the *P*-value have become synonymous with significant and very significant. Values of P that are ≤ 0.05 are considered significant. Values of P that are ≤ 0.01 are considered very significant. In the previous discussion of correlation, it was noted that Hansen found a direct association between body weight and BMD at a variety of skeletal sites *(7)*. These associations were expressed as correlation values of r, which ranged from 0.20 to 0.36. It was noted above that these correlations were weak, but statistically significant. In fact, the correlations were very significant, with a *P*-value of <0.001. This value is interpreted as meaning that there is <1 chance in 1000 of obtaining results such as those seen by Hansen, when in fact there is really no association at all between weight and BMD. Statistical significance, of course, does not necessarily imply medical or practical significance. That is for the clinician to decide.

REFERENCES

1. Phillips JL (1982) Interpreting individual measures. In: *Statistical Thinking*. New York: W. H. Freeman, pp. 62–78.
2. Melton LJ, Chrischilles EA, Cooper C, Lane AW, Riggs BL (1992) How many women have osteoporosis? *J Bone Miner Res* 7:1005–1010.
3. Cooper C, Atkinson EJ, O'Fallon WM, Melton LJ (1992) Incidence of clinically diagnosed vertebral fractures: a population-based study in Rochester, Minnesota, 1985–1989. *J Bone Miner Res* 7:221–227.
4. Melton LJ, Atkinson EJ, O'Fallon WM, Wahner HW, Riggs BL (1993) Long-term fracture prediction by bone mineral assessed at difference skeletal sites. *J Bone Miner Res* 8:1227–1233.
5. Cummings SR, Black DM, Rubin SM (1989) Lifetime risks of hip, Colles', or vertebral fracture and coronary heart disease among white postmenopausal women. *Arch Intern Med* 149:2445–2448.
6. Takada M, Engelke K, Hagiwara S, Grampp S, Jergas M, Gluer CC, Genant HK (1997) Assessment of osteoporosis: comparison of radiographic absorptiometry of the phalanges and dual X-ray absorptiometry of the radius and lumbar spine. *Radiology* 202:759–763.
7. Hansen MA (1994) Assessment of age and risk factors on bone density and bone turnover in healthy premenopausal women. *Osteoporosis Int* 4:123–128.
8. Mazess RB, Barden HS (1991) Bone density in premenopausal women: effects of age, dietary intake, physical activity, smoking, and birth-control pills. *Am J Clin Nutr* 53:132–142.

4 The Importance of Precision in Densitometry

CONTENTS

The concept of precision was introduced in Chapter 3. Current bone densitometry technology cannot perfectly reproduce BMD results from test to test, even when there has been no real change in the patient's BMD. If there is any additional error introduced by the failure of the technician to perfectly reposition and correctly analyze the results, the precision of the test will be adversely affected even more. This being the case, how can a physician determine if any measured change in BMD is a real, biologic change, and not simply the error that is inherent in the technique, or the error introduced by the technician? The first step is to determine the short-term precision for each type of scan that is performed at the densitometry facility. Short-term precision implies that the precision has been determined using repeat studies performed within the space of a week to no more than a month. In a medium-term precision study, the scans have been acquired over a period of time that spans 1 to 6 months. A long-term precision study implies data acquisition that spans more than 6 months.

A precision study should be done at least once for all scan types, and, thereafter, if there is a change in technician or a major equipment change.

Table 4-1
Individual and Mean Spine BMD Values
for 14 Patients in a Short-Term Precision Study

Patient	*Scan 1*	*Scan 2*	*Scan 3*	*Mean*
1	1.010	1.019	1.100	1.043
2	0.925	0.940	0.918	0.928
3	1.164	1.160	1.170	1.165
4	0.999	1.010	1.008	1.006
5	0.900	0.920	0.905	0.908
6	0.955	0.960	0.960	0.958
7	1.000	1.010	1.150	1.053
8	0.875	0.849	0.869	0.864
9	0.898	0.920	0.901	0.906
10	1.111	1.009	1.100	1.073
11	0.964	0.949	0.960	0.958
12	1.000	0.985	0.992	0.992
13	1.200	1.185	1.205	1.197
14	1.165	1.170	1.180	1.172

Values are in g/cm^2.

PERFORMING A SHORT-TERM PRECISION STUDY

The following is the method for determining short-term precision as recommended by Gluer et al. *(1)*. First, the technician should scan either 1 patient 28 times, 14 patients 3 times, or 27 patients 2 times.

The patient must be repositioned between each study. All scans of any one type should be completed within 1 month, although they do not need to be completed for any one patient on the same day. The particular combination of the number of patients and the number of scans per patient is necessary for the study to be statistically valid.

In the following example, the short-term precision for AP spine studies was calculated by scanning 14 patients three times each within the space of 1 month. The same technician scanned all of the patients. Between each scan on the same patient, the patient was repositioned. The individual values and the average value for each of the 14 patients are listed in Table 4-1.

In all, 42 AP spine studies have been performed (14 patients × 3 scans per patient = 42 scans).

Mathematical Procedures Used to Calculate Precision

Step 1. The mean, standard deviation (SD), and coefficient of variation (CV) for the set of 3 scans for each of the 14 patients must be calculated. Patient 1 is Mrs. J., for whom this calculation was made in Chapter 3.

Recall that, to calculate the mean value, the individual values were added, and then divided by the number of scans, as follows:

$$(1.010 + 1.019 + 1.100) \div 3 = 1.043$$

The SD for this set of data on patient 1 (Mrs. J.) was found using the formula:

$$SD = \sqrt{\sum \frac{(X-\overline{X})^2}{n-1}}$$

A statistical calculator is an inexpensive investment that dramatically simplifies these types of calculations. In mathematical longhand, the calculation for the SD on patient 1, Mrs. J., is as follows:

$$\mathrm{SD}_{\mathrm{pt.1}} = \sqrt{\frac{(1.010-1.043)^2 + (1.019-1.043)^2 + (1.100-1.043)^2}{3-1}}$$

$$\mathrm{SD} = 0.050\ \mathrm{g/cm^2}$$

In expressing the precision for patient 1, Mrs. J., it would be appropriate to state that the precision for the set of three scans is 0.05 g/cm^2. As noted previously, however, precision is often expressed as the CV, or the percent coefficient of variation, %CV. The CV is defined as the SD divided by the mean. For patient 1, therefore:

$$\mathrm{CV} = (0.050\ \mathrm{g/cm^2}) \div (1.043\ \mathrm{g/cm^2})$$

$$\mathrm{CV} = 0.0479$$

Expressed as a percentage, the %CV would be 4.79%, or 4.8%, with rounding.

Step 2. The mean or average BMD, the SD, and CV, or %CV, should be calculated for each of the remaining 13 patients. These results are shown in Table 4-2.

Step 3. Although the precision for each of the 14 individuals is now known, the precision for the group as a whole must now be calculated. This is done by finding the root-mean–square (RMS) average for the 14 subjects. To calculate the RMS average SD, the following formula is used:

$$SD = \sqrt{\sum_{j=1}^{m} \mathrm{SD}_j^2 \div m}$$

This formula expresses the following mathematical steps. First, square each of the 14 SDs. Then, sum all 14 squared SDs, beginning with Mrs. J., who is patient number 1, and continue through the total number of patients, *m*. Divide the sum by *m*, the number of patients, or 14. Finally, take the

Table 4-2
Mean, SD, CV, and %CV for Each of 14 Patients in a Precision Study

Patient	*Mean (g/cm²)*	*SD (g/cm²)*	*CV*	*%CV*
1	1.043	0.050	0.048	4.8
2	0.928	0.011	0.012	1.2
3	1.165	0.005	0.004	0.4
4	1.006	0.006	0.006	0.6
5	0.908	0.010	0.012	1.2
6	0.958	0.003	0.003	0.3
7	1.053	0.084	0.080	8.0
8	0.864	0.014	0.016	1.6
9	0.906	0.012	0.013	1.3
10	1.073	0.056	0.052	5.2
11	0.958	0.008	0.008	0.8
12	0.992	0.008	0.008	0.8
13	1.197	0.010	0.009	0.9
14	1.172	0.008	0.007	0.7

square root. This is the SD for the entire group in g/cm^2, and is the precision for the entire group.

For these 14 patients, the long-hand calculation of the RMS average SD is as follows:

$$SD = \sqrt{\frac{\begin{matrix}(0.05)^2 + (0.011)^2 + (0.005)^2 + (0.006)^2 + (0.01)^2 + \\ (0.003)^2 + (0.084)^2 + (0.014)^2 + (0.012)^2 + (0.056)^2 + \\ (0.008)^2 + (0.008)^2 + (0.010)^2 + (0.008)^2\end{matrix}}{14}}$$

$$SD = 0.031 \text{ g/cm}^2$$

Because the precision may also be expressed as the CV, the RMS average for the CV for the entire group of 14 patients is determined using the following formula:

$$CV = \sqrt{\sum_{j=1}^{m} CV_j^2 \div m}$$

Each of the 14 CVs that have been previously calculated are squared and then added. This sum is divided by the number of patients, *m*, and then the square root is taken. This is the CV for the entire group. To express it as a percentage, simply multiply by 100. The %CV for the group of 14 patients is 2.9%.

It is appropriate to state the average BMD for the entire group, in addition to the SD, CV, or %CV, when discussing precision. The average BMD for the group of 14 patients is found simply by adding all 42 scan values and dividing by 42. This value is 1.016 g/cm^2. The average BMD for the group should be stated, because the precision will not be as good in osteopenic or osteoporotic populations as it is in normal populations. When the precision is expressed as a CV, part of the poorer precision in osteopenic groups is simply a function of the denominator being smaller (in the calculation of the CV). For example, in the group of 14 patients with an average BMD of 1.016 g/cm^2 shown in Table 4-2, the precision was found to be 0.031 g/cm^2 when the SD is used, and 2.9% when the %CV is used. If a precision study was done in a different group of 14 individuals, and the RMS SD for this group was also 0.031 g/cm^2, it would be correct to conclude that the precision was equal in the two groups. However, if the average BMD in the second group was lower, at, for example, 0.800 g/cm^2, the %CV would appear to be poorer. When the SD is divided by the mean of the group, and multiplied by 100 to obtain a percentage, the %CV in the second group becomes 3.9%.

Part of the poorer precision is also real, however. As the bones become progressively demineralized and the BMD falls, the precision tends not to be as good as the precision in individuals with higher levels of BMD. In ideal circumstances, a precision study would be performed on different groups of individuals, in which the average BMDs of the groups spanned normal-to-osteoporotic values. The appropriate precision value could then be applied in clinical circumstances, based on the BMD of the patient in question. Another approach is to perform a precision study in each individual patient who will be followed. Neither are clinically practical suggestions, however. Therefore, it is important to remember that the precision value obtained in a short-term study of young, normal individuals represents the best possible precision. Medium-term precision studies tend to demonstrate a decline in precision from short-term studies. In one such study from Lees et al. *(2)*, precision for the AP spine declined from a short-term value of 0.86% to a medium-term value of 1.12%. Precision also declined in the femoral neck, from 1.38 to 1.59%, and in the trochanter from 1.93 to 2.83%. Most authorities agree that precision should be expressed as the SD in g/cm^2, rather than as a CV or %CV. Nevertheless, the use of the CV or %CV remains common.

APPLYING THE PRECISION VALUE TO THE INTERPRETATION OF SERIAL MEASUREMENTS

Assume that a patient has undergone two bone density measurements of the AP spine a year apart to determine if a therapy has been effective in

Table 4-3
Calculation of the Change in BMD Between Two Measurements Required for Statistical Confidence at Three Different Levels of Confidence

Confidence level	*Calculation for two measurements*
95% Confidence	(1.96 × Precision)/0.707 = 2.77 × Precision
90% Confidence	(1.65 × Precision)/0.707 = 2.33 × Precision
85% Confidence	(1.30 × Precision)/0.707 = 1.84 × Precision

increasing the bone density. If the baseline spine BMD was 0.725 g/cm^2, and the follow-up BMD was 0.754 g/cm^2, there has been an increase in the BMD over 1 year of 0.029 g/cm^2. This represents an increase of 4% from the baseline value in 1 year. Is this a statistically significant increase, given that the technology cannot perfectly reproduce the results of any bone-density test, even when there has been no real change in the BMD?

For a change in BMD between two measurements to be considered statistically significant, the magnitude of the change must be equal to or exceed the product of the precision value, multiplied by a factor that is determined by the level of confidence that is required. Table 4-3 illustrates this calculation for three different levels of statistical confidence.

At the 95% confidence level, if a figure of 1% is used for the precision value, a change of 2.77% or greater must be seen before the change can be considered significant. For precision values other than 1%, the magnitude of change necessary is simply 2.77, multiplied by the precision value. The magnitude of change that is necessary for statistical significance is less if a lower level of confidence is acceptable. Although 95% confidence is considered ideal, clinicians routinely make decisions using lower levels of confidence. In the case described above, in which the increase in BMD was a change of 4% from the baseline value, assume also that a previously performed precision study for the AP spine revealed a precision value of 1%. The physician can be 95% confident, then, that a real increase has occurred in this patient. This is possible because the increase of 4% in the BMD clearly exceeds the minimum change of 2.77%, which is required to be 95% confident that a biologic change has occurred. If the precision study had indicated a precision of 1.5%, could the physician be equally as confident about the significance of the 4% change? The answer is no. The product of 1.5% × 2.77 is 4.16%. Because the measured change does not equal or exceed this value, the physician cannot be 95% confident that a real change has occurred. Because less change is required for lower levels of statistical confidence, the physician can be 90% confident that a real change has occurred. Tables 4-4 to 4-6 illustrate the minimum change in

Table 4-4
Minimum % Change Needed Between
Two BMD Measurements for Statistical Confidence
at the 95% Confidence Level for Different Values of Precision

Precision as %CV	*Minimum % change in BMD*
0.50	1.39
0.75	2.08
1.00	2.77
1.25	3.46
1.50	4.16
1.75	4.85
2.00	5.54
2.25	6.23
2.50	6.93
2.75	7.62
3.00	8.31
3.25	9.00
3.50	9.70

Table 4-5
Minimum % Change Needed Between
Two BMD Measurements for Statistical Confidence
at the 90% Confidence Level for Different Values of Precision

Precision as %CV	*Minimum % change in BMD*
0.50	1.17
0.75	1.75
1.00	2.33
1.25	2.91
1.50	3.50
1.75	4.08
2.00	4.66
2.25	5.24
2.50	5.83
2.75	6.41
3.00	6.99
3.25	7.57
3.50	8.16

BMD between two measurements at various levels of precision that is required to achieve statistical confidence.

A different, and perhaps more clinically useful, approach is to determine the maximum level of statistical confidence for any magnitude of

Table 4-6
Minimum % Change Needed Between
Two BMD Measurements for Statistical Confidence
at the 85% Confidence Level for Different Values of Precision

Precision as %CV	*Minimum % change in BMD*
0.50	0.92
0.75	1.38
1.00	1.84
1.25	2.30
1.50	2.76
1.75	3.22
2.00	3.68
2.25	4.14
2.50	4.60
2.75	5.06
3.00	5.52
3.25	5.98
3.50	6.44

change between two measurements when the precision of the testing is known. This is shown in Table 4-7. The precision values in this table are expressed as the RMS SD in g/cm^2, rather than as a CV or %CV. The change in BMD is the absolute difference between the two measurements, also expressed in g/cm^2. For example, a precision value of 0.010 g/cm^2 is not unusual for AP spine measurements. If the magnitude of change between two measurements is 0.015 g/cm^2, the physician may be 71% confident that a real change has occurred. It is important to note that this means only that the physician can be 71% confident that a change has occurred. It does not mean that the physician can be 71% confident that a change of 0.015 g/cm^2 has occurred.

THE CONFIDENCE INTERVAL FOR THE CHANGE IN BMD BETWEEN TWO MEASUREMENTS

Once it has been determined that a measured change in BMD is significant at some level of statistical confidence, the question remains what the actual change in BMD really is. As noted in the example above, with a precision of 0.010 g/cm^2 and a measured change of 0.015 g/cm^2, a physician may be 71% confident that a real change has occurred. The physician cannot be 71% confident that a change of 0.015 g/cm^2 has actually occurred. So how can the range of values in which the true change may lie be calculated? Table 4-8 illustrates the range of values for 95, 90, and 85% confidence intervals (CIs) for a change in BMD between two measurements at various levels of precision. The values shown in the table for the various

Table 4-7
Levels of % Statistical Confidence for Various Combinations of Precision and Change in BMD

Change in BMD	*Precision (g/cm²)*									
(g/cm²)	*0.005*	*0.010*	*0.015*	*0.020*	*0.025*	*0.030*	*0.035*	*0.040*	*0.045*	*0.050*
0.005	52	28	19	14	11	9	8	7	6	6
0.010	84	52	36	28	22	19	16	14	12	11
0.015	97	71	52	40	33	28	24	21	19	17
0.020	100	84	65	52	43	36	31	28	25	22
0.025	100	92	76	62	52	44	39	34	31	28
0.030	100	97	84	71	60	52	46	40	36	33
0.035	100	99	90	78	68	59	52	46	42	38
0.040	100	100	94	84	74	65	58	52	47	43
0.045	100	100	97	89	80	71	64	57	52	48
0.050	100	100	98	92	84	76	69	62	57	52
0.055	100	100	99	95	88	81	73	67	61	56
0.060	100	100	100	97	91	84	77	71	65	60
0.065	100	100	100	98	93	87	81	75	69	64
0.070	100	100	100	99	95	90	84	78	73	68
0.075	100	100	100	99	97	92	87	82	76	71
0.080	100	100	100	100	98	94	89	84	79	74
0.085	100	100	100	100	98	95	91	87	82	77
0.090	100	100	100	100	99	97	93	89	84	80
0.095	100	100	100	100	99	97	95	91	86	82
0.100	100	100	100	100	100	98	96	92	88	84

Table reproduced with permission of Ken Faulkner, Ph.D. Oregon Osteoporosis Center, Portland, Oregon.

Table 4-8
Confidence Intervals for Change in BMD Between Two Measurements for Different Values of Precision

Confidence level	*Precision, %CV*								
	1	*1.25*	*1.5*	*1.75*	*2*	*2.25*	*2.5*	*2.75*	*3*
95% Confidence	± 2.77	± 3.46	± 4.12	± 4.85	± 5.54	± 6.23	± 6.93	± 7.62	± 8.31
90% Confidence	± 2.33	± 2.91	± 3.50	± 4.08	± 4.66	± 5.24	± 5.83	± 6.41	± 6.99
85% Confidence	± 1.84	± 2.28	± 2.76	± 3.22	± 3.68	± 4.14	± 4.60	± 5.06	± 5.52

Table 4-9
Interval Between BMD Measurements Required
Before Statistically Significant Change at the 95% Confidence Level
Is Expected with Various Levels of Precision and Expected Rates of Change

		Interval between BMD measurements	
Precision as %CV	*% Change/year*	*Months*	*Years*
0.5%	1	16.7	1.39
	3	5.6	0.46
	5	3.3	0.28
1.0%	1	33.2	2.77
	3	11.0	0.92
	5	6.7	0.55
1.5%	1	50.0	4.16
	3	16.6	1.39
	5	10.0	0.83
2.0%	1	66.5	5.54
	3	22.2	1.85
	5	13.3	1.11
2.5%	1	83.2	6.93
	3	27.7	2.31
	5	16.6	1.39

levels of precision and confidence are added and subtracted from the actual measured change. For example, if the precision of testing is 1.5%, and the measured change is 3%, the actual range of change for the 95% CI is 3 ± 4.12%, or −1.12% to +7.12%. Because the range of possible values contains 0, the measured change of 3%, with a precision of 1.5%, is not statistically significant at the 95% confidence level. On the other hand, if the precision is 1.25%, and the change between two measurements is 4%, then the 95% CI for the change is 4 ± 3.46% or 0.54 to 7.46%. This range of values does not contain 0, and therefore is significant at the 95% confidence level. Obviously, this is a very wide CI. It is perhaps disconcerting to note that, although the measured change is statistically significant, the actual change may range from as little as 0.54% to as much as 7.46%. The 85% CI is narrower. In this case, the range of values is 4 ± 2.76%, or 1.24 to 6.76%.

EFFECT OF PRECISION ON THE TIMING OF REPEAT MEASUREMENTS OF BMD

It is clear that considerations of precision will also affect the timing of repeat BMD measurements for the assessment of therapeutic efficacy or disease effect. The follow-up BMD measurement should not be performed until the physician can reasonably anticipate seeing a change that is likely to be statistically significant. Obviously, it serves no useful purpose to perform a bone-mass measurement to assess change when a significant change is not yet anticipated. The timing is entirely based on the precision of the testing, the anticipated rate of change from the disease or therapeutic intervention, and the magnitude of change necessary for desired level of statistical confidence. Table 4-9 (*see* previous page) illustrates the time interval necessary before a change that is significant at the 95% confidence level can be anticipated for a variety of combinations of precision values and rates of change. The rates of changes for various diseases and therapeutic interventions are discussed in more detail in Chapter 7.

REFERENCES

1. Gluer CC, Blake G, Lu Y, Blunt BA, Genant HK (1995) Accurate assessment of precision errors: how to measure the reproducibility errors of bone densitometry techniques. *Osteoporosis Int* 5:262–270.
2. Lees B, Stevenson JC (1992) An evaluation of dual-energy X-ray absorptiometry and comparison with dual-photon absorptiometry. *Osteoporosis Int* 2:146–152.

5 Quality-Control Procedures for Densitometry

Contents

The original indications for bone-mass measurements from the National Osteoporosis Foundation, published in 1988, and the guidelines for the clinical applications for bone densitometry from the International Society for Clinical Densitometry, published in 1996, called for strict quality control procedures at clinical sites performing densitometry *(1,2)*. Such procedures are crucial to the generation of accurate and precise bone-density data. In spite of inherently superb accuracy and precision in today's X-ray densitometers, alterations in the functioning of the machines will occur. Quality control procedures to detect these alterations in machine function should be utilized by every clinical site performing densitometry, regardless of the frequency with which measurements are performed.

The quality-control procedures used in densitometry today have been derived from procedures originally developed for quality control in analytical chemistry and industry *(3)*. The most commonly applied methods are the multirule Shewhart chart and the cumulative sum chart (CUSUM). The application of either of these methods requires that a phantom be scanned to establish a baseline value, and then, regularly, to establish longitudinal values.

Manufacturers of today's X-ray-based bone densitometers provide phantoms for use with their machines, although some phantoms, such as the anthropomorphic Hologic (Waltham, MA) spine phantom, are often used with densitometers from other manufacturers. Some manufacturers will provide two phantoms to be used for different purposes. One phantom may be used for daily quality-assurance functions, in which the mechanical operation of the machine is tested. The other phantom is generally designed to mimic a region of the skeleton, and is used for quality-control procedures designed to detect drifting of BMD values. For example, on Lunar DXA (Madison, WI) machines, a block phantom is used for daily quality assurance, and a second phantom, an aluminum spine phantom, is used for quality control.

Most daily quality-assurance procedures to detect mechanical failures on today's densitometers are automated. Readouts will simply indicate a passing or failing condition. Before outright mechanical failure occurs, however, regular scanning of the quality-control phantom, and the application of Shewhart charts and rules, or CUSUM charts, can detect drift or change in machine values that require correction, in order to ensure continued accuracy and precision. It has been suggested that such stringent quality-control measures are more important in multicenter research trials using densitometry than in routine clinical practice. This statement does not seem justified, however, when it is recognized that average BMD values from large groups of individuals are evaluated in multicenter trials. Averaging results from large numbers of research subjects can mute the effects of many types of errors. For the individual patient being followed over time at a clinical site, there is no such protection from undetected machine errors.

ESTABLISHING A BASELINE VALUE WITH THE PHANTOM

Manufacturers generally recommend scanning the phantom 10 times on the same day, without repositioning the phantom between studies. This is also the procedure often used as part of quality-control procedures in longitudinal clinical research trials. Subsequent phantom scans are then performed at least 3 times per week and on every day that a patient is scanned.

The average value of the 10 phantom scans should be calculated. The values that represent the average value ±1.5% should also be calculated. Using these values, limits are established within which all subsequent measurements of the phantom should fall. These results are easily tracked by plotting the results on standard graph paper.

Table 5-1 shows the results of 10 scans of the Hologic spine phantom that were performed on a Lunar DPX. The average value was calculated and found to be 1.182 g/cm^2; 1.5% of the average value was calculated to be 0.018 g/cm^2 (1.182 g/cm^2 × 0.015). Therefore, the range of values within which all subsequent phantom scan values should fall is 1.182 ± 0.018 g/cm^2, or between 1.164 and 1.200 g/cm^2. Subsequent scans of the phantom are plotted onto graph paper that reflects the boundaries of the average ±1.5%, as shown in Fig. 5-1. Scan values are expected to fall randomly on either side of the average value over time. If a value falls outside the boundaries, the phantom scan should immediately be repeated. If it falls

Table 5-1
10 Hologic Spine-Phantom Scans Performed on a Lunar DPX on the Same Day to Establish a Baseline Phantom BMD Value for Quality Control

Phantom scan	*Date*	*BMD L1–L4 g/cm²*
Scan 1	4/22/96	1.181
Scan 2	4/22/96	1.173
Scan 3	4/22/96	1.176
Scan 4	4/22/96	1.180
Scan 5	4/22/96	1.190
Scan 6	4/22/96	1.174
Scan 7	4/22/96	1.189
Scan 8	4/22/96	1.192
Scan 9	4/22/96	1.177
Scan 10	4/22/96	1.187

Average value for the 10 phantom scans is 1.182 g/cm^2. The SD is 0.007 g/cm^2 and 1.5% of the average value is 0.018 g/cm^2.

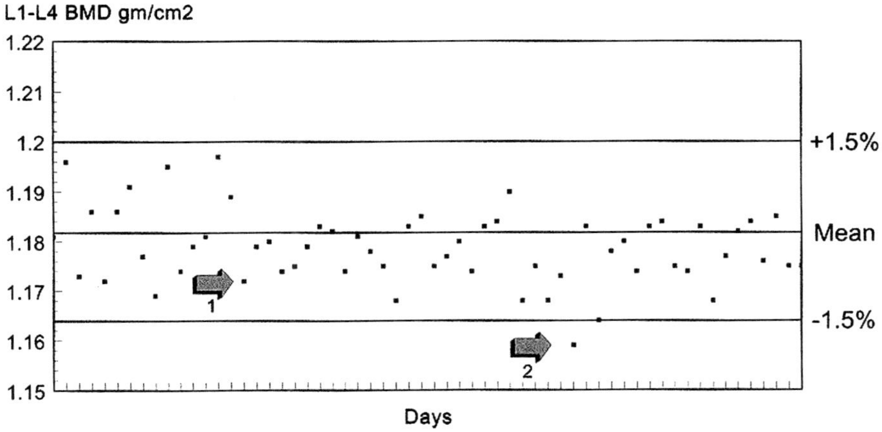

Fig. 5-1. A quality control chart with control limits of ±1.5%. The average BMD of the phantom was established by scanning the phantom 10 times on the same day. Arrow 1 indicates a point at which values appear to be drifting downward. Arrow 2 indicates a violation of the 1.5% rule.

outside the boundaries again, or fails, the manufacturer should be contacted for additional instructions. This constitutes a minimum quality control program that should be in use in every facility performing densitometry.

The creation of an average baseline phantom value by scanning the phantom 10 times on the same day, without repositioning, may not reflect the day-to-day variability in machine values, and the effects of repositioning that would be expected as the phantom is scanned over time. Several groups have consequently recommended that the baseline phantom value be established by scanning the phantom once a day for 25 consecutive days, and then averaging these 25 scans. It is thought that this will more accurately reflect the day-to-day variability in machine values, and result in fewer false-alarm failures. For example, the average BMD of the same Hologic spine phantom, when scanned on 25 consecutive days, as shown in Table 5-2, was 1.177 g/cm^2, resulting in a range for the average ±1.5% of 1.159 to 1.195 g/cm^2. In both cases, 1.5% of the mean value was 0.018 g/cm^2, but the range of acceptable values was different from that seen when the phantom was scanned 10× on the same day, without repositioning. Figure 5-2 is the graph of subsequent scans now plotted against the baseline phantom value obtained after scanning the phantom once on each of 25 consecutive days.

The graphs shown in Figs. 5-1 and 5-2 should be visually inspected for signs that the values are drifting up or down, or for signs that step changes have occurred in the values. Arrow 1 on the graph in Fig. 5-1 indicates a point at which it appears that the phantom values are no longer randomly scattered on either side of the average, but, instead, are concentrated below the average. This suggests that the scan values may be starting to drift downward. These situations can and do occur, even though the absolute BMD values obtained during the phantom scans remain within the established range, and other daily quality-assurance procedures continue to give "pass" indications. Notice that in Fig. 5-2, when the mean was calculated using 25 scans performed on consecutive days, the same phantom values do not give any indication of a loss of random scatter. More sophisticated evaluations of this type of data involve the use of process control charts to determine whether, in fact, there has been a shift in values. Nevertheless, this type of chart is the foundation of a good quality-control program.

SHEWHART RULES AND CUSUM CHARTS

The field of analytical chemistry recognized the need for strict quality control many years ago. Like bone densitometry, analytical chemistry involves the use of machines for quantitative measurements. Techniques had to be developed to determine that the machines continued to function properly over long periods of time, in order to ensure consistency in the results. The methods common to analytical chemistry have been adapted for use in bone densitometry. These methods utilize the BMD values from the phantom scans as described earlier: the average phantom value, and the values from phantom scans performed over time. The two most commonly used methods for tracking machine performance are Shewhart rules and the CUSUM chart.

Table 5-2
25 Hologic Spine-Phantom Scans Performed on a Lunar DPX on 25 Consecutive Days to Establish a Baseline Phantom Value for Quality Control

Phantom scan	*Date*	*BMD L1–L4 g/cm^2*
Scan 1	4/22/96	1.181
Scan 2	4/23/96	1.172
Scan 3	4/24/96	1.176
Scan 4	4/25/96	1.172
Scan 5	4/29/96	1.180
Scan 6	4/30/96	1.185
Scan 7	5/01/96	1.179
Scan 8	5/02/96	1.176
Scan 9	5/06/96	1.177
Scan 10	5/07/96	1.169
Scan 11	5/08/96	1.180
Scan 12	5/09/96	1.167
Scan 13	5/13/96	1.179
Scan 14	5/14/96	1.189
Scan 15	5/15/96	1.174
Scan 16	5/16/96	1.186
Scan 17	5/20/96	1.181
Scan 18	5/21/96	1.170
Scan 19	5/22/96	1.179
Scan 20	5/23/96	1.178
Scan 21	5/28/96	1.180
Scan 22	5/29/96	1.181
Scan 23	5/30/96	1.168
Scan 24	6/03/96	1.182
Scan 25	6/04/96	1.172

The average value for the 25 phantom scans is 1.177 g/cm^2. The SD is 0.006 g/cm^2 and 1.5% of the average value is 0.018 g/cm^2. Compare these values to those shown in Table 5-1.

Shewhart Rules

Shewhart* rules have been used in analytical chemistry since the 1950s. In order to utilize Shewhart rules, it is necessary to establish a baseline value for the phantom measurement. In this context, establishment of the

*Dr. William Andrew Shewhart (1891–1967), as a scientist with Western Electric, devised the basis for the application of statistical methods to quality control. In 1931, his book, *Economic Control of Quality of Manufactured Product,* was published, in which he presented his methods for statistical sampling.

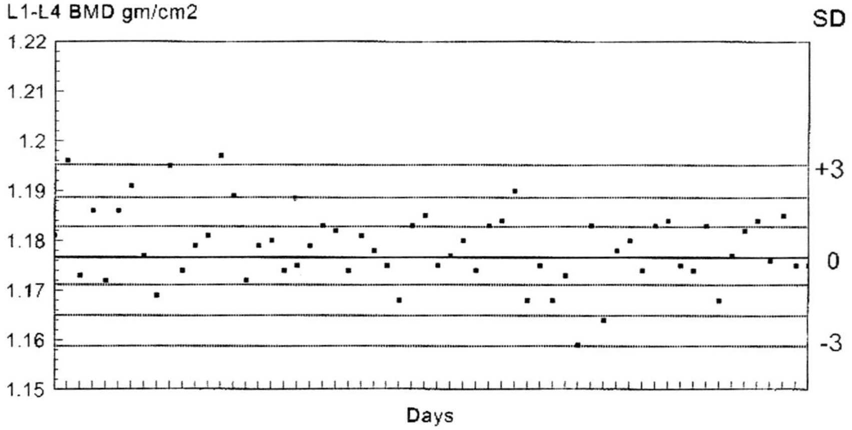

Fig. 5-2. A Shewhart chart for quality control. The average BMD of the phantom was established by scanning the phantom once on 25 consecutive days.

baseline value by scanning the phantom once on 25 consecutive days, rather than 10 times on the same day, is recommended. Once the average value of the 25 phantom scans is determined, the standard deviation (SD) for the set of 25 scans should be calculated. A graph can then be created onto which the BMD data from subsequent phantom measurements is plotted, much as was done in Fig. 5-2. The *y*-axis of the graph should reflect both the actual BMD values and SD units, as shown in Fig. 5-2. To utilize SD units, the average BMD is assigned a value of 0 on the *y*-axis of the graph, and the SD tics are labeled +1 or –1, +2 or –2, and so on. In other words, the *y*-axis reflects both the measured BMD and the *z*-score* of the phantom BMD measurements. The average phantom value used to construct the Shewhart chart in Fig. 5-2 was previously found to be 1.177 g/cm^2. The SD was also previously found to be 0.006 g/cm^2 for this set of measurements. It is not necessary to calculate the *z*-score for each of the subsequent phantom measurements. When the measured BMD is plotted on the graph, it becomes visually apparent how many SDs from the mean the value actually lies, because of the SD, or *z*-score scale, on the *y*-axis. In a normally functioning machine, the values plotted on the graph are expected to be randomly scattered on either side of the mean (that is, above and below the mean).

As these values are being plotted, rules are applied to detect trends or failures that may indicate a change in machine performance. These are

**See* Chapter 4 for a discussion of *z*-scores. In this context, *z*-score has nothing to do with reference population BMD data.

called Shewhart rules, or they may be called sensitizing rules *(4)*. Different combinations of rules have been tested in densitometry, in order to minimize false alarms and increase the ability of the Shewhart rules to detect true alterations in machine performance *(5–7)*.

Shewhart rules are usually set at a certain level. In other words, a control level or limit is selected. When the limit is exceeded, the Shewhart rules are applied. For example, Shewhart rules may be set at a control level or limit of the mean ± 2 SDs. If the phantom BMD value exceeds these limits, the Shewhart rules are applied to detect potential machine failures.

For example, a machine failure may be deemed to have occurred if the phantom value exceeds the mean ± 2 SDs, and any one or more of the following Shewhart rules are confirmed:

1. A phantom BMD value exceeding the mean ± 3 SDs.
2. Two consecutive phantom BMD values on the same side of the mean exceeding the mean ± 2 SDs.
3. Two consecutive phantom BMD values differing by more than 4 SDs.
4. Four consecutive phantom BMD values on the same side of the mean exceeding the mean ± 1 SD.
5. Ten consecutive phantom BMD values falling on the same side of the mean, regardless of their distance from the mean.

Not all violations of the rules will be found to be machine failures that require correction. In order to reduce the false alarms, a filter is sometimes applied to the sensitizing rules. One such filter is to calculate the average BMD for 10 consecutive phantom measurements, after a violation of one of the sensitizing rules has occurred. If this 10-scan average differs by more than 1 SD from the baseline average value, the violation is confirmed. Another method is to set the triggering of the rules at a different level, such as the 3-SD deviation level. When this approach is employed, the occurrence of a single value outside the 3-SD limits then triggers the application of the other rules.

Without such filters or triggers, Shewhart rules, although easy to use, produce a high false-alarm rate. Even if a machine is in perfect working order, a violation of the Shewhart rules is expected to occur once every 39 scans *(6)*. When the filter is added, the false-alarm rate drops to once every 631 scans. Unfortunately, although the addition of the filter to Shewhart rules reduces the number of false alarms, it may also have the undesirable effect of delaying detection of true shifts in machine performance.

Shewhart rules may also be utilized by calculating the mean ± a percentage of the mean, as was done in the quality control chart in Fig. 5-2. For most of the central DXA scanners in clinical use today, repeat phantom measurements will generally result in a SD for the baseline set of phantom measurements that is roughly 0.5% of the mean value. Consequently,

1.5% of the mean value for the phantom BMD will equal approximately 3 SD. For example, when the statistics were calculated for the 10 phantom measurements performed on the same day shown in Table 5-1, the mean was 1.182 g/cm^2, with a SD of 0.007 g/cm^2; 1.5% of the mean was found to be 0.018 g/cm^2. In this case, 1.5% of the mean is equal to 2.6 SDs. In the case of the 25 phantom scans shown in Table 5-2, with a SD of 0.006, the 1.5% value of 0.018 g/cm^2 is equal to 3 SDs. The % values can be used to invoke the Shewhart rules. Using a value of 0.5% of the mean as equaling 1 SD, the Shewhart rules would be applied if a phantom value exceeded the baseline mean value ± 1% (instead of the mean ± 2 SDs). A violation would be deemed to have occurred in any of the following circumstances if:

1. A phantom BMD value exceeds the mean ± 1.5%.
2. Two consecutive phantom BMD values on the same side of the mean exceed the mean ± 1%.
3. Two consecutive phantom BMD values differ by more than 2%.
4. Four consecutive phantom BMD values on the same side of the mean exceed the mean ± 0.5%.
5. Ten consecutive phantom BMD values fall on the same side of the mean, regardless of their distance from the mean.

The 10-scan average filter described above would confirm a failure, if the 10-scan average differed from the baseline average by more than 0.5% (instead of 1 SD).

In quality control jargon, each of these rules has its own name. In the order listed above, the rules are known as the:

1. 3 SD, or 1.5%, rule.
2. 2 SD twice, or 1.0% twice, rule.
3. Range of 4 SD, or range of 2%, rule.
4. 4 ± 1 SD, or 4 ± 0.5%, rule.
5. Mean × 10 rule.

When any of the Shewhart rules are confirmed, the manufacturer should be consulted to determine the cause.

CUSUM Charts

CUSUM charts are not as easy to use as Shewhart rules, but these are the types of charts employed by most professional densitometry quality-control centers. This technique was originally developed for use in industry *(8)*. It was subsequently adapted for use in bone densitometry. In order to utilize the CUSUM chart, a baseline spine-phantom value must again be established by scanning the phantom once per day on 25 consecutive days, as was done previously for the application of Shewhart rules. For all subsequent scans, the difference between the average value and the subsequent value is calculated. The differences are progressively summed and plotted on the CUSUM chart. Mathematically, this is expressed as:

$$\mathrm{CS}_n = \sum_{p=1}^{n} (BMD_p - BMD_{\mathrm{Mean}})$$

where CS is the cumulative sum, n is the total number of measurements, $\mathrm{BMD}_{\mathrm{Mean}}$ is the average phantom value, and $\mathrm{BMD}_{\mathrm{p}}$ is the phantom value for each of the n measurements. Each sequential value of CS is plotted on the graph. The vertical axis of the graph is marked in SD units of the average value. For a properly functioning machine, the values plotted on the CUSUM chart should be scattered in a horizontal pattern around 0 (0 is equal to the mean phantom value). If the pattern is rising or falling, the machine is not functioning properly.

The construction of a CUSUM chart begins again with the data in Table 5-2. The phantom was scanned once each day for 25 consecutive days. The average value of the phantom was found to be 1.177 g/cm^2, and the SD was calculated to be 0.006 g/cm^2. Table 5-3 illustrates the calculations of the cumulative sum for the next 10 phantom measurements. Figure 5-3 illustrates the CUSUM plot for these 10 measurements, and for 30 additional measurements that followed. In Fig. 5-3, instead of BMD on the vertical axis, SD units, or *z*-scores, are utilized. The CUSUM plot for these 40 phantom scans clearly appears to be rising rather than being horizontal.

Although the CUSUM chart is inspected visually to determine machine malfunction indicated by the nonhorizontal plot, two methods have been developed to determine mathematically when control limits have been exceeded. One method involves the superimposition of a V-mask, in which the slope of the arms on the mask is determined mathematically *(9)*. The slope is normally some multiple of the standard error of the mean phantom value. The stringency of the mask can be changed by increasing or decreasing the slope of the V-mask. The other method, called tabular CUSUM, involves the mathematical calculation of upper and lower control limits *(6)*. In either case, when values fall outside the control limits, or the arms of the mask, an alarm is triggered, indicating that the manufacturer should be contacted.

The calculation of the control limits for tabular CUSUM is more tedious than complex, although the equations used for these calculations appear somewhat intimidating at first. The upper control limit is calculated using the following equation:

$$CS_{H\max(i)} = [(X_i - \mu_0)/\sigma] - k + \mathrm{CS}_{H\max(i-1)}$$

In other words, to calculate the upper limit of the maximum cumulative sum for scan i ($\mathrm{CS}_{\mathrm{Hmax}}$), subtract the average phantom value (μ_0) from the phantom value for scan i (X_i), and then divide this difference by the SD (σ)

Table 5-3
Calculation of Cumulative Sum for Sequential Phantom Scans

Date	*Phantom BMD g/cm²*	*Difference from average phantom value g/cm²*	*Cumulative sum of the differences g/cm²*	*Cumulative sum of differences expressed in SD units (z-score)*
6/5/96	1.181	0.004	0.004	0.67 (0.004 ÷ 0.006)
6/6/96	1.196	0.019	0.023 (0.004 + 0.019)	4.33 (0.023 ÷ 0.006)
6/10/96	1.173	–0.004	0.019 (0.019 – 0.004)	3.17 (0.019 ÷ 0.006)
6/11/96	1.186	0.009	0.028 (0.019 + 0.009)	4.67 (0.028 ÷ 0.006)
6/12/96	1.172	–0.005	0.023 (0.028 – 0.005)	3.83 (0.023 ÷ 0.006)
6/13/96	1.186	0.009	0.032 (0.023 + 0.009)	5.33 (0.032 ÷ 0.006)
6/17/96	1.191	0.014	0.046 (0.032 + 0.014)	7.66 (0.046 ÷ 0.006)
6/21/96	1.169	–0.008	0.038 (0.046 – 0.008)	6.33 (0.038 ÷ 0.006)
6/24/96	1.195	0.018	0.056 (0.038 – 0.003)	9.33 (0.056 ÷ 0.006)
6/25/96	1.174	–0.003	0.053 (0.056 – 0.003)	8.83 (0.053 ÷ 0.006)

The *z*-score of the cumulative sum is plotted on the CUSUM chart. The average phantom value is 1.177 g/cm² and the SD is 0.006 g/cm².

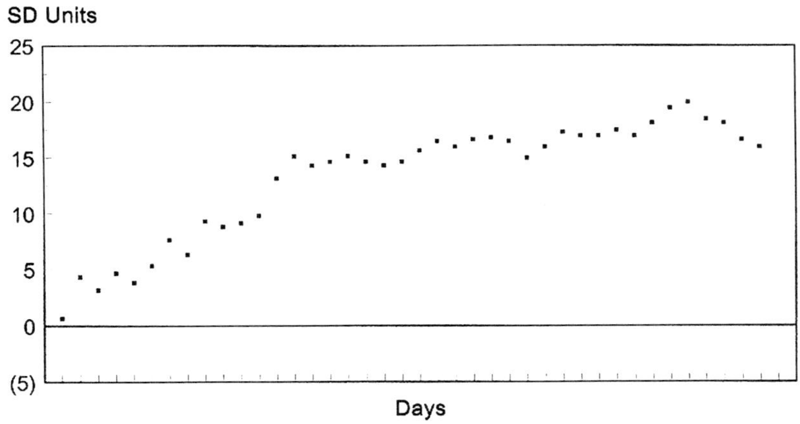

Fig. 5-3. A CUSUM chart. The values are clearly rising, rather than being horizontal.

from the baseline phantom data. Now subtract the value of *k*, which is taken to be 0.5 (this has the effect of subtracting half a SD). The resulting value is then added to the value of $CS_{H\max}$, which had been calculated for the previous phantom scan (scan $i-1$). The lower limit of the maximum cumulative sum is calculated in an analogous fashion, using the equation shown below:

$$CS_{L\max(i)} = [(\mu_0 - X_i)/\sigma] - k + CS_{L\max(i-1)}$$

The process is identical, except that, in this case, the value for phantom scan *i* is subtracted from the average phantom value, which is the opposite of what was done in order to calculate the upper control limit. When either of the two control limits falls below 0, the CS for that limit is set back to 0, the value that is then used for subsequent calculations for that CS. When either of the CS limits exceeds a value of 5, a possible machine failure is deemed to have occurred. Table 5-4 illustrates the calculation of the upper and lower CS control limits for 10 scans that were performed after the initial establishment of the baseline phantom mean value and SD previously shown in Table 5-2.

CUSUM charts or tabular CUSUM are quality-control methods often employed by professional quality-control centers. They are most easily utilized with the help of sophisticated statistical software programs. There is no reason, however, that clinical densitometry centers cannot employ CUSUM methodology, although it is certainly less intuitive to use than Shewhart charts and rules.

AUTOMATED QUALITY CONTROL PROCEDURES

Manufacturers have automated the quality-control process using variations of Shewhart charts and rules. A quality-control graph from a Norland

Table 5-4
Tabular CUSUM Limits for the 10 Phantom Scans Shown in Table 5-3

Date	*Phantom BMD g/cm²*	CS_{Hmax}	CS_{Lmax}
6/5/96	1.181	0.167	0
6/6/96	1.196	2.834	0
6/10/96	1.173	1.667	0.167
6/11/96	1.186	2.667	0
6/12/96	1.172	1.334	0.333
6/13/96	1.186	2.334	0
6/17/96	1.191	4.167	0
6/21/96	1.169	2.334	0.833
6/24/96	1.195	4.834	0
6/25/96	1.174	3.834	0

The CS_{Hmax} approached but did not exceed 5. The CS_{Lmax} was reset to 0 on 7 occasions because the value fell below 0. The mean and SD for the baseline phantom values used in these calculations are 1.177 and 0.006 g/cm², respectively.

XR-Series densitometer (Fort Atkinson, WI) is shown in Fig. 5-4. The upper graph reflects the precision of the system *(10)*. In the upper graph, the solid horizontal line reflects the mean value for the 16 most recent scans. The dashed horizontal lines indicate ±2 SDs about the mean. The value of the SD used to establish this range is a value for the phantom that is entered into the computer during the setup of the system. The BMD values of the individual scans are plotted on the graph. Approximately 1 of every 20 scans is expected to fall outside the range defined by the mean ± 2 SDs simply because, statistically, this range will contain only 95% of the values. The computer will also calculate the SD for each set of 16 scans. This value is not plotted, but is used by the computer. Clearly, the mean and SD will change as new phantom scans are performed and added to the set of the 16 most recent scans. This type of calculation is called a "moving average." The results are monitored for changes in the BMD, as well as increases in the SD. Shewhart rules are applied to detect unacceptable changes in the BMD. The acceptable limits for an increase in the SD are calculated mathematically. If the system passes all tests, the notation "OK" is seen after "PRECISION" at the bottom of the graph. Other messages may be seen, however, which should prompt a call to the manufacturer. For example, an "OUT OF RANGE" notation indicates that the SD from the most recent 16 scans has increased beyond acceptable limits. A "WARNING 1" notation indicates that a single phantom BMD value is more than 3 SDs from the mean. This is a violation of the Shewhart 3 SD rule. "WARNING 2" is a violation of either the Shewhart 2 SDs twice or Range of 4 SDs rule, and "WARNING 3" is a violation of the Shewhart 4 ± 1 SD rule.

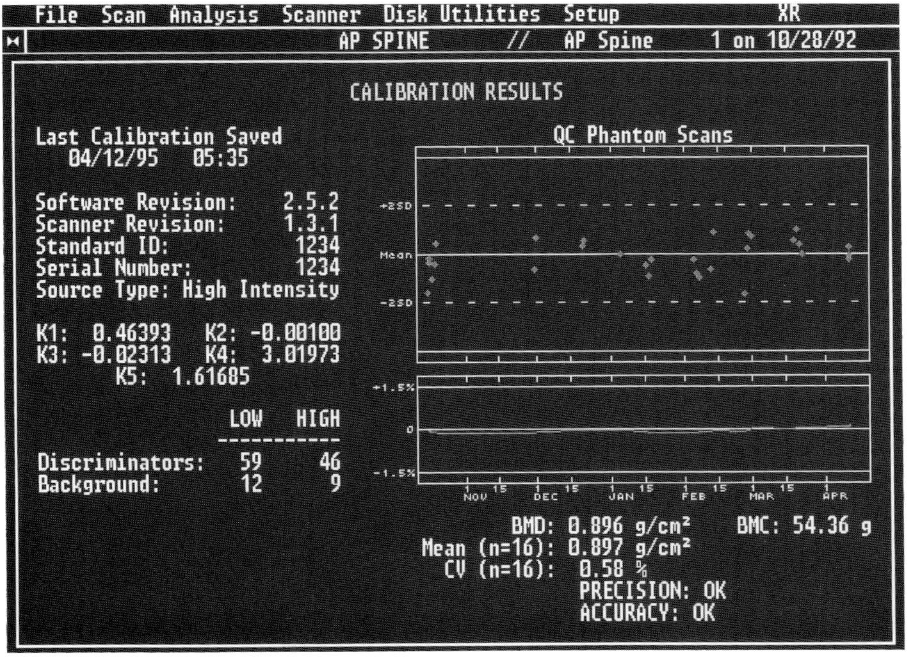

Fig. 5-4. The Norland XR-36 quality-control screen. The upper Shewhart chart tracks the precision of the machine; the lower Shewhart chart tracks accuracy. Courtesy of Norland, Ft. Atkinson, WI. (*see* color plate 13 appearing after p. 174).

The lower graph reflects the accuracy of the system *(10)*. The solid horizontal line represents the correct BMD value of the phantom, which was entered into the computer during the setup of the system. The dashed horizontal lines indicate a range of ±1.5% about this value. The values plotted on this graph are the mean values for BMD for the last 16 phantom scans. If the mean value for the 16 most recent phantom scans falls within ±1.5% of the true phantom value, "OK" will be seen next to the word "ACCURACY" at the bottom of the graph. An "OUT OF RANGE" message will appear if the value falls outside those limits. If eight consecutive values fall on the same side of the true phantom value, a "TREND WARNING" message will appear.

The quality control graphs and calculations for the Norland pDEXA® are very similar to those of the XR-Series. The control limits for the accuracy of the pDEXA system are ±2.5%, instead of 1.5% *(11)*.

Hologic (Waltham, MA) scanners also provide automated quality-control graphing procedures *(12)*. The BMD of a phantom is established during the initial calibration procedures for the scanner. The control limits of

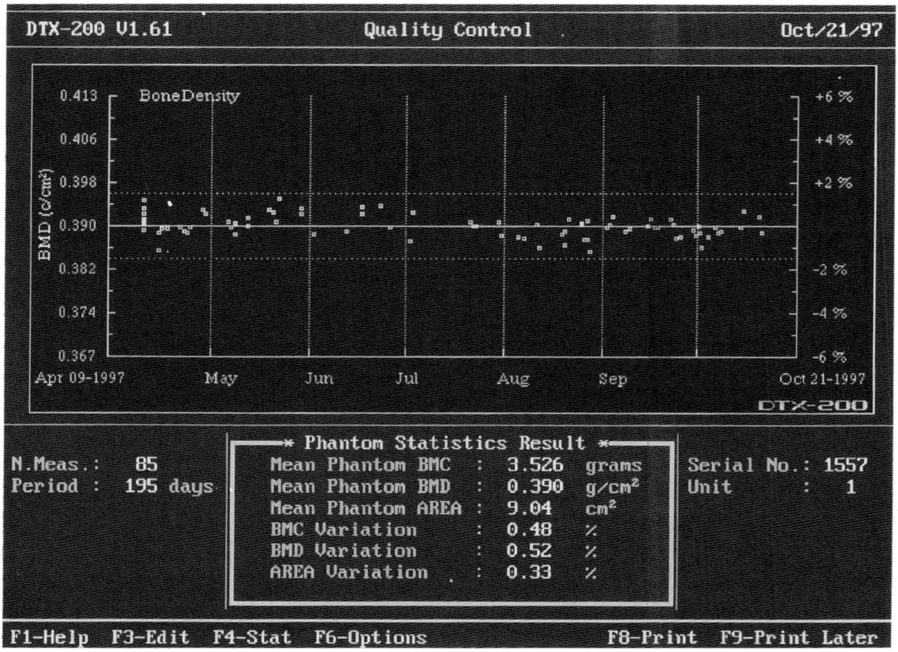

Fig. 5-5. The DTX-200 quality-control screen. This is a Shewhart chart with control limits of ± 1.5%. (*see* color plate 14 appearing after p. 174).

±1.5% of the phantom BMD value are defined on a graph onto which subsequent spine-phantom BMD data is plotted. Beneath the graph, two tables are displayed. The table titled "Reference Values" lists the mean value and SD for the spine phantom established during machine calibration. The table titled "Plot Statistics" lists the number of phantom scans plotted (*n*), the mean, SD, and %CV for those scans. There are no sensitizing rules built into the quality-control program in the computer. With this automated plot, however, Shewhart rules are easy to apply.

Other manufacturers have automated charting of phantom values. Figure 5-5 is such a chart from the Osteometer DTX-200 (Roedovre, Denmark), a dedicated DXA forearm scanner. The dashed horizontal lines on the graph represent control limits of ±1.5%. None of the 85 phantom values has fallen outside the control limits, and the values appear to be randomly scattered about the mean value.

If such charts are not available, they are easily created using the information in this chapter. All densitometry centers should implement quality-control procedures that minimally consist of control charts with defined limits of the mean of phantom scans performed on 25 consecutive days

±1.5%. Shewhart rules with a filter can then be implemented, using rules defined on the basis of % or SD, to further strengthen the quality-control program. The application of CUSUM charts and calculations, as performed at professional quality-control centers, is labor intensive and best utilized with the aid of computerized statistical software programs.

REFERENCES

1. Johnston CC, Melton LJ, Lindsay R, Eddy DM (1989) Clinical indications for bone mass measurements: a report from the scientific advisory board of the National Osteoporosis Foundation. *J Bone Miner Res* 4:S1–S28.
2. Miller PD, Bonnick SL, Rosen CJ (1996) Consensus of an international panel on the clinical utility of bone mass measurements in the detection of low bone mass in the adult population. *Calcif Tissue Int* 58:207–214.
3. Westgard JO, Barry PL, Hunt MR, Groth T (1981) A multirule Shewhart chart for quality control in clinical chemistry. *Clin Chem* 27:493–501.
4. Montgomery DC (1992) *Introduction to Statistical Quality Control.* New York: Wiley.
5. Orwoll ES, Oviatt SK, Biddle JA (1993) Precision of dual-energy X-ray absorptiometry: development of quality control rules and their application in longitudinal studies. *J Bone Miner Res* 8:693–699.
6. Lu Y, Mathur AK, Blunt BA, Gluer CC, Will AS, Fuerst TP, et al. (1998) Dual X-ray absorptiometry quality control: comparison of visual examination and process-control charts. *J Bone Miner Res* 11:626–637.
7. Orwoll ES, Oviatt SK, and the Nafarelin Bone Study Group (1991) Longitudinal precision of dual-energy X-ray absorptiometry in a multicenter trial. *J Bone Miner Res* 6:191–197.
8. British Standards Institution (1980) BS5703: Guide to data analysis and quality control using Cusum techniques. London.
9. Pearson D, Cawte SA (1997) Long-term quality control of DXA: a comparison of Shewhart rules and CUSUM charts. *Osteoporosis Int* 7:338–343.
10. Norland Medical Systems (1993) *XR-Series X-Ray Bone Densitometer Operator's Guide*. Ft. Atkinson, WI.
11. Norland Medical Systems (1996) *Model pDEXA Forearm X-ray Bone Densitometer Operator's Guide*. Ft. Atkinson, WI.
12. Hologic *QDR 4500 X-Ray Bone Densitometer User's Guide,* Revision C. Waltham, MA.

6 The Prediction of Fracture Risk with Densitometry

CONTENTS

In Chapter 3 it was noted that there are several ways to assess the risk of any outcome. The more commonly used measures of risk are prevalence, incidence, absolute and relative risk, and odds ratios. All of these measures can be employed in the specific context of the assessment of fracture risk. In densitometry, new measures of risk are being employed as well, such as the fracture threshold, lifetime risk, and remaining-lifetime fracture probability. A physician may choose to use whichever measure of risk best conveys the clinical importance of the patient's BMD.

PREVALENCE OF FRACTURE AT DIFFERENT LEVELS OF BMD

Prevalence describes the ratio of the number of individuals with a disease at a given point in time, in a particular population, to the number of individuals who are at risk for the disease. Prevalence can be used to answer the question of how common a disease is in a population considered to be at risk for the disease. In the context of this volume, prevalence is used to answer the question, how common is fracture at a given level of BMD? This question was addressed by Mazess *(1)* in a study of 590 Caucasian women, ages 50 to 89 years, who underwent AP spine and proximal femur

Table 6-1
Prevalence of Spine or Hip Fracture, or Both, at Varying Levels of Spine BMD, Measured with DPA

L2–L4 BMD (g/cm^2)	*N*	*Spine fracture %*	*Hip fracture %*	*Either/Both %*
>1.10	100	6.0	3.0	7.0
1.00–1.09	111	9.9	5.4	13.5
0.90–0.99	159	17.0	6.3	22.0
0.80–0.89	134	23.1	9.7	29.9
0.70–0.79	49	40.8	12.2	44.8
0.60–0.69	20	50.0	15.0	60.0

Adapted with permission from Mazess RB. (1990) Bone densitometry for clinical diagnosis and monitoring, in DeLuca HF, Mazess R (eds.), *Osteoporosis: Physiologic Basis, Assessment and Treatment,* pp. 66, Elsevier Science Inc., 655 Avenue of the Americas, New York, NY 10010-5107.

bone density studies with DPA. Approximately 25% of these women had spine or hip fractures. The prevalence of either spine or hip fracture, or both, at varying levels of BMD at L2–L4 or the femoral neck, is shown in Tables 6-1 and 6-2. This type of risk assessment can be useful to a physician who is trying to determine the clinical significance of any given level of BMD in his or her patient, even if the patient has not yet fractured. The data shown in Tables 6-1 and 6-2 were based on measurements made with DPA. The ranges for spine BMD and for femoral neck BMD (depending on the type of DXA device) should be adjusted downward, in order to compare DXA measurements to this data. The equations for converting DPA data to DXA data are given in Chapter 8.

FRACTURE-RISK PREDICTION

Site-Specific and Global Fracture-Risk Prediction

Fracture risk predictions fall into two general categories. The prediction may be a site-specific fracture risk prediction, or it may be a global fracture risk prediction. A site-specific fracture-risk prediction is the prediction of the risk of fracture at a specific site. For example, the prediction of spine fracture risk is a type of site-specific fracture-risk prediction. Similarly, the prediction of hip-fracture risk is a type of site-specific fracture-risk prediction. Site-specific fracture-risk prediction does not by definition mean that the measurement is being performed at a specific site. A global fracture risk prediction is the prediction of the risk of having any and all types of osteoporotic fractures. Again, the terminology does not imply the measurement of bone density at a particular site.

Table 6-2
Prevalence of Spine or Hip Fracture, or Both, at Varying Levels of Femoral Neck BMD, Measured with DPA

Femoral neck BMD (g/cm^2)	*N*	*Spine fracture* %	*Hip fracture* %	*Either/Both* %
>0.80	133	3.8	0.0	3.8
0.70–0.79	178	10.6	3.4	12.9
0.60–0.69	164	21.3	10.4	31.1
0.50–0.59	89	32.6	29.2	51.7
0.40–0.49	26	38.5	46.2	76.9

Adapted with permission from Mazess RB. (1990) Bone densitometry for clinical diagnosis and monitoring, in DeLuca HF, Mazess R (eds.), *Osteoporosis: Physiologic Basis, Assessment and Treatment,* pp. 66, Elsevier Science Inc., 655 Avenue of the Americas, New York, NY 10010-5107.

Relative-Risk Fracture Data

The studies that conclusively established the predictive capabilities of bone-mass measurements for fracture risk generally reported the data as the increase in relative risk per standard deviation (SD) decline in bone density. In Chapter 3, it was noted that relative risk is the best indicator of the strength of the relationship between a risk factor (in this case, low bone mass or density) and an outcome (fracture). It is understandable, therefore, that much of the information in the medical literature about the prediction of fracture risk from bone-mass measurements is presented in the form of relative-risk values. Relative risk is calculated from absolute-risk data that is collected during prospective fracture trials. The ratio of the absolute risk for fracture between two groups constitutes the relative risk for fracture between the two groups. If the relative risk is 1, this implies that there is no difference in risk between the groups. It is possible that both groups have an increased absolute risk, but the risk of one group is no greater than the risk of the other group. Relative-risk data also obscures the actual magnitude of the absolute risk for either group. For example, if the absolute risk for fracture in group A is 50%, compared to the absolute risk for fracture of 25% in group B, the relative risk of group A compared to group B is 2 (50% ÷ 25% = 2). This would be interpreted to mean that the risk in group A is twofold greater than group B's. The relative risk would also be 2, however, if the absolute risk in group A was 2% and the absolute risk in group B was 1% (2% ÷ 1% = 2). The interpretation would still be that group A has a twofold greater risk of fracture than group B.

Relative-risk data can also be used to establish which skeletal sites have the best predictive power for certain types of fracture-risk predictions. The site that has the greatest increase in relative risk for fracture per SD decline in bone mass or density will be the skeletal site that has the best predictive power for that type of fracture-risk prediction.

Global Fracture-Risk Prediction

The sites on the forearm have been used in several classic fracture trials to assess global fracture risk, as well as site-specific assessments of spine, hip, or forearm fracture risk. Hui et al. *(2)* evaluated radial bone mass in 386 community-based women and 135 retirement-home-based women, using SPA (Norland-Cameron). Bone mass was measured at the midradius at baseline, and the women were subsequently followed for the development of nonspine fractures for 1 to 15 years. During that time, 89 women had 138 nonspine fractures of various types. The statistical analysis revealed that for each SD decline in bone mass at the midradius, the relative risk for any type of nonspine fracture was 2.2 in the community-based women and 1.5 in the retirement-home women.

Gardsell et al. *(3)* also used the radius to evaluate global fracture risk in a study of 332 women over an average period of 14.6 years. The distal and midradius were measured using SPA. During the follow-up period, 100 women had one or more fragility fractures. The relative risk for fracture, when measured at the distal radius, was 2.6, and at the midradius, 3.2.

The lumbar spine, femoral neck, and trochanter are also useful for global fracture-risk prediction *(4)*. In a study of 304 women, aged 30 to 94 years, who were followed for a median of 8.3 years, 93 women experienced 163 new fractures. Bone mass was measured at baseline at five sites, which included the AP lumbar spine, femoral neck, and trochanter by DPA, and the distal and midradius by SPA. The relative risk for fracture, as measured at the spine, femoral neck, and trochanter, was 1.5, 1.6, and 1.5, respectively, when only those fractures that resulted from mild-to-moderate trauma were considered. The midradius was also predictive of global fracture risk for fractures resulting from mild-to-moderate trauma, with a relative risk of 1.5.

Other studies have quantified the increase in relative risk per SD decline in bone mass or density measured at different skeletal sites for the prediction of global fracture risk. In the Study of Osteoporotic Fractures, a 1 SD decrease in BMC at the midradius resulted in an age-adjusted increase in relative risk of 1.3, and, at the distal radius, 1.4 *(5)*. Measurements of BMD at the lumbar spine and femoral neck were also predictive of global fracture risk, with comparable relative risk values of 1.35 and 1.41, respectively. The calcaneus was equally predictive of global fracture risk, with a relative risk of 1.51 for each SD decline in bone density. In another study of

Table 6-3
Age-Adjusted Increase in Relative Risk for Fracture for Global Fracture-Risk Prediction per SD Decrease in Bone Mass, Measured at Various Skeletal Sites

Site	*Global fracture risk RR*
AP Lumbar spine	1.5[b], 1.35[b]
Total femur	1.40[b]
Femoral neck	1.6[b], 1.41[b]
Trochanter	1.5[b], 1.38[b]
Midradius	1.5[a], 1.32[b], 3.2[a]
Distal radius	1.42[b], 2.6[a]
Calcaneus	1.51[b]

[a]Per SD decrease in BMC.
[b]Per SD decrease in BMD.
From refs. *2–5*.

1098 women followed for an average of 4.5 years, a decrease of 2 SDs in BMC at the midradius resulted in an increase in relative risk of 2.8 for any type of nonspine fracture *(6)*. The relative risk values for global fracture-risk prediction are summarized in Table 6-3.

Site-Specific Spine Fracture-Risk Prediction

It appears that several sites may also be useful for the site-specific prediction of spine fracture risk. In the study by Melton et al. *(4)*, the increase in relative risk for spine fracture resulting from mild-to-moderate trauma for each SD decline in BMD or BMC was statistically significantly different from 1 at the spine itself, but also at the femoral neck, trochanter, and midradius *(4)*. The relative-risk values were 2.2, 2.0, 1.7, and 2.5, respectively. The greatest increase in relative risk of 2.5 was seen at the midradius, suggesting that this was the preferred site to measure for spine fracture-risk prediction. However, a statistical analysis suggested that each of these four sites actually performed equally well.

Data presented in abstract form at the 19th Annual Meeting of the American Society for Bone and Mineral Research suggests that the phalanges and metacarpals, as measured by radiographic absorptiometry (RA) can be useful predictors of spine fracture risk. In a study of 251 women, whose average age at baseline was 74 years, 18 spine fractures occurred during an average follow-up of 2.7 years *(7)*. Based on RA measurements (Osteogram Analysis Center, Manhatten Beach, CA) of the phalanges, the increase in relative risk per SD decline in BMD was 3.4. In another study of 509 postmenopausal women, with an average age of 74 at baseline, 37 spine fracture cases were observed during an average follow-up of

2.7 years *(8)*. The relative risk for spine fracture from RA (Bonalyzer, Teijin, Tokyo) of the metacarpals in this study was 1.9.

Site-Specific Hip Fracture-Risk Prediction

There are several studies in the medical literature that have evaluated different skeletal sites for site-specific hip fracture-risk prediction. In the study from Melton et al. *(4)* noted above, 10 fractures of the proximal femur from mild-to-moderate trauma occurred during the study. Statistically significant increases in relative risk for hip fracture could be determined for BMD measured at the femoral neck, trochanter, and distal radius. The increases in relative risk for hip fracture from BMD measured at the spine or midradius did not reach statistical significance. In what is considered a sentinel study for determining hip fracture risk, Cummings et al. *(9)* evaluated 8134 women aged 65 and over. During an average follow-up period of 1.8 yr, 65 hip fractures occurred (33 femoral neck, 32 intertrochanteric). BMD was measured at the lumbar spine and proximal femur with DXA (Hologic QDR-1000, Waltham, MA) and at the distal and midradius and os calcis with SPA (OsteoAnalyzer, Norland Medical Systems, Inc., Ft. Atkinson, WI). Within the proximal femur, the total femur, femoral neck, trochanter, intertrochanteric, and Ward's triangle were measured. All of these sites had statistically significant increases in relative risk for hip fracture for each SD decline in BMD. In this study, the sites in the proximal femur were clearly stronger predictors of hip fracture than the AP lumbar spine or radial sites. The os calcis (os calcis and calcaneus are used interchangeably) was also an excellent predictor of hip-fracture risk, being outperformed by the proximal femur regions of interest by the narrowest of margins. The age-adjusted increases in relative risk for hip fracture in the total femur, femoral neck, Ward's, and trochanteric and intertrochanteric regions were all very similar. They were 2.7, 2.6, 2.8, 2.7, and 2.5, respectively. The increase in relative risk at the os calcis was 2.0. The lumbar spine and distal radius both had a relative risk of 1.6 per SD decline in BMD; the midradius had a relative risk of 1.5 per SD decline.

In the previously described study from Hui et al. *(2)*, 30 hip fractures occurred in the retirement-community women. Based on measurements of the midradius with SPA in this group, the relative risk for hip fracture per SD decline in bone mass was 1.9.

Phalangeal bone density also appears to be useful as a predictor of hip fracture risk. During the National Health and Nutrition Examination Survey I, between 1971 and 1975, 3481 subjects underwent radiographic photodensitometry studies of the hand *(10)*. At baseline, the ages of the subjects ranged from 45 to 74. During the follow-up period through 1987, 72 hip fractures occurred. The relative risk for hip fracture, as calculated

Table 6-4
Increase in Age-Adjusted Relative Risk for Spine or Hip Fracture per SD Decrease in Bone Mass, Measured at Various Skeletal Sites

Site	*Spine fracture risk RR*	*Hip fracture risk RR*
AP Lumbar spine	2.2[b]	1.6[b]
Total femur		2.7[b]
Femoral neck	2.0[b]	2.6[b], 2.8[b]
Ward's		2.8[b]
Trochanter	1.7[b]	2.7[b], 2.4[b]
Distal radius		1.6[b], 3.1[b]
Midradius	2.5[a]	1.5[b], 1.9[a]
Calcaneus		2.0[b]
Phalanges	3.4[c]	1.8[c]
Metacarpals	1.9[c]	

[a]Per SD decrease in BMC.
[b]Per SD decrease in BMD.
[c]Per SD decrease in RA units.
From references *2,4,7–10.*

from radiographic photodensitometry measurements of the middle phalanx of the small finger, was 1.57 for all subjects. When the analysis was restricted to Caucasian women only, the relative risk was 1.56. The radiographic photodensitometry films were reanalyzed using the more modern technique of radiographic absorptiometry. When the films were analyzed in this manner, the relative risk for each SD decline in RA bone density was 1.81 for all subjects, and 1.79 for Caucasian women only. Table 6-4 summarizes the increases in relative risk per SD decline in bone mass for site-specific fracture risk prediction, when the bone mass is measured at different skeletal sites.

Applying Relative-Risk Data in Clinical Practice

The values for relative risk discussed above were derived from specific study populations. The characteristics of each study population, such as the mean age and the mean and SD for BMD, make the increase in relative risk per SD decline in BMD unique for that population. Applying such relative risk data to an individual patient, and utilizing the SD for the reference population supplied by the manufacturer to calculate the relative risk for the patient in question, is clearly an extrapolation of the data that may not be appropriate. Nevertheless, with this caution in mind, relative risk fracture data is being applied in this fashion in clinical practice today.

The actual calculation of a patient's relative risk for various types of fracture is not difficult. The relationships between absolute risk, relative risk, and the magnitude of the SD decline in bone density, which were discussed in Chapter 3, are the key to this calculation and its interpretation. For example, Mrs. M. M., whose spine bone-density report is shown in Fig. 3-1, has an L2–L4 average BMD of 0.747 g/cm^2. As noted in Chapter 3, her young-adult *z*-score of –3.78 indicates that this average BMD is 3.78 SDs below the average peak BMD of the young adult. Her age-matched *z*-score of –1.73 indicates that the L2–L4 average BMD is 1.73 SDs below the average BMD predicted for her age. How does the physician calculate her global fracture relative risk or site-specific spine-fracture relative risk? The age-adjusted increases in relative risk for fracture from Melton et al. *(4)* can be used to calculate these values. Melton et al. found that, for each SD decline in bone density when measured at the spine, the increase in relative risk for any type of low-to-moderate trauma fracture was 1.5. Therefore, the relative risk for global fracture in this patient compared to the individual who still has an average peak bone density, based on this measurement of bone density at the lumbar spine, is $1.5^{3.78}$ or 4.6. This is the increase in relative risk per SD decline in bone density, raised to the power of the young-adult *z*-score or *T*-score. Compared to the individual who has a spine bone density that would be predicted for the patient's age, her global-fracture relative risk would be $1.53^{1.73}$, or 2.1. This is the increase in relative risk raised to the power of the age-matched *z*-score.

The relative risks for the site-specific spine-fracture prediction are calculated in a similar fashion. Using an increase in relative risk per SD decline in BMD of 2.2 for spine fracture when measured at the spine, the calculation would be $2.2^{3.78}$ or $2.2^{1.73}$, depending on the comparison the physician wishes to make.

The relative risk for global fracture from BMD measurements at other sites can be calculated using data from Melton, as well as other authors. Similarly, the relative risk for a site-specific spine-fracture risk prediction can be calculated from bone density measured at other sites, using Melton's and other's data. The data from Cummings et al. *(9)* is most commonly used for the calculation of relative risk for a site-specific hip fracture-risk prediction.

LIFETIME RISK OF FRACTURE

In 1992, Black et al. *(11)* proposed a method for calculating a woman's lifetime risk for hip fracture. The prediction was based on the woman's bone mass at menopause, expressed as a percentile for her age, estimations of bone mass at subsequent ages, and then estimating her risk for hip fracture at each age. The risk of hip fracture at each age was based on two factors: the risk of fracture at a particular age derived from population-based data, and the risk of fracture at a particular bone mass from prospective fracture trials. Based on a review of the literature at the time, an

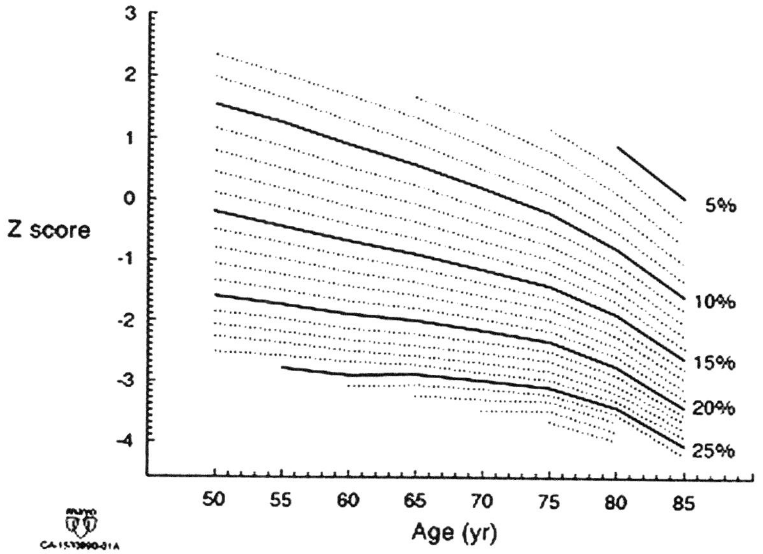

Fig. 6-1. Lifetime hip fracture risk as predicted from age and radial bone density. *z*-scores are based on the average BMD of the 50-year-old woman. Reprinted with permission from Suman VJ, et al. A nonogram for predicting lifetime hip fracture risk from radius bone mineral density and age. *Bone* 16:843–846, Elesevier Science, Inc., 655 Avenue of the Americas, New York, NY 10010-5107.

increase in relative risk for hip fracture of 1.65 for each SD decline in bone mass at the radius was used in the calculation of risk based on the level of bone mass. Using this method, the lifetime risk of hip fracture for a 50-year-old Caucasian woman, whose midradial bone mass was at the tenth percentile, was calculated to be 19%. If her bone mass was at the ninetieth percentile, her lifetime risk of hip fracture was 11%. The gradient of risk, therefore, between the ninetieth and tenth percentile, was 1.7 (19% ÷ 11% = 1.7). This model is obviously dependent on the value chosen for the increase in relative risk per SD decline in bone mass. The authors noted that, if the increase in relative risk was 2.0 instead of 1.65, the lifetime risks for the tenth and ninetieth percentiles would be 21% and 9%, respectively. The gradient of risk would therefore increase to 2.3.

In 1993, Suman et al. *(12)* developed a nomogram for predicting lifetime risk of hip fracture that was derived from the model developed by Black et al. *(11)*. This nomogram is shown in Fig. 6-1. The *z*-scores utilized in the nomogram are based on the mean and SD for bone mass for 50-year-old Caucasian women. Like the concept of remaining lifetime fracture probability, which is discussed next, lifetime fracture risk goes beyond the prediction of current fracture risk. A young individual with a slightly low bone mass and low current fracture risk will be identified as having a higher lifetime-fracture risk. Similarly, an older individual with a low bone mass and high current-fracture risk may have a lower lifetime-fracture risk, because of a shorter life expectancy.

REMAINING-LIFETIME FRACTURE PROBABILITY

Remaining-lifetime fracture probability, or RLFP, is a type of future global fracture risk prediction that was proposed by Ross et al. *(13)*. The concept of RLFP is based on the recognition that the risk of fracture increases in an exponential fashion as BMD falls, and that survival decreases markedly after age 75. Therefore, although a 50-year-old woman and an 80-year-old woman may both have the same low bone density, and therefore the same current fracture risk, their RLFP will be quite different. Because the expected life span of the 80-year-old woman is much shorter than that of the 50-year-old, the RLFP for the 80-year-old will be less. RLFP is calculated based on the individual's current age and bone density, life expectancy, and anticipated rate of bone loss. These values are entered into a statistical model that predicts the number of osteoporotic fractures that the individual is expected to experience in her lifetime. If the RLFP value is 5, for example, this means that the individual is expected to suffer five osteoporotic fractures in her lifetime, if no intervention is undertaken to slow the anticipated rate of bone loss. The site of the fractures cannot be specified. RLFP is thus a global fracture-risk prediction. RLFP is one of the most concrete and easily understood modalities for expressing future fracture risk.

The fracture incidence and bone-loss rate data on which the RLFP model was originally based were derived from the Kuakini Osteoporosis Study. The original implementation of RLFP was based on measurements of bone mass at the calcaneus. Bone-density measurements performed at other sites had to be converted to an equivalent calcaneal measurement. Using nomograms, the physician could find the calcaneal BMC on one scale and the patient's age on a second scale *(14)*. By connecting the two values, the physician could then read the RLFP from a third scale. RLFP predictions have now been recalculated for DXA measurements of the skeleton.*

RLFP is based on a statistical model. When the RLFP model is applied to the United States population, the estimates of vertebral and nonvertebral fracture incidence are comparable to actual observations of fracture inci-

*RLFP calculations are available as a commercial service through the Internet at http:\\www.medsurf.com.

dence *(15)*. This observation provides an external validation of the theory and application of RLFP.

FRACTURE THRESHOLD

Many experts in the field object strenuously to discussions of the concept of a fracture threshold, noting that it is more appropriate to emphasize that there is a gradient of risk for fracture, with risk increasing as the bone density declines. They correctly observe that there is no arbitrary level of bone density above which no one fractures, and below which everyone fractures. Nevertheless, the concept of a fracture threshold exists, and can be useful in the clinical setting. It suggests a cutoff level of bone density above which it is desirable to stay, in order to keep fracture risk at a minimum. It also emphasizes that bone density need not be returned to normal levels to reduce the risk of fracture.

In 1982, Riggs et al. *(16)* proposed a fracture threshold level for BMD in the spine and proximal femur, based on studies of 205 subjects (123 women, 82 men). Of these 205 subjects, 31 subjects (26 women, 5 men) had hip fractures, and 84 women had vertebral fractures. BMD was measured with DPA in the AP spine and proximal femur. The fracture threshold was defined as the ninetieth percentile for BMD in the proximal femur for subjects with hip fracture and in the spine for women with spine fracture. For women, the fracture threshold was 0.95 g/cm^2 in the femoral neck, 0.92 g/cm^2 in the intertrochanteric region, and 0.97 g/cm^2 in the lumbar spine.

Ross et al. *(17)* proposed that the fracture threshold be defined as the BMC or BMD at which the risk of fracture doubles in comparison to premenopausal women. This recommendation was based on a prospective study of 1098 women, who participated in the Kuakini Osteoporosis Study, beginning in 1981. These women underwent BMC and BMD measurements at the proximal and distal radius and os calcis yearly with SPA, and, beginning in 1984, lumbar-spine BMD measurements with DPA. Four hundred eight women had spine films at baseline that were used to calculate spine fracture incidence during 4 years of follow-up. Spine-fracture prevalence was calculated based on data from subjects who had fractures prior to the first bone-density measurements. The authors looked at a variety of different ways of defining the fracture threshold, and the resulting BMC or BMD levels at the various sites that resulted. These findings are shown in Table 6-5. The authors concluded that the most appropriate definition of a fracture threshold would be the level of bone mass or density at which the risk of fracture doubles in comparison to premenopausal women. They observed that these levels of BMC and BMD corresponded to the levels that would also result if different definitions for the fracture threshold were used, such as the tenth percentile of young normals, the

Table 6-5
Comparison of Different Definitions for the Fracture Threshold

Definition	*Proximal radius (g/cm)*	*Distal radius (g/cm)*	*Calcaneus* (g/cm^2)	*Lumbar spine* (g/cm^2)
Based on young normals				
10th percentile	0.78	0.76	0.33	0.97
2 SDs below mean	0.71	0.66	0.28	0.90
Based on postmenopausal women				
10th percentile	0.59	0.52	0.22	0.74
2 SDs below mean	0.49	0.42	0.17	0.60
Based on prevalent fracture cases				
80th percentile	0.78	0.75	0.33	0.94
Based on incident fracture cases				
95th percentile	0.78	0.67	0.31	0.94
Based on increased fracture risk				
Absolute risk of 5%/decade	0.78	0.74	0.32	0.97
Doubling of risk relative to age 45	0.77	0.78	0.32	0.94
Reference values (mean and SD)				
Young normals[a]	0.88 ± 0.08	0.89 ± 0.11	0.41 ± 0.07	1.13 ± 0.12
Postmenopausal women[b]	0.73 ± 0.11	0.70 ± 0.13	0.31 ± 0.08	0.92 ± 0.15

[a]Premenopausal women, ages 30–45. Mean age 38 years, $n = 128$.
[b]Postmenopausal women, mean age 64, $N = 1083$.

Reprinted with permission from Ross PD, et al. (1987) Definition of a spine fracture threshold based upon prospective fracture risk. *Bone* 8:271–278, Elsevier Science Inc., 655 Avenue of the Americas, New York, NY 10010-5107.

eightieth percentile of prevalent spine-fracture cases, or an absolute risk of fracture of 5% per decade.

Vega et al. *(18)* calculated a fracture threshold for femoral neck and trochanteric hip fractures, based on cross-sectional data from 75 women with atraumatic fractures of the proximal femur, and 51 age-matched nonfractured controls. The average age of the women was 70.1 years. In the hip-fracture group, there were 36 femoral neck fractures and 39 trochanteric fractures. BMD was measured at the lumbar spine and proximal femur with DPA (Lunar DP3), and at the midradius with SPA. The average BMD and SD in the femoral neck of the femoral-neck-fracture patients were 0.624 and 0.055 g/cm^2, respectively. For the trochanteric-fracture patients, these values in the femoral neck were 0.548 and 0.066 g/cm^2. The authors defined the fracture threshold as the mean BMD plus 2 SDs at the femoral neck, as calculated from the BMD measurements in the fracture group. For fractures of the femoral neck, this value was 0.73 g/cm^2. For trochanteric fractures, this value was 0.68 g/cm^2. Using a spine-fracture threshold of 0.98 g/cm^2 from Riggs et al. *(16)*, these authors observed that 94% of the patients with trochanteric fracture, and 74% of the patients with femoral neck fracture, had spine BMD values that were also below the spine-fracture threshold.

The fracture threshold concept can also be utilized to assess the benefit of any particular therapy. For example, a 57-year-old woman may have a bone density that is currently above the fracture threshold at a particular site. It is anticipated, however, that her bone density will fall below the fracture threshold in the future at a point in time that will be determined by the rate of bone loss. Using statistical models, it can be anticipated that if the patient loses bone mineral density at a rate of 1%/yr, she will fall below the threshold by age 64. If the rate of bone loss is reduced to 0.5%, she will not reach the fracture threshold until age 72, gaining 8 years of relative protection from fracture.

OTHER RISK ASSESSMENTS DERIVED FROM, OR COMBINED WITH, DENSITOMETRY

Pre-Existing Fractures

The presence of a vertebral fracture, or what is called a prevalent vertebral fracture, was demonstrated to increase the risk of future or incident vertebral fractures by Ross et al. *(19)*. This study was performed in the same group of women from the Kuakini Osteoporosis Study who were described earlier in the discussion of the definition of a spine-fracture threshold. In this study, the presence of one vertebral fracture at baseline resulted in a fivefold increase in the risk for new vertebral fractures. If two vertebral fractures were present at baseline, the risk for new vertebral fractures was increased 12-fold.

Pre-existing vertebral fractures have also been shown to be predictive of nonvertebral fractures *(20)*. Two hundred fifty subjects (225 women, 25 men), with an average age of 74 years, were evaluated for the presence of vertebral deformity at baseline, and the subsequent development of nonvertebral fracture during a follow-up period of 3 years. During this period, 39 subjects suffered nonvertebral fractures, of which 10 were hip fractures, 17 were forearm fractures, and 13 were at a variety of other skeletal sites. Twenty-seven of the 39 subjects who developed nonvertebral fractures had spine deformities at baseline. Spinal deformities were graded as mild or severe, based on the number of vertebrae affected and/or the degree of deformity. After adjusting for age, sex, and BMD in the femoral neck (DXA), subjects with severe spinal deformities at baseline had a fourfold increase in the risk of nonvertebral fracture (relative risk 4.1; 95% confidence interval 1.3–12.4). Subjects with mild spinal deformities had a relative risk of 1.5 for the development of nonvertebral fractures, but this increase in relative risk was not significant at the 95% confidence level.

Increasing Number of Low Bone-Mass Sites

Davis et al. *(21)* observed that the risk of new spine fractures increased 1.3-fold for each additional low bone-mass site, after the observation of low bone mass at an initial site. This data was derived from a study of 744 postmenopausal women from the Kuakini Osteoporosis Study who underwent bone mass measurements at the os calcis, proximal, and distal radius (SPA), and at the AP lumbar spine (DPA) at the same examination, and who had at least two follow-up spine radiographs. The average age of these women was 66.6 years. The women were classified into the lower, middle, or upper tertiles of bone mass or density at each of the four skeletal sites. In the women who had at least one skeletal site in the lower tertile of bone mass or density, the odds ratio for new spine fractures was 1.3 for each additional site in the lower tertile.

Hip-Axis Length

Hip-axis length has been demonstrated to be a predictor of hip-fracture risk that is independent of BMD *(22)*. As part of the Study of Osteoporotic Fractures, 8074 women aged 65 and older were evaluated with DXA (Hologic QDR-1000) measurements of the proximal femur. Hip-axis length was measured in 134 women without fractures, and in 64 women who experienced hip fractures during 1.6 years of follow-up. This dimension was measured from the printout of the DXA study, using a goniiometer. The hip-axis length was defined as the distance from the inner pelvic brim to the outer edge of the greater trochanter along the femoral neck axis. Odds ratios for BMD and the risk of hip fracture, and for hip-axis length and the risk of hip fracture, were calculated. Using femoral neck BMD, each SD decline in BMD resulted in a 2.7-fold increase in the risk of hip fracture. For hip-axis length, each SD increase in length resulted in a 1.8-fold increase in the risk of fracture.

REFERENCES

1. Mazess RB (1990) Bone densitometry for clinical diagnosis and monitoring. In: DeLuca HF, Mazess R, eds. *Osteoporosis: Physiologic Basis, Assessment and Treatment*, New York: Elsevier, pp. 63–85.
2. Hui SL, Slemenda CW, Johnston CC (1989) Baseline measurement of bone mass predicts fracture in white women. *Ann Intern Med* 111:355–361.
3. Gardsell P, Johnell O, Nilsson BE (1991) The predictive value of bone loss for fragility fractures in women: a longitudinal study over 15 years. *Calcif Tissue Int* 49:90–94.
4. Melton LJ, Atkinson EJ, O'Fallon WM, Wahner HW, Riggs BL (1993) Long-term fracture prediction by bone mineral assessed at different skeletal sites. *J Bone Miner Res* 8:1227–1233.
5. Black DM, Cummings SR, Genant HK, Nevitt MC, Palermo L, Browner W (1992) Axial and appendicular bone density predict fractures in older women. *J Bone Miner Res* 7:633–638.
6. Wasnich RD, Ross PD, Heilbrun LK, Vogel JM (1985) Prediction of postmenopausal fracture risk with use of bone mineral measurements. *Am J Obstet Gynecol* 153: 745–751.
7. Huang C, Ross PD, Yates AJ, Wasnich RD (1997) Prediction of vertebral fractures by radiographic absorptiometry. Abstract. *J Bone Miner Res* 12:S496.
8. Huang C, Ross PD, Davis JW, Imose K, Emi K, Wasnich RD (1997) Prediction of single and multiple vertebral fractures by metacarpal BMD using poisson regression. Abstract. *J Bone Miner Res* 12:S496.
9. Cummings SR, Black DM, Nevitt MC, Browner W, Cauley J, Ensrud K, et al. (1993) Bone density at various sites for prediction of hip fracture. *Lancet* 341:72–75.
10. Mussolino ME, Looker AC, Madans JH, Edelstein D, Walker RE, Lydick E, Epstein RS, Yates AJ (1997) Phalangeal bone density and hip fracture risk. *Arch Intern Med* 157:433–438.
11. Black DM, Cummings SR, Melton JL (1992) Appendicular bone mineral and a woman's lifetime risk of hip fracture. *J Bone Miner Res* 7:639–645.
12. Suman VJ, Atkinson EJ, O'Fallon WM, Black DM, Melton LJ (1993) A nomogram for predicting lifetime hip fracture risk from radius bone mineral density and age. *Bone* 14:843–846.
13. Ross PD, Wasnich RD, MacLean CJ, Vogel JM (1987) Prediction of individual lifetime fracture expectancy using bone mineral measurements. In: Christiansen C, Johansen JS, Riss BJ, eds. *Osteoporosis 1987*, Copenhagen, Denmark: Osteopress ApS, pp. 288–293.
14. Wasnich RD, Ross PD, Vogel JM, Davis JW (1989) *Osteoporosis: Critique and Practicum*. Honolulu: Banyan.
15. Wasnich RD (1996) Vertebral fracture epidemiology. *Bone* 18:179S–183S.
16. Riggs BL, Wahner HW, Seeman E, Offord KP, Dunn WL, Mazess RB, Johnson KA, Melton LJ (1982) Changes in bone mineral density of the proximal femur and spine with aging. *J Clin Invest* 70:716–723.

17. Ross PD, Wasnich RD, Heilbrun LK, Vogel JM (1987) Definition of a spine fracture threshold based upon prospective fracture risk. *Bone* 8:271–278.
18. Vega E, Mautalen C, Gomez H, Garrido A, Melo L, Sahores AO (1991) Bone mineral density in patients with cervical and trochanteric fractures of the proximal femur. *Osteoporosis Int* 1:81–86.
19. Ross PD, Davis JW, Epstein RS, Wasnich RD (1991) Pre-existing fractures and bone mass predict vertebral fracture incidence in women. *Ann Intern Med* 114:919–923.
20. Burger H, van Daele PLA, Algra D, Hofman A, Groobbee DE, Schutte HE, Birkenhager JC, Pols HAP (1994) Vertebral deformities as predictors of non-vertebral fractures. *Br Med J* 309:991,992.
21. Davis JW, Ross PD, Wasnich RD (1994) Evidence for both generalized and regional low bone mass among elderly women. *J Bone Miner Res* 9:305–309.
22. Faulkner KG, Cummings SR, Black D, Palermo L, Gluer CC, Genant HK (1993) Simple measurement of femoral geometry predicts hip fracture: the study of osteoporotic fractures. *J Bone Miner Res* 8:1211–1217.

7 Effects of Age, Disease, and Drugs on Bone Density

CONTENTS

When the clinician must quantify the effects of a disease process on the skeleton, the sites affected by that disease process must be known in order to choose the appropriate skeletal region to measure. Similarly, if the effect of a disease process on the skeleton is to be followed over time with densitometry, the expected magnitude of the change must be known in order to choose the appropriate interval between measurements.* The sites expected to be affected by certain drugs and the magnitude of changes with time must also be appreciated for similar reasons. All of this must be appreciated against the background of the expected age-related changes in bone density. Brief summaries of the effects of age, disease, and drugs on the skeleton follow. The reader is referred to the cited references for more detailed descriptions of the actual studies.

AGE-RELATED CHANGES IN BONE DENSITY

There is general agreement that bone density peaks relatively early in life, and then tends to decline from a process that is called age-related bone loss. The exact age of attainment of peak bone density at the various skeletal sites remains controversial, as does the age at which age-related bone loss begins at each site. Most studies that have evaluated these issues have been, of necessity, cross-sectional rather than prospective in design. In addition, there is no single study that has attempted to span childhood to

**See* Chapter 4 for a discussion of the interval between measurements as determined by the precision of testing and the expected magnitude of change.

old age, or to evaluate every skeletal site within a defined age range. As a consequence, many studies must be reviewed to obtain an overview of changes in bone density with age at the various skeletal sites being measured today.

Bone Density in Children

In a cross-sectional study of 110 boys and 124 girls ranging in age from 8 to 17 years, bone mineral density (BMD) in the proximal femur, AP lumbar spine, and total body was measured using DXA (Hologic QDR-2000, Waltham, MA) *(1)*. For both the boys and girls, BMC and BMD increased at the spine, proximal femur, and total body, between the ages of 8 and 17. The BMD values of the 17-year-old girls were also compared to BMD values from a separate group of healthy 21-year-old women. No significant difference was seen in BMD at any site between the 17-year-old girls and the 21-year-old women, suggesting that peak bone density had been reached by the age of 17 in the girls.

In a cross-sectional study of 266 subjects (136 boys, 130 girls) ages 4 to 27 years, BMD was measured in the total body, AP spine, and femoral neck, using DXA (Lunar DPX, Madison, WI) *(2)*. The average age of the subjects was 13 years. BMD increased at all sites in boys until the age of 17.5 years. In girls, BMD increased at the total body and spine until the age of 15.8 years, and in the proximal femur, until the age of 14.1 years.

In a very large, cross-sectional study of 778 Caucasian children (433 girls and 345 boys), ages 2 to 20, BMD was measured in the total body, AP and lateral spine, radius, and proximal femur with DXA (Norland XR-26, Fort Atkinson, WI) *(3)*. BMD increased significantly at the AP lumbar spine and proximal femur until age 14 in girls. In boys, BMD in the proximal femur increased until age 16. BMD in the AP lumbar spine increased throughout the age range in boys. Total body BMC and BMD increased until age 16 in girls, and continued to increase in boys throughout the age range in this study. Radial bone density increased until age 16 in girls, and throughout the age range in boys.

BMD was measured in the AP and lateral spine using DXA (ODX-240, Oris, Gif-sur Yvette, France) in 574 girls and young women, ages 10 to 24 years, and in the AP spine only in 333 women aged 27 to 47 years *(4)*. AP spine and lateral spine BMD increased markedly between ages 10 and 14, or until 1 year after menarche. There were additional increases in BMD and BMC at the AP spine between the ages of 14 and 17, but not in the lateral spine. After age 17, or 4 years after menarche, BMD did not increase significantly, and did not differ from the BMD seen in the older group of women. The authors estimated that 86% of peak adult bone density in the spine is achieved by age 14, or the second year after menarche.

The BMD in the spine and distal radius was measured with DXA in 121 normal children (69 boys, 52 girls), ages 3 to 18 years *(5)*. BMD increased at both sites throughout this age range. The correlation between the BMD at the spine and distal radius was significant at $r = 0.83$.

A study of 247 girls and young women, ages 11 to 32, was performed using DXA (Lunar DPX-L) to measure BMD in the total body *(6)*. The investigators found that 99% of total body BMD was achieved by age 22.1 ± 2.5 years, and that 99% of peak BMC is attained by age 26.2 ± 3.7 years.

Bone Density in Premenopausal Women

Mazess and Barden studied 300 young women between the ages of 20 and 40 *(7)*. BMD was measured in the AP spine and proximal femur, using dual-photon absorptiometry (DPA), and at the ultradistal and 33% radial sites, using single-photon absorptiometry (SPA). BMD did not change significantly with age at any site. BMD tended to decrease with age at the femoral neck and Ward's area, but the change was not statistically significant. Additional BMD measurements were obtained at the spine and midradius after 2 years *(8)*. In this longitudinal extension of the original study, there was no evidence of age-related bone loss at either the spine or 33% radial site.

Hansen evaluated 249 healthy premenopausal women whose average age was 39 years, measuring BMD at the distal forearm, using SPA, and at the AP spine and proximal femur, using DXA (Hologic QDR-1000) *(9)*. In this study, no decline in BMD was seen at any site after age 30, and peak BMD appeared to be reached prior to age 30.

Two other large cross-sectional studies have suggested that BMD in the proximal femur does decline in women prior to menopause. Rodin et al. *(10)*, found a significant premenopausal decline in femoral neck BMD in a study of 225 women who ranged in age from 18 to 52. Similarly, Bonnick et al. *(11)* found a decline in proximal femoral BMD after the age of 30 in a study of 237 premenopausal women, ages 20 to 45. In this latter study, no increase in BMD in the spine or proximal femur was seen in any age group, suggesting that peak BMD in both regions was achieved prior to the age of 20. There was no significant change in spine BMD, again suggesting that spine BMD does not change appreciably prior to age 45 in premenopausal women after the achievement of peak BMD.

Dissimilar BMDs Between Skeletal Sites at Peak and Prior to Menopause

Two hundred thirty-seven premenopausal women between the ages of 20 and 45 were evaluated with DXA (Lunar DPX) measurements of the AP spine and proximal femur, to determine if differences exist in *z*-scores for

Table 7-1
Dissimilar Spine and Femoral *z*-Scores in Premenopausal Women

Site comparison	*20–29 yr (n = 122)*	*30–45 yr (n = 115)*
Lumbar vs femoral neck		
FN > L (1+)	11.5%	6.9%
FN > L (0–1)	39.3%	15.7%
L > FN (0–1)	36.9%	38.3%
L > FN (1+)	12.3%	39.1%
Lumbar vs Ward's		
W > L (1+)	11.4%	5.2%
W > L (0–1)	39.3%	20.9%
L > W (0–1)	39.3%	35.8%
L > W (1+)	9.8%	39.1%
Lumbar vs troch		
T > L (1+)	9.8%	6.1%
T > L (0–1)	37.7%	24.3%
L > T (0–1)	42.6%	43.4%
L > T (1+)	9.8%	26.1%

Note: FN > L (+1) indicates that the femoral neck *z*-score is greater than the lumbar spine *z*-score by more than 1; (0–1) indicates the *z*-scores differ by 1 or less.

Reproduced with permission of the publisher from Bonnick SL, et al. (1997) Dissimilar spine and femoral *z*-scores in premenopausal women. *Calcified Tissue International* 61:263–265.

the spine and proximal femur *(11)*. The reference population for the calculation of the mean BMD and the SD were the 20- to 29-year-old women of the study population. Twenty to 24% of the 20- to 29-year-old women had differences in *z*-scores of >1 between the lumbar spine and any of the three sites in the proximal femur (neck, Ward's, trochanter). In the 30- to 45-year-old women, however, this percentage increased to 32 to 46%. In the younger age group, the percentage of women having higher *z*-scores in the spine, or higher *z*-scores in the proximal femur, was roughly equally split. In the older age group, however, there was clearly a shift in percentages favoring a higher *z*-score in the spine. This appeared to be the result of the earlier onset of bone loss from the proximal femur in this age group. Table 7-1 gives these findings in greater detail.

Bone Density in Perimenopausal Women

Changes in spine BMD in pre-, peri-, and postmenopausal women were evaluated in a longitudinal study by Pouilles et al. *(12)*. The subjects were 230 Caucasian women ranging in age from 45 to 66 years. Menopausal status was determined by menstrual history, and estradiol and LH levels. Based on these determinants, 71 women, ages 45 to 51, were premenopausal throughout the study, 42 women, ages 47 to 57, experienced menopause during the study and were considered perimenopausal, and 117 women were postmenopausal throughout the study. BMD in the AP spine was assessed using DPA. The women were followed for an average of 27 months. Bone loss in the premenopausal women averaged 0.8% per year. In the perimenopausal women, bone loss was 2.3% per year. In the postmenopausal women, bone loss was again 0.5% per year. The authors noted that approximately half the bone loss observed in the first 10 years after menopause was seen in the first 3 years after menopause. There was no difference in the rates of bone loss between the perimenopausal women and the postmenopausal women 3 years past menopause.

Changes in radial BMD in perimenopausal women, compared to premenopausal women, were studied by Gambacciani et al. *(13)*. BMD was measured in the distal radius, using DPA. The measurements were repeated every 6 months for 2 years. At the onset of the study, there was no significant difference in distal radial BMD between the two groups. In the premenopausal women, radial BMD did not change significantly during the 2 years of the study. BMD was 436.5 ± 19.8 mg/cm^2 at baseline, and 434.6 ± 15.8 mg/cm^2 at 24 months. In the perimenopausal group, however, there was a significant decline in distal radial BMD. At baseline, the BMD was 428.5 ± 10.5, compared to the 24-month value of 410.1 ± 8.2 mg/cm^2. This represented an overall decline from baseline of 4.3% in 2 years in the perimenopausal group.

Dissimilar Spine and Femoral BMD in Perimenopausal Women

Eighty-five Caucasian women between the ages of 45 and 60, who were within 6 months to 3 years past menopause, underwent spine and proximal femur bone density testing using DXA (Lunar DPX) *(14)*. These values were compared with reference values (mean and SD) from a group of 30 healthy women between the ages of 40 and 45. Thirty-nine women had both spine and femoral neck *z*-scores that were better than –1. Seventeen women had both spine and femoral neck *z*-scores that were both poorer than –1. Twenty-two women out of the 85, or 26%, had dissimilar spine and femoral neck *z*-scores. Eight had spine *z*-scores that were better than –1, but femoral neck *z*-scores that were poorer than –1. Fourteen had femoral neck *z*-scores that were better than –1, but spine *z*-scores that were poorer than –1.

In a similar study, Lai et al. evaluated 88 Caucasian women, ages 44 to 59, who were within 5 years past menopause *(15)*. BMD measurements of the lumbar spine and proximal femur were made using DXA (Hologic QDR-1000). The subjects' BMDs were compared to the manufacturer's young-adult reference data, in order to calculate the *T*-scores for the subjects. In this study, 18 women had both spine and femoral neck *T*-scores that were better than –1. Thirty-nine had spine and femoral neck *T*-scores that were both poorer than –1. Thirty-one of the 88 women, or 35%, had dissimilar spine and femoral neck *T*-scores. Twenty-eight had spine *T*-scores better than 1, but femoral neck *T*-scores poorer than –1. Three women had femoral neck *T*-scores that were better than –1, and spine *T*-scores that were poorer than –1.

Because the dissimilarity in either the *T*-scores or *z*-scores seen in these two studies could lead to an incorrect diagnosis, the authors of both these studies concluded that the choice of the measurement site could clearly affect patient management decisions. Both groups suggested that measurement of either the spine or proximal femur alone in the perimenopausal woman might not be appropriate.

Changes in Bone Density in Postmenopausal Women

BMD of the AP and lateral spine and proximal femur was measured in 353 Caucasian women ranging in age from 20 to 84, using DXA (Lunar DPX-L) *(16)*. One hundred fifty-four of these women were age 50 or older. Between 50 and 80 years of age, BMD in the AP spine and femoral neck decreased 18%, or 0.6% per year. BMD in the lateral spine decreased 35 to 40%, or 1.4% per year; BMD in Ward's area decreased 30%, or 1.1% per year.

Changes in BMC at the distal radius were followed in 307 women who were an average of 10 years postmenopausal. The average age of these women was 59 years, with a range of 39 to 72 years. BMC was measured with SPA at the beginning and end of the 5-year period. BMC declined in these postmenopausal women at the distal radius, at a rate of approximately 1.0% per year.

As in young adults and perimenopausal women, dissimilarities in BMD among skeletal sites has also been reported in elderly women. Davis et al. studied 744 women with a mean age of 66.6 years *(17)*. BMD was measured in the AP spine, calcaneus, and distal and proximal radius. A combination of SPA and DPA was used to obtain these measurements. The women were classified by tertiles of BMD at each of the four skeletal sites. Fifteen percent of these women demonstrated marked heterogeneity in BMD among the four sites, having one or more sites in both the lowest and highest tertiles. Fourteen percent were in the lowest tertile at all four sites, and 14% were in the highest tertile at all four sites. Of all of the women who had one site in the lowest tertile, 85% had at least one other site in the lowest tertile, but only 24% were low at all four sites. In women who were classified as being in a middle tertile at any one site, there was marked heterogeneity in classification of the other sites. Slightly more than one-half had other sites that would be classified in the lowest tertile, but more than one-half of these women were in the lowest tertile at only one site. Women

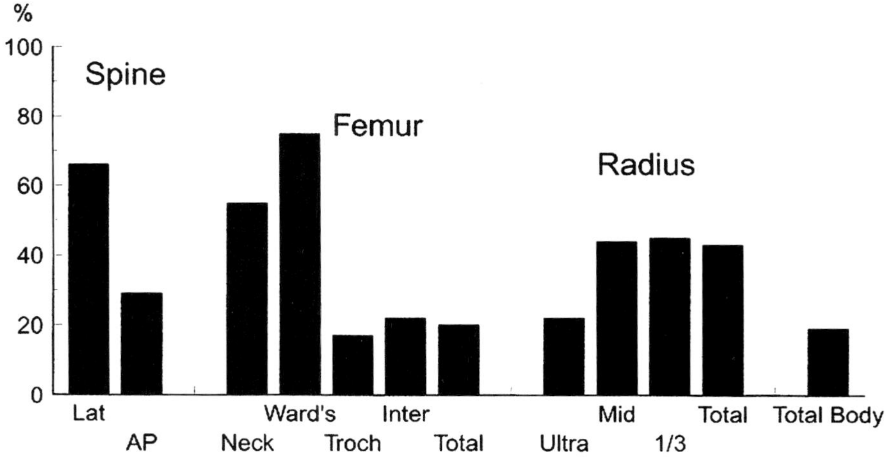

Fig. 7-1. The percentage of women diagnosed with osteoporosis, depending on which skeletal site is measured. Reproduced with permission of the publisher from Greenspan SL, et al. (1996) Classification of osteoporosis in the elderly is dependent on site-specific analysis. *Calcified Tissue International* 58:409–414.

classified in the upper tertile at any one site were infrequently found to have another site that would be classified in the lowest tertile.

Not surprisingly, then, the diagnosis of osteoporosis may depend on which skeletal site is measured. Greenspan et al. *(18)* studied 120 women 65 years of age and older. BMD was measured in the AP and lateral spine, total body, forearm, and proximal femur, using DXA (Hologic QDR-2000). Using the WHO criteria for the diagnosis of osteoporosis, the percentage of individuals who would be classified as osteoporotic at the various skeletal sites was noted. The largest percentage of individuals (66%) was identified as being osteoporotic when the lateral spine BMD was used. The AP spine identified only 29% as osteoporotic. The femoral neck identified 55% as osteoporotic, and the one-third radial site identified 45.4% as osteoporotic. This is graphically represented in Fig. 7-1.

Rates of bone loss in this elderly population were also determined by Greenspan et al. *(18)*. A loss of 1% per year was seen at the lateral spine, but the AP spine demonstrated no significant change. Femoral bone loss occurred at a rate of 0.7 to 1% per year; bone loss at the radial sites occurred at a rate of 0.7 to 0.8% per year.

Changes in Bone Density in Men

BMD measurements of the AP spine (n = 315) and proximal femur (n = 282) were made in men ranging in age from 20 to 89, using DPA *(19)*. The rate of loss from the AP spine was extremely small, at 0.001 g/cm^2 per year, or approximately 1% per decade. Losses from the trochanteric region were also very small, at 0.002 g/cm^2 per year, or approximately 2% per decade. In the femoral neck and Ward's area, the rate of loss was greater, at 0.005 and 0.007 g/cm^2 per year, respectively. This would result in a decrease of 21% from the femoral neck and 34% from Ward's area between the ages of 20 and 70 in men.

DISEASES KNOWN TO AFFECT BONE DENSITY

Acromegaly

Forty-five subjects (24 women and 21 men) with acromegaly for an average of 11.4 years underwent AP spine, proximal femur, and total body bone density studies with DXA (Lunar DPX) *(20)*. The subjects ranged in age from 21 to 77 years, with a median age of 43 years. Twenty-five individuals were Caucasian, and 20 were Black. Twenty percent of the individuals had age-matched *z*-scores in the spine of −1 or poorer, but only 8.8% had similar age-matched *z*-scores in the proximal femur. Osteopenia in the spine was correlated with duration of disease and hypogonadism. Total body calcium was increased, even in osteopenic patients, suggesting that excess GH/IGF-1 caused a positive bone balance except in the spine. Thirteen percent of subjects in this study had BMD values in the spine that were 2 or more SDs above the age-matched mean BMD value.

Sixteen patients (10 women, 6 men) with acromegaly were studied by Kotzmann et al. *(21)*. BMD measurements of the AP lumbar spine, femoral neck, and Ward's area were obtained with DXA (Norland XR-26), and compared to BMD measurements in 16 sex- and age-matched controls. The average age of the subjects with acromegaly was 49.1 years. BMD in the lumbar spine was not significantly different between the subjects with acromegaly and the controls. BMD in the femoral neck and Ward's area, however, was statistically significantly higher in the subjects with acromegaly.

Alcoholism

The effect of chronic alcoholism on lumbar spine BMD was evaluated in 76 Caucasian men, using DPA (Lunar DP3) *(22)*. The average age of the subjects was 47 years. Twenty-two of the 76 men had spine BMD measurements more than 2 SDs below the young adult mean BMD for healthy men. As a group, the alcoholic subjects had significantly lower spine BMDs than a group of 62 healthy men who served as controls. Thirty-six percent of the alcoholic subjects were found to have vertebral fractures. Sixty-one percent had a history of nonvertebral fracture, with rib fractures occurring in 26%.

Amenorrhea

Hyperandrogenic Amenorrhea

Nine women with androgenic amenorrhea and 30 women with androgenization, and either eumenorrhea or oligomenorrhea, underwent BMD measurements of the AP lumbar spine with DPA (Scan Detectronic Diagnostic A/S Lab 23) *(23)*. Results were compared to 22 healthy women who served as controls. BMD in the lumbar spine in the nonamenorrheic androngenized women was significantly higher than controls and the amenorrheic androgenized women. BMD was not different between controls and the amenorrheic androgenized women. Serum levels of DHEAS were negatively correlated with BMD in the androgenized women. The authors postulated that the high levels of androgens had a positive effect on bone that was negated in the women with amenorrhea.

Exercise-Induced Amenorrhea

Fourteen amenorrheic athletes whose average age was 24.9 years underwent BMD measurements at the AP lumbar spine with DPA, and at the distal radius with SPA (Norland-Cameron Model 178) *(24)*. The results were compared to those obtained in 14 eumenorrheic athletes with an average age of 15.5 years. The average duration of amenorrhea was 41.7 months. Bone mineral density was significantly lower in the amenorrheic athletes, compared to the eumenorrheic athletes, at the lumbar spine. The mean difference was 13.9%. There was no significant difference in BMD at the distal radius between the two groups.

Anorexia Nervosa

Eighteen women with anorexia nervosa underwent radial bone-mass measurements at the 33% site, with SPA *(25)*. The results were compared to those from 28 healthy women. All of the women with anorexia had been amenorrheic for at least 1 year, and had not been taking estrogens, progestins, or corticosteroids. The age of the women with anorexia ranged from 19 to 36 years, with an average age of 25 years. The women with anorexia had significantly lower radial bone density than the controls (0.64 ± 0.06 vs 0.72 ± 0.04 g/cm^2, respectively). When the subjects were divided on the basis of the level of physical activity, only the inactive anorectic women continued to have a significantly lower radial bone density than the controls, suggesting that exercise might be protective. Two of the women with anorexia had multiple vertebral compression fractures.

Hay et al. evaluated 69 women with anorexia in varying stages of recovery *(26)*. BMD was measured at the spine by QCT. Results were compared to 31 controls. Bone density was significantly lower in the anorectic subjects, compared to the controls (120 vs 148 mg/cm^3). These authors did not find any protective effect of exercise on the skeletons of the anorectic women. Bone density in these subjects was significantly associated with the duration of illness and amenorrhea, and with weight.

Fifty-one women with anorexia, who had been followed for an average of 11.7 years, were evaluated with BMD measurements in the lumbar spine with DPA (NOVO Lab 22a, Novo Diagnostic, Bagsvaerd, Denmark), and at the midradius with SPA (Nuclear Data ND 1100A, Nuclear Data Co., Frankfurt, Germany) *(27)*. The subjects were classified into three groups, based on their disease outcome. A good outcome meant that the subjects had regular menses, and did not weigh less than 85% of their predicted weight. A poor outcome meant that the subject had not resumed normal menses, and weighed less than 85% of predicted. An intermediate outcome indicated that the subject had either not resumed normal menses, or weighed less than 85% of predicted. Subjects with a good outcome had significantly higher lumbar and radial bone densities than either of the other two groups. Subjects with an intermediate outcome had higher lumbar bone densities than the subjects with a poor outcome. Subjects with a poor outcome had a lumbar spine *z*-score of –2.18 and a midradial *z*-score of –1.73, compared to a control group of healthy women. Subjects with a good outcome also had negative *z*-scores, compared to the control group, of –0.26 in the spine and –0.68 at the radius. The authors suggested that recovery of trabecular bone density might be possible with successful treatment of anorexia, but that cortical bone recovered more slowly, if at all.

Cirrhosis

Fifty-five cirrhotic patients (6 with primary biliary cirrhosis, 14 with alcoholic cirrhosis, and 38 with posthepatic cirrhosis), who were referred for liver transplantation, underwent bone-density testing of the AP spine and proximal femur with DXA (Lunar DPX-L) *(28)*. The subjects were 39 men and 19 women, with an average age of 50 ± 7.6 years. Compared to age- and sex-matched controls, 15 patients had spine *z*-scores of –2 or poorer; only 5 had *z*-scores in the femoral neck that were –2 or poorer. An additional 13 patients were found to have fractures in the spine that were judged to be atraumatic. The authors observed that the more severe the liver dysfunction, the greater the reduction in femoral bone mass. A significant number of patients were found to have vitamin D deficiency, reduced serum PTH levels, and hypogonadism.

Diabetes

Insulin-Dependent Diabetes Mellitus

Ninety-four subjects (45 men, 49 women) with insulin-dependent diabetes mellitus underwent bone-density measurements of the AP spine and proximal femur with DXA (Hologic QDR-1000) *(27)*. The subjects ranged in age from 20 to 56 years, with a mean age of 30 years. Disease duration ranged from 1 to 35 years. Diabetic patients had reduced BMD at all sites in comparison to age- and sex-matched controls. *Z*-scores were –0.89 for the spine, –0.99 for the femoral neck, and –1.05 for Ward's; 19.1% met WHO diagnostic criteria for osteoporosis. The presence and severity of diabetic complications was associated with lower BMD.

NONINSULIN-DEPENDENT DIABETES MELLITUS (NIDDM)

Forty-seven women with NIDDM underwent BMD measurements of the spine and proximal femur with DXA (Hologic QDR-1000), and of the spine with QCT (Toshiba 600 HQ, Toshiba Medical Systems) and were compared to 252 healthy nondiabetic women *(30)*. The average age of the NIDDM patients was 61.3 years. There was no significant difference in BMD at either site, by either technique, between the women with NIDDM and the controls.

Hyperinsulinemia has been postulated to be an osteogenic factor. In a study of 411 men and 559 women aged 50 to 89, who were not diabetic by history or oral glucose tolerance test, BMD was measured in the lumbar spine and proximal femur, using DXA (Hologic QDR-1000), and in the midradius by SPA (Lunar SP2) *(31)*. Fasting insulin levels were positively associated in women only with BMD in the spine and radius. For each 10 μU/mL increase in fasting insulin levels in women, BMD in the spine and radius increased by 0.57 and 0.33 g/cm^2, respectively.

Estrogen Deficiency (Postmenopausal)

Ninety-three healthy women, who had experienced a natural menopause 6 to 60 months earlier, were followed prospectively for two consecutive 22-month periods *(32)*. BMD was measured in the spine and proximal femur, using DXA (Lunar DPX). The average decline in BMD in the spine was 1.46% per year (+2.6% to –6.9%) in the first period, and 1.28% per year (+2.8% to –5.3%) in the second period. In the proximal femur, the average decline in the first period was 1.41% per year (+4.8 to –6.8%), and 1.35% per year (+1.8 to –7.0%) in the second. Individual rates of bone loss were not stable over time. Only 20 to 30% of women retained their initial classification as fast, intermediate, or slow losers during both observation periods. Of 24 women classified as fast losers during the first observation period, 5 remained fast, 12 became intermediate, and 5 became slow losers during the second period. The mean rate of loss in the fast-loser group initially was –3.9%. Women who were originally classified as slow losers at the spine, during the initial observation period, were reclassified as intermediate or fast losers during the second observation period. Similar patterns were seen at the femoral neck.

BMD measurements were made at the AP spine, lateral spine, and distal forearm, using DXA (Hologic QDR-2000), in a cross-sectional study of 363 women who were 6 months to 10 years postmenopausal *(33)*. The most rapid decline in bone density was initially seen in the lateral spine, followed by the AP spine, and then the forearm. Ten years after menopause, however, the overall percent decrease at all three sites was approximately the same, at 12% at the AP spine and 13% at the lateral spine and forearm.

Gastrectomy

BMD, as measured in the os calcis by DPA, was found to be significantly lower in men who had previously undergone partial gastrectomy, compared to controls *(34)*. The average of the subjects was 72.1 years, and the average time since surgery was 28.5 years. Men who underwent Billroth-II procedures had significantly lower BMDs than men who underwent Billroth-I procedures. Billroth-II-operated subjects had BMDs that were 20% lower than controls. Billroth-I-operated subjects had BMDs that were 8% lower than controls; this difference was not statistically significant. Nineteen percent of the men who had undergone partial gastrectomy were found to have vertebral fractures, compared to only 4.4% of the control group. The relative risk for vertebral fracture in the partial gastrectomy group was calculated to be 4.3.

Gaucher Disease, Type 1

Sixty-one adults (32 men, 29 women) with type 1 Gaucher disease were evaluated with DXA (Hologic QDR-1000W) of the lumbar spine, femoral neck, trochanter, and distal radius *(35)*. They ranged in age from 22 to 77, with a mean age of 45.5 years. Mean bone density at each site was significantly below that predicted for age and sex, when compared to the manufacturer's reference data. The greatest decrease in BMD was seen in the patients with splenectomy or severe hepatomegaly.

Gluten-Sensitive Enteropathy

Eight subjects with biopsy-proven gluten-sensitive enteropathy and magnesium depletion underwent bone-density testing of the lumbar spine and proximal femur with DXA (Hologic QDR-1000) *(36)*. Four of 8 had lumbar spine *T*-scores ≤ -2.5. Five had femoral neck *T*-scores and 5 had total hip *T*-scores ≤ -2.5. All but 2 had *T*-scores less than 0 at all three sites, and only 4 had *z*-scores greater than 0 at any of the three sites.

Forty-four subjects with celiac disease underwent BMD measurements of the AP lumbar spine, femoral neck, and total body with DXA (Lunar DPX-L) *(37)*. Thirty-four of the subjects were considered as having been successfully treated. The remaining 10 were either newly diagnosed or untreated. Compared to the manufacturer's reference data, subjects with newly diagnosed or untreated celiac disease had BMDs that were significantly lower than age-matched controls at all sites. Subjects with successfully treated celiac disease had BMDs that were not significantly different from predicted age-matched values.

Human Immunodeficiency Virus Infection

The effect of human immunodeficiency virus (HIV) infection on BMD was studied in 45 men *(38)*. BMD measurements of the total body, AP spine, and proximal femur were obtained with DXA (Lunar DPX). Twenty-one subjects had additional BMD measurements 15 months later. BMD results were compared to sex- and age-matched means supplied by the manufacturer. The average age of the subjects was 36 years and the mean CD4 count was 90. At baseline, BMD in the lumbar spine was 3% lower than controls. This value had borderline statistical significance. BMD values in the other regions were not statistically different from controls. In the subjects followed over time, there was a decrease in total body BMD of 1.6%, which was statistically significant. The other sites did not demonstrate significant change.

Hypercalciuria

Fifty adults (30 premenopausal women and 20 men under the age of 55) with idiopathic hypercalciuria and nephrolithiasis, and 50 age- and sex-matched controls, underwent bone densitometry of the lumbar spine, using DPA (Norland 2600) *(39)*. BMD in the lumbar spine in the subjects with idiopathic hypercalciuria was significantly lower than in controls. The authors postulated that this difference was the result of a negative calcium balance sustained over time.

The BMDs in 62 subjects (42 men, 20 women) with absorptive hypercalciuria, 27 subjects with fasting hypercalciuria, and 31 nonhypercalciuric subjects with nephrolithiasis were evaluated using DXA of the lumbar spine (Lunar DPX and Hologic QDR-1000) and SPA of the 33% radial site (Norland-Cameron) *(40)*. The values were compared to the age- and sex-matched reference values supplied by the manufacturers. Radial bone density did not differ among the three groups, and was not different from age- and sex-matched normal values. Compared to sex- and age-matched reference values, lumbar BMD was 9% lower in the subjects with absorptive hypercalciuria and stones, and 11% lower in the subjects with fasting hypercalciuria and stones. Lumbar BMD in the subjects with nonhypercalciuric nephrolithiasis was not different from reference values.

Hyperparathyroidism

In a study of patients with mild primary hyperparathyroidism, 22 of 143 patients had lumbar spine BMDs more than 1.5 SDs below the sex- and age-matched mean *(41)*. Fourteen of these 22 patients underwent surgery, and 8 were followed medically. BMD measurements were performed annually for 4 years, using DXA (Hologic QDR-1000) or a combination of DPA and SPA (Lunar DP3 and SP2) at the AP lumbar spine, proximal femur, and distal radius. After surgery, BMD in the lumbar spine rose an average of 15% in the first year, reaching 21% by the fourth year. In the patients not undergoing surgery, BMD did not change significantly over the 4 years.

At baseline in this study, the patients with lumbar spine *z*-scores poorer than –1.5 had an average *z*-score of –2.285. They also had femoral neck and distal radius *z*-scores of –1.695 and –1.522, respectively. The majority of patients with hyperparathyroidism in this study (85%), with lumbar spine *z*-scores better than –1.5, had an average spine *z*-score of –0.061. In this group, BMD was decreased most severely in the distal radius, with an average *z*-score poorer than –1. BMD in the femoral neck was also decreased in this group, but not as severely as the distal radius, when compared to sex- and age-matched controls.

Thirty-three postmenopausal women with mild primary hyperparathyroidism were followed prospectively for 2 years with BMD measurements of the total body, AP lumbar spine, proximal femur, and proximal forearm by DXA (Lunar DPX-L) *(42)*. Seventeen of the women received hormone replacement therapy and 16 received a placebo. In the women receiving placebo with untreated mild hyperparathyroidism, BMD decreased at all sites over the 2 years. Total body BMD decreased 2.3%. BMD in the lumbar spine decreased 1.4%, although this change was not statistically significant. BMD decreased 3.5% in the proximal forearm, and 1.4% in the femoral neck.

McDermott et al. *(43)* evaluated 59 women with mild asymptomatic primary hyperparathyroidism with BMD measurements at the distal and midradius with SPA (Norland), and at the AP lumbar spine and femoral neck with DPA (Norland). Forty-three of the 59 women had never taken estrogen replacement therapy (ERT); 16 were current users of ERT. Results were compared to a control group of 84 healthy women, who were not on ERT, and 45 healthy women who were current users of ERT. The women with primary hyperparathyroidism who were never users of ERT had lower BMC at the distal and midradius, and lower BMD at the lumbar spine and femoral neck, compared to controls (20, 20, 17, and 11%, respectively). The women with primary hyperparathyroidism who were current users of ERT had BMCs and BMDs that were not significantly different from controls, and that were significantly higher than the hyperparathyroid subjects who had never used ERT. Among the control group, estrogen users had BMCs in the distal and midradius, and BMDs in the spine and femoral neck, that were higher than the hyperparathyroid estrogen users (13, 8, 11, and 8%, respectively), although only the difference at the distal radius reached statistical significance.

Hyperprolactinemia

BMD of the lumbar spine was evaluated in 13 women with hyperprolactinemia, with an average age of 29.2 years by QCT (GE 8800 CT/T, General Electric Medical Systems, Milwaukee, WI), and compared to sex- and age-matched controls *(44)*. Seven of the women had idiopathic hyperprolactinemia, and 6 had prolactin-secreting pituitary tumors. The average duration of amenorrhea in the hyperprolactinemic women was 98.9 months. The average BMD of the spine was 10% less in the hyperprolactinemic women, compared to controls.

Forearm and vertebral BMD was evaluated by Schlechte et al. *(45)* in 26 women, aged 24 to 43 years, with histologically confirmed prolactin-secreting pituitary tumors, 7 to 10 years after transsphenoidal surgery. Ten of the women had persistent amenorrhea and increased prolactin levels; 16 had regular menses and normal prolactin levels. An addition 17 amenorrheic women, aged 24 to 42, with untreated hyperprolactinemia, were studied. Eleven of these women were amenorrheic on the basis of a pituitary tumor; in 6, the cause was unknown. Forty healthy women served as controls. BMD in the spine was measured by QCT (Picker International Inc., Highland Heights, OH) and at the 33% radius by SPA (Norland). In women with hyperprolactinemia, the spine bone density was 25% lower than in the healthy controls. Women who were considered cured, on the basis of normalized serum prolactin levels and resumption of menses, also had significantly lower spine BMD than the controls, but slightly higher spine BMD than the untreated or noncured women with hyperprolactinemia. BMD at the 33% radius did not differ between the untreated or noncured hyperprolactinemic women and the healthy controls.

Hyperthyroidism

Fifty-two patients (32 women, 20 men) with hyperthyroidism underwent BMD studies of the lumbar spine and proximal femur with DXA (Hologic QDR-1000) *(46)*. Values were compared to a control population. Hyperthyroidism in these patients was caused by Graves' disease. The average age of the men with hyperthyroidism was 45.6 years, and of the women, 43.8 years. BMD in the lumbar spine was 92.6% of sex- and age-matched reference values in the hyperthyroid subjects. There was no difference in this comparison between the men and women, or between the pre- and postmenopausal women with hyperthyroidism. Proximal femur BMD data was not reported.

Fifty-six women with Graves' disease, multinodular toxic goiter, or nodular toxic goiter were evaluated with DXA (Hologic QDR-1000) of the lumbar spine and proximal femur *(45)*. Three hundred fifty healthy women served as controls. In women with active, untreated hyperthyroidism, lumbar spine *z*-scores averaged –1.50, and femoral neck *z*-scores averaged –0.67. In women who had been treated in the past for hyperthyroidism, but who had been in remission without treatment for an average of 8.5 months, *z*-scores were significantly lower in the spine and femoral neck in the postmenopausal women only. The *z*-scores in premenopausal women did not differ from controls. In women being treated with nonsuppressive doses of L-thyroxine, the postmenopausal women again had significantly lower *z*-scores in the spine and femoral neck when compared to controls (–1.39 and –0.18, respectively). *Z*-scores in the premenopausal women did not differ from controls. The authors noted that postmenopausal women appeared to be at greatest risk for bone loss caused by a hyperthyroid state, and that trabecular regions of the skeleton were more affected than predominantly cortical regions.

Inflammatory Bowel Disease

Thirty-five patients (17 women and 18 men) with inflammatory bowel disease (IBD) were followed prospectively for 19 months with BMD measurements at the AP lumbar spine and proximal femur with DXA (Hologic QDR-1000) *(48)*. Fourteen patients had Crohn's disease, and 21 had ulcerative colitis. They ranged in age from 17 to 60 years, with a mean age of 36 years. Crohn's disease patients lost 3.08 ± 4.91% per year in the lumbar spine and 6.91 ± 6.57% per year in the femoral neck. Ulcerative colitis patients without ileoanal anastomosis lost 6.42 ± 7.5% per year in the lumbar spine and 5.59 ± 11.12% per year in the femoral neck. No ulcerative colitis patient with ileoanal anastamosis had a significant bone loss from either site. Patients on steroids had mean bone loss of 6.23 ± 7.04% per year in the spine and 8.97 ± 9.57% per year in the femoral neck. Patients not on steroids had gains of 0.87 ± 0.002 per year in the spine and 0.20 ± 5.78% per year in the femoral neck.

In another study of 79 patients with IBD (34 men, 45 women), bone density was measured with DXA in the AP lumbar spine and proximal femur with DXA (Norland XR-26) *(49)*. Forty-four patients had Crohn's disease, and 35 had ulcerative colitis. The mean age of the subjects was 39 years. Nineteen of the patients were taking corticosteroids. A high prevalence of low BMD was found at all sites, but the proximal femur sites were affected more often than the spine. At the spine, 54% had *T*-scores poorer than –1, and 18% had *T*-scores that were poorer than –2.5. At the femoral neck, 78%

had *T*-scores poorer than –1, and 29% had *T*-scores that were poorer than –2.5. The authors found no significant difference between the *T*-scores for Crohn's disease patients and ulcerative colitis patients.

Sixty patients with Crohn's disease were compared to 60 patients with ulcerative colitis and 60 controls *(50)*. Each of the three groups consisted of 36 women and 24 men, ranging in age from 21 to 75 years. The mean age of the Crohn's disease patients and controls was 36 years, and of the ulcerative colitis patients, 38 years. AP lumbar spine, femoral neck, and total-body bone density were measured using DXA (Lunar DPX). Patients with Crohn's disease had age-matched *z*-scores that were significantly lower than either the normal subjects or ulcerative colitis patients. The patients with ulcerative colitis had BMDs that were similar to controls.

Intravenous Drug Abuse

A syndrome of diffuse osteosclerosis was first reported with intravenous drug abuse in St. Louis *(51)*. The syndrome is considered rare, and its cause is unknown. Patients have presented with aching limbs and a generalized increase in density throughout the skeleton. One such subject, a 38-year-old Caucasian man, underwent BMD measurements with DXA (QDR-2000) of the spine and proximal femur, and of the spine using QCT (General Electric HiSpeed Advantage) *(52)*. The BMD in all regions was dramatically increased, compared to age- and sex-adjusted normal values. Spine values by DXA were 160% of predicted, and, by QCT, 185% of predicted. Values in the proximal femur ranged from 188 to 246% of predicted. Bone biopsy in this patient demonstrated dense lamellar bone. Skeletal X-rays demonstrated diffuse osteosclerosis that spared only the calvarium and facial bones.

Klinefelter's Syndrome

BMD in the lumbar spine and proximal femur in 32 patients with Klinefelter's syndrome was compared to 24 age-matched male controls *(53)*. The average age of the Klinefelter's syndrome subjects was 25.4 years, and the average age of the controls was 25.5 years. BMD was measured with DXA (Hologic QDR-1000). There was no significant difference found between the two groups in BMD at the AP lumbar spine, femoral neck, Ward's area, or total hip.

Marfan's Syndrome

Thirty-two women and 16 children (9 boys, 5 girls) with Marfan's syndrome underwent BMD measurements of the AP lumbar spine and proximal femur with DXA (Hologic QDR-1000W) *(54)*. The women ranged in age from 23 to 58 years, and the children ranged in age from 9.9 to 17.5 years. BMD in the spine and proximal femur in both the adults and children was found to be decreased when compared to sex- and age-matched controls. The authors concluded that patients with Marfan's syndrome have decreased BMD in both the axial and peripheral skeleton, which may be the result of inadequate development of peak bone density.

Mastocytosis

Sixteen patients (6 men and 10 women) with mastocytosis underwent bone density measurements of the AP spine, hip, and total body with DXA (Lunar DPX), and of the distal right radius and ulna with SPA (Osteometer DT 100, Roedovre, Denmark) *(55)*. BMD results from the patients with mastocytosis were compared to a reference population of 317 men and 1123 women from the local population. Both low bone density and increased bone density were found in the patients with mastocytosis. Bone density in the proximal femur was increased in both men and women with mastocytosis, if there was increased methylimidazoleacetic acid excretion. In patients with moderately increased mast cell mass, low bone density in the proximal femur and vertebral fractures were seen. Fractures are thought to occur in approximately 16% of patients with mastocytosis *(56)*. In patients with only urticaria pigmentosa, no change in bone density is apparent. In patients with systemic disease, however, the changes in bone density range from severe osteoporosis to osteosclerosis.

Multiple Myeloma

A prospective study of BMD in 34 patients (19 women and 15 men) with newly diagnosed multiple myeloma was performed using DXA (Hologic QDR-1000) of the lumbar spine and proximal femur *(57)*. The myeloma patients ranged in age from 43 to 83 years, with a median age of 71 years. Controls were 289 healthy volunteers. Lumbar spine BMD was significantly reduced in comparison to age-matched controls, but proximal femur BMD was not. The average age-matched *z*-score in the lumbar spine was –0.56. Multiple myeloma patients with vertebral fractures had age-matched *z*-scores poorer than –1 on average. Fifteen of the 34 patients had vertebral fractures at the start of the study (defined as a reduction in height of >20%). There was no correlation between lumbar spine BMD values and the type of paraproteins identified in the myeloma patients. In an another study, however, demineralization was found to be more common in IgA myeloma than in IgG myeloma *(58)*.

Multiple Sclerosis

Low bone density has been reported in multiple sclerosis (MS). Seventy-one women with MS underwent total body BMD measurements with DXA (Norland XR-26) *(59)*. Seventy-one healthy women served as controls. Total-body BMC was reduced in the women with MS by approximately 8%. When the women with MS were evaluated based on their ambulatory status, only nonambulatory women with MS were found to have lower total body BMC when compared to controls. The authors concluded that physical disuse is the major contributing factor in reduced bone mass in MS, although corticosteroid use also contributes.

Osteoarthritis

Studies of the effects of osteoarthritis on BMD in various regions of the skeleton are challenging. In the presence of osteophytes, joint-space narrowing, and sclerosis caused by osteoarthritis, accurate measurement of the BMD of the presumably nondiseased bone can be difficult. Nevitt et al. *(60)* reported a study of 4090 women who underwent pelvic radiographs, which were assessed for the presence of unilateral or bilateral hip osteoarthritis. A subset of 1225 women also underwent spine radiographs. All of the women underwent AP spine and proximal femur bone-density studies with DXA (Hologic QDR-1000) and studies of the os calcis and proximal and distal radius with SPA (OsteoAnalyzer, Norland Medical Systems, Inc., Ft. Atkinson, WI).

A grading scale was devised for the presence and severity of osteoarthritic changes in the hip joint, which ranged from 0 to 4, with 0 indicating that no osteoarthritis was present. An assignment of grade 2 or greater required that the subject have osteophytes or joint-space narrowing, and at least one other feature, such as subchondral sclerosis or cysts, or femoral head deformity. Grade 2 was considered as indicative of radiographic osteoarthritis in the hip, and grades 3 to 4 indicative of moderate or severe disease.

Women with grade 3 or 4 osteoarthritis in either hip had significantly higher bone densities at all sites, even after adjustment for age, compared to women with no evidence of osteoarthritis, or only grade 1. The increase in BMD was approximately 8 to 10% at the femoral neck, Ward's area, and lumbar spine, and about 3 to 5% at the os calcis, distal radius, and trochanteric region. At the femoral neck, women with grade 3 or 4 hip osteoarthritis had a BMD that was 0.092 ± 0.011 g/cm^2 higher than women without osteoarthritis, or only grade 1 findings. Women with grade 2 osteoarthritis also had significant elevations in BMD after adjustment for age at all sites, although the increases were smaller, in the range of 2 to 4%. The elevation in BMD at the femoral neck in these women averaged 0.037 ± 0.008 g/cm^2. The authors recognized that the inability to adequately rotate the femur internally, because of osteoarthritis, might artifactually increase the BMD,* but correcting for this did not alter the finding of significantly

**See* Chapter 2 for a discussion of the effects of femoral rotation on BMD measurements of the proximal femur.

increased BMD in the proximal femur in the women with grades 2 to 4 osteoarthritis. The authors also considered the effects of osteophytes and sclerosis in the spine from osteoarthritis as a potential cause of increased spine BMD. After adjusting the spine BMD for these findings, there was still a strong association between grade 3 or 4 osteoarthritis in the hip and increased spine BMD.

The authors postulated that a possible explanation for increased BMD in the femoral neck of subjects with osteoarthritis of the hip might be bone remodeling, with thickening of the medial cortex and trabecular hypertrophy from altered mechanical stress. This would not account for the increased BMD at other sites.

Preidler et al. *(61)* evaluated 68 adults with plain radiography and DXA studies of the proximal femur, in order to evaluate the influence of thickening of the medial cortex on bone density in the femoral neck, Ward's area, and trochanter, in subjects with osteoarthritis. They found that the BMD in the femoral neck and Ward's area was highly correlated with the cortical thickness, but that BMD in the trochanter was not. The authors suggested that the trochanteric region of the proximal femur might be the best region of interest for evaluation of bone density in subjects with osteoarthritis of the hip.

Paralysis

Hemiplegia

Eighty-seven hemiplegic stroke patients (50 men, 37 women) and 28 age-matched controls underwent radiographic photodensitometry of the hands *(62)*. Bone mass was significantly reduced on the hemiplegic side in the stroke patients. Vitamin D deficiency and disuse were thought by the authors to be the most likely explanations. In another study, this same group observed a significant decrease in bone mass in the hand on the hemiplegic side, compared with the contralateral side, in 93 hemiplegic stroke patients *(63)*. The authors attributed this difference to a combination of weakness and immobilization. They postulated that this decreased bone mass may explain why hip fractures occur almost exclusively on the hemiplegic side in stroke patients.

One hundred twelve subjects (53 women, 59 men), with hemiplegia from cerebral infarction or hemorrhage, underwent BMD measurements of both femurs with DXA (Hologic QDR-1000) *(64)*. The mean age of these subjects was 68.3 years. The mean period after the onset of hemiplegia was 45.7 months. Sixty-three subjects were affected on the right side and 49 subjects were affected on the left. BMD measurements were compared to reference population data supplied by the manufacturer. BMD in the total femur, femoral neck, Ward's, and trochanter was significantly decreased on the paretic side, compared to the nonparetic side (8.8, 6.6, 10.3, and 10.4%, respectively). BMD in both proximal femurs was significantly decreased in comparison to reference population values. BMDs in the paretic femur were approximately 20 to 24% below reference values; BMDs in the nonparetic femur were 14 to 17% below reference values.

Paraplegia

Fifty-three patients (11 women, 42 men) with complete traumatic paraplegia of at least 1 year duration underwent BMD studies of the AP lumbar spine and proximal femur with DXA (Hologic QDR-1000/W), and at the forearm by SPA (Nuclear Data 1100A) *(65)*. These subjects were wheelchair bound, but not bedridden. They ranged in age from 21 to 60, with a median age of 35.9 years. Compared to age-matched controls, there was no significant difference in BMD at the lumbar spine. BMD for the total hip was reduced by 33%, and was reduced at the femoral shaft by 25%. There was no significant difference in BMD at the cortical forearm site described as being at the junction of the distal and midthird of the forearm.

Parkinson's Disease

In a study of 52 subjects with Parkinson's (28 men and 24 women), using DXA (Norland XR-26) to measure total-body BMC, bone mineral content was found to be significantly decreased when compared to controls *(66)*. The *z*-score for men with Parkinson's averaged –0.47, and for women, –0.84. In this same study, metacarpal radiogrammetry did not reveal any significant differences between Parkinson's disease patients and controls.

A brief report in abstract form from Turc et al. *(67)*, noted that, in 19 men with Parkinson's disease, BMD in the AP spine, as measured with DXA, was significantly reduced in comparison to age-matched controls. BMD averaged 0.965 ± 0.146 g/cm^2 in the Parkinson's disease subjects, and 1.063 ± 0.146 g/cm^2 in the controls. Although femoral bone density was also reduced in the Parkinson's disease subjects, the difference from age-matched controls was not significant.

Kao et al. *(68)* also measured AP spine bone density with DPA (M&SE OsteoTech 300, Medical and Scientific Enterprises, Sudbury, MA) in 22 Parkinson's disease subjects (3 women, 19 men) aged 58 to 76. All of the Parkinson's disease subjects had lower AP spine bone densities than healthy age-matched controls. Sixty-eight percent of the Parkinson's disease subjects had spine BMDs that were more than 2 SDs below the age-matched mean BMD.

Pregnancy

Controversy exists regarding whether a separate entity of pregnancy-induced osteoporosis exists, or whether pregnancy is an incidental or precipitating factor in persons who already have osteoporosis. The syndrome is considered rare, with about 80 cases documented in the literature. The women who are affected often present with vertebral fractures in the third trimester, or shortly after delivery. Densitometry has demonstrated markedly low bone density in both the spine and proximal femur *(69)*. Five cases of postpregnancy osteoporosis have been reported by Yamamoto et al. *(70)*. These women ranged in age from 24 to 37 years. Four of the five women were diagnosed after their first pregnancy. The fifth was diagnosed after her second pregnancy. All of the women presented with back pain and vertebral compression fractures, most within 1 month of delivery. BMD measurements were made at the 33% radial site with SPA (Norland-Cameron), and at the spine by either QCT or DXA (Hologic QDR-1000). Measurements were made at various times in the evaluation and management of these patients. BMD at the 33% radial site was not decreased in these women when compared to a reference population. BMD at the spine by either QCT or DXA revealed values lower than expected for the population.

Renal Failure

Eighty-nine patients with chronic renal failure underwent bone density testing of the spine, using QCT. Sixty-six were receiving long-term hemodialysis *(71)*. In the 23 patients not on dialysis, spine BMD was 9% lower than predicted normal values, but this difference was not statistically significant. In patients receiving dialysis, however, the average *z*-score was –1.3. In 42 patients on dialysis who were followed over 8 months, spinal BMD by QCT decreased an average of 2.9%. Osteosclerosis was found in 11 patients on dialysis.

In a cross-sectional study, 45 patients on continuous ambulatory peritoneal dialysis (CAPD) were evaluated using DXA *(72)*. Total body, spine, and proximal femur bone densities were assessed. BMDs were not significantly different from an age-matched control population. The authors concluded that the prevalence of decreased bone density was not increased in CAPD patients. They also noted that BMD in the lumbar spine, femoral neck, and Ward's area was increased, compared to controls, in patients with evidence of hyperparathyroid disease. The authors observed that the utility of DXA regional studies to detect osteodystrophy is limited by the confounding effects of hyperparathyroid osteosclerosis.

Rheumatoid Arthritis

BMD of the distal and midradius was measured by DXA (Norland XR-26) in 34 women with rheumatoid arthritis, and compared to 40 controls *(73)*. The women with rheumatoid arthritis ranged in age from 40 to 79 years, with a mean age of 61 years. The average duration of disease was 12 years. BMD in both the distal and midradius was reduced in the women with rheumatoid arthritis, who were in their fifties and sixties, compared to controls. Women with rheumatoid arthritis in their forties and seventies did not have BMDs that were significantly lower than controls. The authors suggested that postmenopausal bone loss may amplify the bone loss seen in rheumatoid arthritis.

Forty-six postmenopausal women with rheumatoid arthritis, with a disease duration of 2 to 35 years, underwent bone density testing at a variety of skeletal sites *(74)*. The ultradistal radius was evaluated with pQCT (Stratec XCT-960, Birkenfeld, Germany), the os calcis with ultrasound (McCue CUBA, McCue Ultrasonics Ltd., Winchester Hampshire, UK), and the spine and proximal femur with DXA (Norland XR-26 Mark II). Results were compared to 29 healthy postmenopausal women who served as controls. The postmenopausal women with rheumatoid arthritis had significantly lower bone density at all sites when compared to controls, except at the lumbar spine and in the cortical measurement at the ultradistal radius. The total ultradistal BMD was 15.6% lower and the trabecular ultradistal BMD was 36.1% lower than controls. Femoral neck BMD was 15.4% lower than controls. Os calcis broadband ultrasound attenuation was 31.7% lower, and the velocity of sound was 6.6% lower. BMD at the lumbar spine in the women with rheumatoid arthritis was 6.7% lower than controls, but this difference was not statistically significant.

BMD measurements of the hand, AP spine, and proximal femur were performed on 202 subjects (61 men, 141 women) with rheumatoid arthritis, using DXA (Lunar DPX-L) *(75)*. The average age of the subjects was 58 years, and the median disease duration was 1.8 years. BMD measurements of the hand were significantly correlated with BMD at lumbar spine and femoral neck ($r = 0.67$ and $r = 0.63$, respectively). In a separate study of 56 subjects with rheumatoid arthritis, hand BMC was shown to be significantly reduced in subjects with rheumatoid arthritis, compared to controls *(76)*. In another 42 subjects with recent onset of rheumatoid arthritis, who were followed prospectively with hand BMC, losses of 5.36% in men and 2.14% in women were noted in 1 year *(77)*.

Lane et al. *(78)* evaluated 120 postmenopausal women with rheumatoid arthritis, measuring BMD at the AP lumbar spine and proximal femur with DXA (Hologic QDR-1000), and at the distal radius and os calcis with SPA (OsteoAnalyzer). The women with rheumatoid arthritis were divided into three groups, based on corticosteroid use: never users, current users, and past users. Results were compared to 7966 age-matched controls. All of the women were 65 years of age or older. Women with rheumatoid arthritis were found to have significantly lower BMD at all measurement sites when compared to controls. Women with rheumatoid arthritis who were never users had significantly lower BMD at the distal radius, os calcis, and total femur, compared to controls. Women with rheumatoid arthritis who were current users had the lowest BMD at the distal radius, os calcis, and total femur. The authors concluded that postmenopausal women with rheumatoid arthritis have lower appendicular and axial bone densities that cannot be attributed to corticosteroid use.

In 1996, Deodhar and Woolf reviewed bone densitometry studies in patients with rheumatoid arthritis *(79)*. They concluded that patients with rheumatoid arthritis have lower bone density in both the appendicular and axial skeletons when compared with controls, and that the most rapid bone loss occurred within the first year after the onset of disease. They also noted that the evidence suggested that doses of oral corticosteroids >5 mg per day were associated with significant bone loss in patients with rheumatoid arthritis.

Thalassemia Major

Seventeen patients (9 men, 8 women) with thalassemia major were studied to determine the effects of the disease process on BMC and BMD *(80)*. The average age of the subjects was 24 years. Bone density at the distal radius was measured by Compton scattering, and at the distal and midradius by SPA (Norland). Cortical indices of the third metacarpal were also measured. At the distal radius, BMC was found to be 34% lower than controls, and, at the midradius, BMC was 24% lower than controls. The metacarpal cortical indices were 36% lower in the thalassemia subjects than controls. Higher BMC and cortical indices were seen in patients who had received more blood transfusions and longer treatment with desferrioxiamine, but this difference was not statistically significant.

Transient Osteoporosis of the Hip

This disorder was first described in women in the third trimester of pregnancy. It has been reported in both sexes, however, usually occurring in young to middle-aged patients *(81)*. In men, both hips are affected with equal frequency, but in women, the disease is seen almost exclusively in the left hip. The disease presents with progressive pain, loss of range of motion, and a limp, without any preceding history of trauma. Localized demineralization is seen in the femoral head, neck, and intertrochanteric region. Radionuclide bone scans demonstrate increased uptake in the regions that are demineralized. The disease is self-limited, with spontaneous resolution in 6 to 12 months.

Transplantation

Cardiac Transplantation

Twenty-five patients (21 men, 4 women) were evaluated after orthoptic cardiac transplant, with DXA (Lunar DPX-L) of the lumbar spine and total body *(82)*. Bone density testing was performed immediately posttransplant, and at 6 and 12 months posttransplant. All patients received immunosuppressive therapy with prednisolone, cyclosporine, azathioprine, and antithymocyte globulin. The mean cumulative dose of prednisolone was 9.2 g during the first 6 months, and 2.8 g during the second 6 months. Lumbar spine bone loss was rapid, with a mean of –6.7% at 6 months, and –8.8% at 12 months. Total body calcium fell at 6 months by –2.4%, and at 12 months by –2.8%.

Marrow Transplantation

Twenty-seven women who underwent bone marrow transplant underwent bone density testing of the AP lumbar spine with DXA (Hologic QDR-1000) *(83)*. Conditions leading to bone marrow transplant were: acute nonlymphoblastic leukemia (10), chronic myeloid leukemia (8), acute lymphoblastic leukemia (3), non-Hodgkin's lymphoma (2), Hodgkin's disease (2), aplastic anemia (1), and refractory anemia with excess blasts (1). All the subjects had experienced ovarian failure, with amenorrhea of an average duration of 35.4 ± 36.1 months. Their average age was 31.3 ± 9.9 years. The average time between marrow transplant and the bone density studies was 33.5 ± 34.5 months. Using WHO criteria*, 9 had osteopenia and 5 had osteoporosis. The authors postulated that immunosuppressive therapy and ovarian failure were the principal factors in bone loss after bone marrow transplantation.

In another study of both men and women with allogenic bone marrow transplantation, lumbar and femoral neck BMD were reported to be 8 to 13% lower, respectively, than age-matched controls *(84)*.

Renal Transplantation

BMD measurements of the AP lumbar spine, proximal total femur, and total body were performed on 34 renal transplant recipients (19 men, 15 women) with DXA (Hologic QDR-1000W) *(85)*. Measurements were compared to those made in 34 healthy controls. The average age of the subjects was 45 years. The cause of renal failure was glomerulonephritis in 12, analgesic nephropathy in 6, reflux nephropathy in 3, polycystic kidney disease in 5, nephroangiosclerosis in 2, chronic pyelonephritis in 4, oculorenal syndrome in 1, and Fabry's disease in 1. Immediately after transplant, total body and lumbar spine BMD was decreased in comparison to controls. In women receiving transplants, total femoral BMD was also decreased in comparison to controls. The difference in total femur BMD

**See* Chapter 9 for a discussion of World Health Organization criteria for the diagnosis of osteoporosis.

in men was not statistically different from controls. In the 5 months following transplantation, total body BMD and BMC decreased in both men and women, as did BMD in the lumbar spine and total femur. The decrease in total body BMC was 41 g. Lumbar BMD decreased at a rate of 1.6% per month. The authors suggested that the bone loss seen after transplantation may be a result of corticosteroid administration to prevent graft rejection.

EFFECT OF DRUGS ON BONE DENSITY

Alendronate Sodium

The effect of varying doses of alendronate sodium on lumbar spine and proximal femur bone density was evaluated in 994 women with postmenopausal osteoporosis *(86)*. The women were followed for 3 years, during which time they received either placebo, 5 mg alendronate daily, 10 mg alendronate daily for 3 years, or 20 mg alendronate daily for 1 year, followed by 5 mg daily for the remaining 2 years. All of the women received 500 mg calcium per day. Bone density measurements were obtained at the lumbar spine, proximal femur, midforearm, and total body, using DXA (Hologic QDR-1000, Lunar DPX-L, Norland XR-26). The placebo group receiving calcium alone lost BMD at all sites. In the alendronate-treated groups, there were significant gains at the spine, femoral neck, trochanter, and total body. Significant increases from baseline in BMC or BMD at the midforearm site were not seen in the alendronate-treated groups. The increase in BMD was most rapid in the first 6 months of treatment. The 10 mg dose of alendronate produced greater gains in BMD than the 5 mg dose, and was as effective as the 20 mg/5 mg regimen. Over 96% of the women receiving 10 mg of alendronate daily had measurable gains in spine BMD. The gain in BMD at the end of 3 years in this group was approximately 8% in the lumbar spine and 5% in the femoral neck. At the end of 1 year, the gain in spine BMD in the 10 mg per day alendronate-treated group was approximately 5%.

A second study of 2 years duration, of 188 postmenopausal women with low BMD in the spine, confirmed a gain of 7.21% in the spine in women taking 10 mg alendronate per day at the end of 2 years *(87)*. In the total hip, the gain was 5.27% at the end of 2 years. No significant change was seen at any forearm site. BMD measurements were made with DXA (Hologic QDR-1000).

Calcitriol

Fifty postmenopausal women with nontraumatic vertebral fractures were followed for 2 years with bone density measurements of the AP spine and total body, using DPA *(88)*. All women received 400 IU of vitamin D_2

and 1000 mg of calcium per day. Half of the women received 0.25 μg of calcitriol twice a day and half received a placebo. Calcium intake and the dose of calcitriol were adjusted during the study, in order to keep serum and urine levels of calcium within specified ranges. At the end of 2 years, women receiving calcitriol had an increase in lumbar spine BMD of 1.94%; the placebo group lost 3.92%. Total body BMD increased in the calcitriol-treated group by 0.21%; the placebo group lost 1.86%.

Calcium and Vitamin D

The effects of calcium supplementation and vitamin D_3 on bone density were evaluated by Dawson-Hughes et al. *(89)* in a 3-year study of 176 men and 213 women aged 65 and over. BMD was measured by DXA (Lunar DPX-L) in the AP spine, proximal femur, and total body. The subjects received either a double-placebo at bedtime or 500 mg of calcium citrate malate and 700 IU of vitamin D_3. At the end of 3 years, subjects receiving calcium and vitamin D_3 demonstrated an increase in BMD at the femoral neck of 0.50%, at the spine of 2.12%, and of the total body of 0.06%. Subjects receiving the double placebo had an increase in BMD at the spine of 1.22%, a loss in BMD at the femoral neck of –0.70%, and a loss in total body BMD of –1.09%. At the end of the first year of the study, the differences in BMD between the placebo group and the calcium–vitamin D_3 group were significant at all sites. At the end of the third year, however, only the difference in BMD of the total body was significant. Thirty-seven subjects experienced nonvertebral fractures during the 3-year trial. Twenty-six of the 37 were in the placebo group. The relative risk for fracture in the calcium–vitamin D_3 group, compared to the placebo group, was 0.4 (95% confidence interval of 0.2 to 1.0).

Chapuy et al. *(90)* followed 3270 ambulatory women, with an average age of 84 years, for 18 months. Half the women received 1200 mg of elemental calcium as tricalcium phosphate and 800 IU of vitamin D_3, and half received a double placebo. One thousand seven hundred sixty-five women completed the study. BMD of the proximal femur was measured by DXA (Hologic QDR-1000) at baseline and after 18 months in 56 women. At the end of 18 months, BMD in the total femur region of interest had increased 2.7% in the calcium–vitamin D_3 group, and had declined 4.6% in the placebo group. This difference was highly statistically significant. Bone density increased in the femoral neck in the calcium–vitamin D_3 group by 2.9%, and decreased in the trochanter by 1%. In the double placebo group, the BMD declined by 6.4% in the trochanter, and increased by only 1.8% in the femoral neck. During the 18-month study, 151 nonvertebral fractures occurred in the calcium–vitamin D_3 group, compared to 204 in the placebo group. There were 32% fewer nonvertebral fractures and 43% fewer hip fractures in the calcium–vitamin D_3 group, compared to the placebo group. In addition, there was a marked increase in the incidence of hip fracture with time in the placebo group; the incidence remained stable in the calcium–vitamin D_3 group.

Corticosteroids

Oral Corticosteroids

The decrease in BMD at the AP lumbar spine and proximal femur was quantified, using DXA (Lunar DPX), in 31 asthmatic subjects (18 men, 13 women) receiving glucocorticoid therapy, and compared with BMD at those sites in age-matched controls *(91)*. The average dose and duration of corticosteroid therapy in these subjects was 16 mg of prednisone equivalents per day for 10 years. BMD of the lumbar spine was 80% of the sex- and age-matched controls. The BMD of the femoral neck, Ward's area, and trochanter were also reduced in comparison to sex- and age-matched controls at 83, 78, and 86%, respectively. The dose and duration of corticosteroid therapy did not correlate significantly with BMD in this study.

Laan et al. *(92)* evaluated the effects of low-dose prednisone on BMD in subjects with rheumatoid arthritis. Forty subjects (28 women, 12 men) with active rheumatoid arthritis, all of whom were receiving gold salts, were begun on 10 mg prednisone per day or placebo. The prednisone was gradually discontinued between weeks 12 and 20 of therapy. BMD was measured in the spine by dual-energy QCT (Somatom DR3, Siemens, Erlangen, Germany). There was an 8.2% decline in BMD in the first 20 weeks of therapy in the trabecular region of interest in the spine in the prednisone-treated group; the BMD in the placebo group did not change. No changes were seen in either group in the BMD in the cortical region of interest in the spine in the first 20 weeks of therapy. In the patients who discontinued corticosteroid therapy after 20 weeks, BMD in the trabecular region of interest in the spine increased 5.3% over the next 24 weeks.

BMD in the AP lumbar spine, as measured by DPA (Lunar DP3), decreased at a rate of 4.3% per year in the first year, and at a rate of 2.3% per year in the second year, in subjects who began corticosteroid therapy at the start of the study period *(93)*. These subjects received 1000 mg of calcium per day during the 2-year follow-up as part of a larger study evaluating the effects of calcitriol and calcitonin on the prevention of corticosteroid-induced bone loss. The mean daily dose of prednisone or prednisolone was 13.5 mg in the first year and 7.5 mg in the second year.

Inhaled Corticosteroids

The effect of inhaled corticosteroids on BMD was evaluated by Marystone et al. *(94)* in a cross-sectional study of 78 Caucasian subjects.

The subjects ranged in age from 56 to 91. Forty-four subjects (27 women, 17 men) had used inhaled corticosteroids, and 34 (19 women, 15 men) had used oral corticosteroids. BMD was measured at the ultradistal and midradius with SPA (Lunar SP2), and at the lumbar spine and proximal femur with DXA (Hologic QDR-1000). These subjects were drawn from a larger study of 1673 subjects, with the nonusers of corticosteroids serving as controls. Among the men, BMD did not differ significantly at any site by corticosteroid usage. Among the women, users of oral corticosteroids had BMDs that were 7.2% lower at the midradius, 8.0% lower at the spine, and 9.4% lower at the total hip than the nonusers. These differences were statistically significant. Women using inhaled corticosteroids had BMDs at the ultradistal radius, proximal femur, and spine that were intermediate between the oral corticosteroid users and the nonusers. Although the differences were not statistically significant, BMD was 2.3% lower at the total hip, and 3.7% lower at the spine, in women using inhaled corticosteroids, compared to controls.

A comparison of the effects of inhaled budesonide and inhaled beclomethasone on BMD at the spine was performed by Packe et al. *(95)*. Twenty subjects with asthma, receiving inhaled budesonide in a median daily dose of 800 μg, and 20 subjects receiving inhaled high-dose beclomethasone in a median daily dose of 1000 μg, underwent BMD measurements of the spine with QCT. These results were compared to those of 17 asthmatics who had never received any kind of corticosteroid therapy. The average BMD of the budesonide subjects of 139.5 mg/cm^3 was significantly lower than the BMD of 160.6 mg/cm^3 in the asthmatics who had never used steroids. The mean BMD of the beclomethasone subjects of 127.5 mg/cm^3 was not different from the budesonide subjects. The authors noted that the subjects receiving inhaled budesonide or beclomethasone had received previous courses of oral corticosteroids, which could account for the decreased BMD.

Estrogen/Hormone Replacement

The effects of cyclic hormone replacement, with either transdermal estrogen or oral estrogen, on BMD in the spine and proximal femur were compared to controls by Hillard et al. *(96)*. Ninety-six Caucasian women, between 6 months and 7 years postmenopausal, participated in this study. Thirty women served as controls. Sixty-six women received either 0.05 mg transdermal 17β-estradiol continuously, and 0.25 mg per day of norethisterone for 14 days of each cycle, or oral-conjugated equine estrogen 0.625 mg per day and 0.15 mg per day of DL-norgestrel for 12 days of each cycle. BMD measurements of the AP spine and proximal femur were obtained every 6 months for 3 years with DPA (Lunar DP3). In the control group, BMD in the spine declined by 4%, and in the femoral neck by 5% at the end of 3 years. BMD increased at both sites in the two groups receiving some form of hormone replacement, with no significant difference between the two groups. The average increase in BMD at the spine in the transdermal-estrogen-treated group at the end of the first year was 0.033 g/cm^2, and at the end of the third year was 0.046 g/cm^2. In the conjugated-estrogen-treated group, the average increase in spine BMD was 0.032 g/cm^2 at the end of the first year, and 0.038 g/cm^2 at the end of the third year. At the femoral neck, the average increase in the transdermal-estrogen-treated group was 0.015 g/cm^2 at the end of the first year, and 0.020 g/cm^2 at the end of the third year. In the conjugated-estrogen-treated group, the average gain in femoral neck BMD was 0.003 g/cm^2 at the end of the first year, and 0.009 g/cm^2 at the end of the third year. Six of the women receiving hormone replacement had significant losses in BMD from the femoral neck during the 3 years of treatment, despite good compliance.

The effects of hormone replacement on BMD in women just beginning therapy were compared to the effects on BMD in women on established hormone replacement by Lees et al. *(97)*. Twenty-nine women who had never taken hormone replacement therapy and 19 women who had been taking hormone replacement were begun on micronized estradiol 2 mg per day orally, and dydrogesterone 10 mg per day orally for 14 days of each cycle. BMD measurements of the AP lumbar spine and proximal femur were obtained with DXA (Lunar DPX) at yearly intervals for 2 years. In the women just beginning hormone replacement, BMD increased at the spine by 5.3% at the end of 12 months, and by 6.4% at the end of 14 months. In the women who had been on hormone replacement, BMD increased to a lesser degree in the spine, by 2.1% at the end of 12 months, and by 2.3% at the end of 24 months. Femoral neck BMD increased in both groups, but there was no difference between the two groups. At the end of 2 years, BMD had increased at the femoral neck in the women beginning hormone replacement by 3.27%, and in the women continuing hormone replacement by 2.28%.

The effect of estrogen replacement on BMD in women at least 10 years past menopause was evaluated by Kohrt and Birge *(98)*. Twenty-four women, ranging in age from 61 to 74 years, and who were 10 to 33 years postmenopausal, underwent BMD studies with DXA (Hologic QDR-1000/W) of the total body, AP spine, proximal femur, and ultradistal radius and ulna. Measurements were made at baseline and every 3 months for 1 year. One-half the women received 0.625 mg per day conjugated estrogen and 5 mg per day medroxyprogesterone acetate for 13 consecutive days every 3 months. The other 12 women served as controls. A calcium intake of 1500 mg per day was maintained by all the subjects. In these late postmenopausal women receiving hormone replacement, BMD increased in the total body, lumbar spine, femoral neck, trochanter, and Ward's triangle, and declined insignificantly at the ultradistal radius and ulna. Compared to the placebo group, the differences were significant at all sites, with the exception of the ultradistal radius and ulna. In the hormone-replacement group, BMD at the total body increased 0.013 g/cm^2, or 1.4%; at the lumbar spine by 0.041 g/cm^2, or 5.0%; at the femoral neck by 0.019 g/cm^2, or 3.1%; at the trochanter by 0.017 g/cm^2, or 3.0%; and at Ward's triangle by 0.026 g/cm^2, or 5.8%. The decline at the ultradistal radius and ulna was 0.001 g/cm^2, or 0.3%.

Dose-response studies of four estrogen preparations indicate that there are doses of estrogen replacement that are ineffective in preserving skeletal mass. The minimum effective dose of Premarin® (Wyeth-Ayerst, Philadelphia, PA) is considered to be 0.625 mg *(99)*. For Estrace® (Bristol-Myers Squibb, New York, NY), the minimum dose is 0.5 mg *(100)*. The minimum effective dose of Ogen® (Pharmacia & Upjohn, Kalamazoo, MI) is 0.625 mg, and for Estraderm® (Novartis, East Hanover, NJ), 0.05 mg *(101,102)*.

The effects of the withdrawal of estrogen replacement on forearm BMC were studied by Christiansen et al. *(103)* in 94 women who were 6 months to 3 years postmenopausal. Women who stopped hormone replacement after 2 years lost BMC from the distal radius, as measured by SPA, at virtually the same rate as those who did not begin hormone replacement. The loss of BMC occurred at approximately 2.3% per year from the distal radius in the women stopping hormone replacement.

Etidronate

The effects of etidronate alone, or etidronate preceded by phosphate, were evaluated in a double-blind, placebo-controlled trial of 429 postmenopausal women with 1 to 4 vertebral compression fractures and radiographic demineralization *(104)*. The women received either a double placebo; 1 g phosphate orally twice daily on days 1 through 3, followed by 400 mg etidronate orally daily on days 4 through 17; placebo on days 1 through 3, followed by etidronate on days 4 through 17; or phosphate on days 1 through 3, followed by placebo on days 4 through 17. All women received calcium 500 mg per day on days 18 through 91. The treatment cycles were repeated eight times. BMD was measured at the lumbar spine and proximal femur with DPA (Lunar DP3, Norland 2600). BMC was measured at the distal and midradius with SPA (Lunar SP2, Nuclear Data 1100, Norland Model 178, OsteoAnalyzer). At the end of 24 months, significant gains in BMD at the spine were seen in the etidronate and etidronate–phosphate-treated groups. The average increase in spine BMD in the etidronate-alone group was 4.2% and in the etidronate–phosphate group, 5.2%. The women receiving etidronate alone had a significant gain at the femoral neck at the end of 2 years of approximately 3.5%. No significant change in BMC at the distal or midradius was seen in any treatment group during the 24 months of observation.

GnRH Agonists

Twenty-eight women with endometriosis, who ranged in age from 22 to 44 years, were treated with 3.6 mg of goserelin acetate depot every 28 days for 6 months *(105)*. BMD measurements of the AP lumbar spine were obtained with DXA (Hologic) at baseline, 6, 12, and 30 months. Results were compared to those in 25 healthy women who served as age-matched controls. There was a significant decrease of 4% in lumbar spine BMD in the treated group after 6 months that persisted for the second 6 months, during which no goserelin was administered. Values in the control group did not change during this period. At 30 months, however, BMD values in the treated group had returned to baseline levels.

Eleven women with endometriosis were treated with 3.6 mg goserelin every 28 days for 6 months, and 12 women with endometriosis were treated with oral danazol 600 mg for 6 months *(106)*. BMD measurements of the lumbar spine and proximal femur were performed in both groups using DPA (Lunar DP3) at the beginning and end of therapy. During the treatment period, BMD did not change at any site in the danazol-treated group. In the women receiving goserelin, there was a 2.5% decline in spinal BMD, and a 1.7% decline in femoral neck BMD at the end of 6 months.

The effects of buserelin on BMC at the 10% and 33% radial sites were evaluated in 18 women who were being treated for 6 months for uterine fibroids *(107)*. BMC measurements at the radius were performed with SPA (Norland Cameron). The women ranged in age from 28 to 49 years. Eighteen healthy women served as controls. Buserelin was administered in a dose of 0.5 mg subcutaneously three times per day for the first 10 days, followed by 200 μg intranasally four times per day for 6 months. No significant changes in BMC were observed in the treated group in the first 6 months, or at the end of a 6-month treatment-free observation period.

Twenty-five women with endometriosis were treated with nafarelin, and followed for 12 months with BMD measurements of the AP lumbar spine by DPA, and measurements of the distal and midradius by SPA *(108)*. Sixteen of the women received nafarelin in a dose of 200 μg per day; 9 of the women received 400 μg per day. During 6 months of treatment, women receiving the lower dose of nafarelin had no significant change in bone density; women receiving the higher dose experienced losses of 2 to 6%. These values returned to baseline levels 6 months after discontinuation of therapy. An additional study of 17 women with endometriosis was performed by Riis et al. *(109)*. These women were treated with nafarelin 400 μg per day, plus 1.2 mg per day norethindrone for 6 months. BMC was again measured at the distal and midradius with SPA, and BMD was measured at the lumbar spine and total body by DPA. There was no significant change in BMC or BMD during the treatment period, except in the distal forearm. Six months after treatment, this value had returned to baseline levels.

Heparin

Sixty-one premenopausal women, who had been previously treated with subcutaneous or intravenous heparin for at least 1 month, were evaluated with bone-density measurements of the spine with DPA (Norland 2600), and of the distal third of the radius with SPA (Norland 278A) *(110)*. The average duration of heparin therapy was 26.7 weeks, and the average total dose was 4.1×10^6 U. Sixty-one healthy women served as age-matched controls. The mean BMD at the spine and radius did not differ significantly between the two groups. The authors also evaluated the proportion of women in each group whose bone densities fell below either the presumed fracture threshold* of 1.000 or 0.840 g/cm^2 (2 SDs below young normals) at the spine and below 0.690 g/cm^2 at the radius (2 SDs below young normals). A significantly greater proportion of women who had been treated with heparin fell below these cutoff levels.

Ipriflavone

Ipriflavone is a synthetic flavonoid that is being investigated for its effects on bone density. Passeri et al. *(111)* studied 28 postmenopausal women over the age of 65 with at least one vertebral fracture and a BMD at the distal radius that was more than 2 SDs below the young adult peak BMD. The women received either 200 mg of ipriflavone or placebo three times daily. BMD was measured at the 10% radial site with DPA (Osteoden P, NIM, Verona, Italy) at baseline and after 12 months. Women receiving ipriflavone increased BMD at the 10% radial site by 6% after 12 months; the women receiving placebo had an insignificant loss of 0.3%.

In a larger study of 255 postmenopausal Caucasian women, the effects of ipriflavone on the BMD of the distal radius as measured by DPA (Osteoden P) were reported by Adami et al. *(112)*. These women ranged in age from 50 to 65 years, and had a BMD at the distal radius that was at least 1 SD below the age-matched mean BMD. The women received 200 mg of ipriflavone orally, or placebo three times daily. All women received 1 g calcium during the 2 years of the study. At the end of 2 years, women

*See Chapter 6 for a discussion of the fracture threshold.

receiving ipriflavone maintained their baseline bone density at the distal radius, and women receiving placebo lost slightly more than 3%.

Medroxyprogesterone Acetate

Thirty women receiving injectable depot medroxyprogesterone acetate for contraception for at least 5 years were evaluated by Cundy et al. *(113)*. BMD was measured at the AP lumbar spine and femoral neck, and compared to BMD in 30 premenopausal women and 30 postmenopausal women who served as controls. Compared to the premenopausal women, the women who received depot medroxyprogesterone had BMDs that were 7.5% lower in the lumbar spine and 6.6% lower in the femoral neck. Compared to the postmenopausal women, however, women who received depot medroxyprogesterone acetate had BMDs that were 8.9% higher in the lumbar spine and 4% higher in the femoral neck.

Nandrolone Decanoate

Nandrolone decanoate is an anabolic steroid. Twenty postmenopausal women with osteoporosis were followed with bone-mass measurements at the AP lumbar spine and femoral shaft with DPA (Novo Diagnostic) for 12 months *(114)*. One-half of the women received 50 mg of nandrolone decanoate IM every 3 weeks; the remainder received placebo injections. All the women received 1 g calcium daily. In the lumbar spine, women receiving nandrolone had an increase in BMC of 9.8%; the women receiving placebo lost 3.2%. The increase in spinal BMC from baseline was significant, and the difference between groups was also significant. In the femoral shaft, women receiving nandrolone had an increase of 3.5%, compared to the placebo group, which lost 3.3%. This difference in the femoral shaft did not reach statistical significance.

Raloxifene

The effects of raloxifene on BMD in 143 postmenopausal women with one or more prevalent spine fractures, whose average age was 68.4 years, was reported by Lufkin et al. *(115)*. The women were treated with 60 or 120 mg per day of raloxifene or placebo for 1 year. BMD was measured at the AP lumbar spine, total femur, ultradistal radius, and total body with DXA. All women received 750 mg of calcium daily and 400 IU of vitamin D. At the end of 1 year, there were significant differences in the change in BMD at the total femur between the 60-mg per day group and the placebo group, and at the ultradistal radius between both raloxifene groups and the placebo group. At the total femur, the 60-mg per day group increased BMD 0.95%; the placebo group decreased BMD 0.71%. At the ultradistal radius, the 60-mg per day group increased BMD 0.22%, the 120-mg per day group decreased BMD 0.19%, and the placebo group decreased BMD 2.70%. There were no significant differences in BMD at the end of 1 year between the two raloxifene groups and the placebo group at the spine or total body. This was a preliminary report in abstract form presented at the 19th Annual Meeting of the American Society for Bone and Mineral Research.

In a study of 601 postmenopausal women between the ages of 45 and 60 years, Delmas et al. also evaluated the effects of raloxifene on BMD with DXA (Hologic QDR-1000 and QDR-2000) *(116)*. The women were treated for 2 years with placebo, 30, 60, or 150 mg of raloxifene. All of the women received 400 to 600 mg of elemental calcium daily. The women had spine BMDs less than 2 SDs below the peak BMD. At the end of 2 years, all three raloxifene groups demonstrated gains in BMD at the lumbar spine, total hip, and femoral neck that were significantly different from the placebo group. The percent increase from baseline at the end of 2 years at the lumbar spine, total hip, and femoral neck for the 30 mg group was 1.3, 1.0, and 0.6% respectively. For the 60 mg group, it was 1.6, 1.6, and 1.2%. For the 150 mg group, the percent change from baseline at 2 years was 2.2, 1.5, and 1.5%.

Risedronate

The efficacy of risedronate in increasing lumbar spine BMD was studied in 648 postmenopausal women for 18 months by McClung et al. *(117)*. The average age of the women was 62 years, and all were at least 1 year postmenopausal, with an average duration of menopause of 16 years. At entry into the study, the lumbar spine *T*-score was ≤–2. BMD was measured by DXA at the AP lumbar spine, proximal femur, and at the distal and midradius. The women received either 2.5 or 5 mg of risedronate daily, or placebo. All of the women received 1 g calcium daily. Risedronate increased BMD at the lumbar spine, femoral neck, and trochanter, and at the distal radius in a dose-dependent fashion. At the lumbar spine, both risedronate groups had significant changes in BMD from baseline, but the placebo group did not change significantly. The 5-mg risedronate group had a significantly greater increase than the 2.5-mg group. The gains in lumbar spine BMD at the end of 18 months for the 2.5- and 5-mg risedronate groups were 2 to 3% and 4 to 5%, respectively. In the femoral neck and trochanter, both risedronate groups again demonstrated significant increases from baseline and significant increases in comparison to the placebo group. The 5-mg risedronate group again demonstrated a significantly greater increase in BMD at both sites than the 2.5-mg group. The average gain in BMD at the femoral neck in the 5-mg group was approximately 3%, and at the trochanter, approximately 5%. At the distal radius, only the 5-mg risedronate group had a significant increase in BMD from baseline, at 18 months, of slightly more than 1%. At the midradius, no group demonstrated a significant change in BMD from baseline values. This data was presented in abstract form at the 19th Annual Meeting of the American Society for Bone and Mineral Research

Salmon Calcitonin

Preliminary data on the effect of salmon calcitonin nasal spray on lumbar spine BMD and vertebral fracture risk was reported at the 19th Annual Meeting of the American Society for Bone and Mineral Research *(118)*. One thousand one hundred seventy-five women, with an average age of 68.3 years, were randomized to receive placebo, 100, 200, or 400 IU of salmon calcitonin nasal spray daily. All of the women also received 1000 mg calcium and 400 IU of vitamin D daily. Each woman had at least one prevalent fracture and a BMD at the lumbar spine that was more than 2 SDs below the young-adult mean value. At the end of 3 years in this 5-year study, no group demonstrated a significant change from baseline in lumbar spine BMD. In the 200 and 400 IU groups, the % change in lumbar spine BMD at the end of 3 years was 1.26 and 1.51%, respectively. Despite the lack of a significant change in lumbar spine BMD, however, there was a 37.4% reduction in the relative risk for vertebral fracture in the 200 IU group.

In a study of 208 postmenopausal women with a distal forearm BMC 2 SDs or more below the young adult mean BMC, the response to nasal-spray salmon calcitonin was evaluated at the end of 2 years, with measurements of BMC at the distal forearm by SPA, and at the AP lumbar spine by DXA (Hologic QDR-1000) *(119)*. The women received placebo, 50, 100, or 200 IU of nasal-spray salmon calcitonin daily, in addition to 500 mg of calcium. BMC increased in the salmon-calcitonin-treated women in a dose-dependent manner. At the end of 2 years, BMC in the lumbar spine had increased 3% in the women receiving 200 IU per day, and 1% in the women receiving placebo. BMC at the distal radius declined in all groups approximately 1% at the end of 2 years.

The effectiveness of nasal spray calcitonin in preventing bone loss from the spine was evaluated in recently postmenopausal women by Reginster et al. *(120)*. Two hundred fifty-one women, who were 6 months to 5 years postmenopausal, were randomized to receive either placebo, 50 IU, or 200 IU of nasal-spray salmon calcitonin daily for 5 consecutive days each week for 2 years. All of the women also received 500 mg calcium daily. BMD measurements of the AP lumbar spine were obtained with DPA (Novo Lab 22A) every 6 months. At the end of 2 years, BMD in the lumbar spine decreased by 6.98% in the placebo group. In the 50- and 200-IU salmon calcitonin groups, BMD in the lumbar spine increased by 0.51 and 2.26%, respectively. The difference in BMD between both salmon calcitonin groups and the placebo group was statistically significant, but the difference between the two salmon calcitonin groups was not.

Sodium Fluoride

Sodium fluoride is a potent stimulator of osteoblastic bone formation. Its effect on BMD in the lumbar spine and proximal femur was evaluated by Riggs et al. *(121)* in 202 women with postmenopausal osteoporosis. Osteoporosis was defined as at least one prevalent vertebral fracture and a spine BMD below the normal range for premenopausal women. The women received placebo or 75 mg of sodium fluoride daily and 1500 mg calcium daily for 4 years. BMD of the AP lumbar spine and femoral neck were measured by DPA. The 33% radial site was measured by SPA. Women receiving placebo increased lumbar spine BMD by 0.4% per year; the women receiving fluoride increased lumbar spine BMD 8.2% per year. At the femoral neck, women receiving placebo lost 0.9% per year; women receiving sodium fluoride increased BMD 1.8% per year. At the radius, the fluoride-treated group had a decline in BMC of 1.8% per year; the placebo group increased 0.4% per year. The difference between the rates of change in the fluoride-treated group and the placebo group was significant at these sites.

A different preparation of sodium fluoride and different regimen was evaluated by Pak et al. *(122)* in 110 Caucasian women with postmenopausal osteoporosis. These women were randomized to receive cyclic treatment with 25 mg of slow-release sodium fluoride or placebo twice daily for 12 months, followed by 2 months withdrawal and 400 mg calcium citrate twice daily continuously. BMD was measured at the AP lumbar spine and proximal femur by DPA and DXA, and at the midradius by SPA (Norland). In this ongoing study, the average subject had completed more than two treatment cycles, with only a few subjects having completed four cycles. In the placebo group, BMC in the lumbar spine did not change significantly over the first four cycles. In the slow-release sodium fluoride group, however, BMC in the lumbar spine increased 4 to 6%. At the femoral neck, the BMD did not change in the placebo group; it increased in the slow-release fluoride group by 4.1% by the end of the first cycle, and 2.1% by the end of the second cycle. The midradial BMD did not change significantly in either group.

Tamoxifen

In a small, uncontrolled trial, eight postmenopausal women beginning tamoxifen 10 mg orally, twice a day, after a diagnosis of breast cancer, were followed every 6 months with BMD measurements of the AP spine with DPA (Lunar) *(123)*. At the end of 6 months, BMD in the lumbar spine had increased an average of 0.0456 g/cm^2, and at 12 months, 0.0565 g/cm^2. All eight subjects had increases in BMD in the lumbar spine.

The effect of tamoxifen on lumbar spine BMD and the 33% radial site was determined in 70 women receiving 10 mg twice daily after a diagnosis of breast cancer, and compared to the findings in 70 women with similar-stage breast cancer who served as controls *(124)*. BMD at the lumbar spine was measured with DPA (Lunar DP3), and at the 33% radius, by SPA (Lunar SP2). The women were followed for 2 years. Women receiving tamoxifen increased lumbar spine BMD 0.61% per year, but lost BMD at the 33% radial site at a rate of 0.88% per year. The women not receiving tamoxifen lost BMD at both sites at a rate of 1.29% at the radius and 1% at the spine. The differences between the two groups were statistically significant at the spine, but not at the 33% radial site.

Thyroid Hormone

BMD at the distal and 8-mm sites on the radius was measured with SPA (Nuclear Data ND 1100A) in 78 postmenopausal women who had been on thyroid hormone replacement for a minimum of 5 years *(125)*. The average age of the women was 64 years. Hypothyroidism in these women was initially caused by idiopathic hypothyroidism or primary autoimmune hypothyroidism. Forty-four of these women had persistently suppressed TSH values, but 34 did not. One hundred two women served as controls. The women with nonsuppressed TSH values had *z*-scores at the 8-mm and distal radial sites of –0.07 and –0.03; the women with suppressed TSH had *z*-scores of –0.25 and –0.20, respectively. The differences between the three groups were not statistically significant. The authors estimated that a suppressed TSH was associated with, at most, a 5% decrease in BMD.

Affinito et al. *(126)* also measured BMD at the distal radius in a study of 54 postmenopausal women with primary hypothyroidism and suppressed TSH levels during thyroid hormone replacement. Fifty-four healthy postmenopausal women served as controls. *Z*-scores at the distal radius in the women with suppressed TSH in this study were significantly decreased, compared to the women in the control group in this study.

Guo et al. *(127)* conducted a prospective study of 64 postmenopausal women on thyroid hormone replacement. BMD was measured at the total body, AP lumbar spine, and femoral neck with DXA (Lunar DPX). The average age of the women on thyroid hormone replacement was 61 years. The women were divided into three groups, based on their diagnosis and TSH levels. Group 1 consisted of women on replacement, with normal TSH levels. Group 2 consisted of women on replacement, with suppressed TSH levels. Group 3 consisted of women with a history of thyroid cancer, followed by thyroidectomy and suppressed TSH levels. Thirty-six healthy age-matched women served as controls. The women were followed for 2 years. After the baseline BMD measurements, the dose of thyroid hormone replacement was reduced in group 2, to return the TSH levels to normal. At baseline and at follow-up 2 years later, there was no significant difference in BMD at any of the sites among the four groups. In group 2, however, BMD significantly increased at the spine and femoral neck over 2 years, suggesting that the reduction in the dose of thyroid hormone was beneficial.

Seventeen postmenopausal women with subclinical hypothyroidism were randomly assigned to receive thyroid hormone replacement or placebo for 14 months *(128)*. BMD was measured at the 33% radial site with SPA, and at the lumbar spine with DXA (Hologic QDR-1000). In the thyroxine-treated group, the dosage was adjusted to maintain the TSH in the normal range. Over the 14-month period, BMD at the radius decreased in the treated group and the placebo group by 0.5 and 1.8%, respectively. The difference between the two groups was not significant. In the lumbar spine, the BMD increased 0.1% in the treated group, and decreased 0.7% in the untreated group. Again, this difference was not significant. The author concluded that there was no detrimental effect on BMD of levothyroxine treatment that normalized TSH in postmenopausal women with subclinical hypothyroidism.

Tibolone

Tibolone is a synthetic compound with estrogenic, progestational, and androgenic activity. Its potential utility in preventing postmenopausal bone loss was reported 20 years ago *(129)*. In 1994, Rymer et al. *(130)* reported the results of a 2-year nonrandomized prospective study, in which women, between 6 and 36 months after menopause, received either 2.5 mg tibolone or no medication. Bone mineral density was measured in the AP lumbar spine and proximal femur with DXA (Hologic QDR-1000) at baseline, and again at 6, 12, and 24 months. Forty-six women in the tibolone group completed the study and 45 women in the control group completed the study. The average age of the subjects was 49.5 years. At the end of 2 years, women in the tibolone group had significant increases in bone density at the lumbar spine, the femoral neck, Ward's area, and the trochanter, and women in the placebo group had significant losses at those sites. On an individual basis, 39 of the women receiving tibolone increased bone density at the spine, and 33 had increases in bone density in the femur. The average increase in lumbar spine BMD after 2 years in the tibolone-treated group was 2.5%, and in the femoral neck, 3.5%. The control group had losses of 2.9 and 3.7% in the spine and femoral neck, respectively.

A comparison trial of 2.5 mg per day of tibolone, 2 mg per day of estradiol orally, and 50 μg per day of transdermal 17β-estradiol vs no medication was performed in 140 postmenopausal women with a median duration of menopause of 3 years *(131)*. BMD was measured at the lumbar spine, proximal femur, and total body, using DXA (Hologic QDR-1000). At the end of 2 years, all three treatment regimens prevented bone loss, and the women in the control group lost BMD. There was no significant difference in BMD among the three treatment groups. In the control group, there was a loss of 3.4% from the lumbar spine, 2.2% from the total femur, 1.6% from the femoral neck, and no change in total body BMD at the end of 2 years.

REFERENCES

1. Faulkner RA, Bailey DA, Drinkwater DT, McKay HA, Arnold C, Wilkinson AA (1996) Bone densitometry in Canadian children 8–17 years of age. *Calcif Tissue Int* 59:344–351.
2. Lu PW, Briody JN, Ogle GD, Morley K, Humphries IR, Allen J, et al. (1994) Bone mineral density of total body, spine, and femoral neck in children and young adults: a cross-sectional and longitudinal study. *J Bone Miner Res* 9:1451–1458.
3. Zanchetta JR, Plotkin H, Alvarez Filgueira ML (1995) Bone mass in children: normative values for the 2-20-year-old population. *Bone* 16:393S–399S.
4. Sabatier JP, Guaydier-Souquieres G, Laroche D, Benmalek A, Fournier L, Guillon-Metz F, et al (1996) Bone mineral acquisition during adolescence and early adulthood: a study in 574 healthy females 10–24 years of age. *Osteoporosis Int* 6:141–148.
5. Moreira-Andres MN, Canizo FJ, Papapietro K, Rejas J, Hawkins FG (1995) Comparison between spinal and radial bone mineral density in children measured by X-ray absorptiometry. *J Pediatr Endocrinol Metab* 8:35–41.
6. Teegarden D, Proulx WR, Martin BR, Zhao J, McCabe CP, Lyle RM, et al. (1995) Peak bone mass in young women. *J Bone Miner Res* 10:711–715.
7. Mazess RB, Barden HS (1990) Interrelationships among bone densitometry sites in normal young women. *Bone Min* 11:347–356.
8. Mazess RB, Barden HS (1991) Bone density in premenopausal women: effects of age, dietary intake, physical activity, smoking, and birth-control pills. *Am J Clin Nutr* 53:132–142.
9. Hansen MA (1994) Assessment of age and risk factors on bone density and bone turnover in healthy premenopausal women. *Osteoporosis Int* 4:123–128.
10. Rodin A, Murby B, Smith MA, Caleffi M, Fentiman I, Chapman MG, Fogelman I (1990) Premenopausal bone loss in the lumbar spine and neck of femur: a study of 225 Caucasian women. *Bone* 11:1–5.
11. Bonnick SL, Nichols DL, Sanborn CF, Lloyd K, Payne SG, Lewis L, Reed CA (1997) Dissimilar spine and femoral z-scores in premenopausal women. *Calcif Tissue Int* 61:263–265.
12. Pouilles JM, Tremollieres F, Ribot C (1993) The effects of menopause on longitudinal bone loss from the spine. *Calcif Tissue Int* 52:340–343.
13. Gambacciani M, Spinette A, Taponeco F, Cappagli B, Maffei S, Manetti P, Piaggesi L, Fioretti P (1994) Bone loss in perimenopausal women: a longitudinal study. *Maturitas* 18:191–197.
14. Pouilles JM, Tremollieres F, Ribot C (1993) Spine and femur densitometry at the menopause: are both sites necessary in the assessment of risk of osteoporosis? *Calcif Tissue Int* 52:344–347.

15. Lai K, Rencken M, Drinkwater BL, Chesnut CH. (1993) Site of bone density measurement may affect therapy decision. *Calcif Tissue Int* 53:225–228
16. Mazess RB, Barden HS, Eberle RW, Denton MD (1995) Age changes of spine density in posterior–anterior and lateral projections in normal women. *Calcif Tissue Int* 56:201–205.
17. Davis JW, Ross PD, Wasnich RD (1994) Evidence for both generalized and regional low bone mass among elderly women. *J Bone Miner Res* 3:305–309.
18. Greenspan SL, Maitland-Ramsey L, Myers E (1996) Classification of osteoporosis in the elderly is dependent on site-specific analysis. *Calcif Tissue Int* 58:409–414.
19. Mazess RB, Barden HS, Drinka PJ, Bauwens SF, Orwoll ES, Bell NH (1990) Influence of age and body weight on spine and femur bone mineral density in U.S. white men. *J Bone Miner Res* 5:645–652.
20. Kayath MJ, Vieira JGH (1997) Osteopenia occurs in a minority of patients with acromegaly and is predominant in the spine. *Osteoporosis Int* 7:226–230.
21. Kotzmann H, Bernecker P, Hubsch P, Pietschmann P, Woloszczuk W, Svoboda T, Gerer G, Luger A (1993) Bone mineral density and parameters of bone metabolism in patients with acromegaly. *J Bone Miner Res* 8:459–465.
22. Peris P, Guanabens N, Pares A, Pons F, del Rio L, Nomegal A, et al. (1995) Vertebral fractures and osteopenia in chronic alcoholic patients. *Calcif Tissue Int* 57:111–114.
23. Prezelj J, Kocijancic A (1993) Bone mineral density in hyperandrogenic amenorrhoea. *Calcif Tissue Int* 52:422–424.
24. Drinkwater B, Nilson K, Chesnut CH, Bremner WJ, Shainholtz S, Southworth MB (1984) Bone mineral content of amenorrheic and eumenorrheic athletes. *N Engl J Med* 311:277–281.
25. Rigotti NA, Nussbaum SR, Herzog DB, Neer RM (1984) Osteoporosis in women with anorexia nervosa. *N Engl J Med* 311:1601–1606.
26. Hay PJ, Delahunt JW, Hall A, Mitchell AW, Harper G, Salmond C (1992) Predictors of osteopenia in premenopausal women with anorexia nervosa. *Calcif Tissue Int* 50:498–501.
27. Herzog W, Minne H, Deter C, Leidig G, Schellberg D, Wuster C, et al. (1993) Outcome of bone mineral density in anorexia nervosa patients 11.7 years after first admission. *J Bone Miner Res* 8:597–605.
28. Monegal A, Navasa M, Guanabens N, Peris P, Pons F, Martinez de Osaba MJ, Rimola A, Rodes J (1997) Osteoporosis and bone mineral metabolism disorders in cirrhotic patients referred for orthotopic liver transplantation. *Calcif Tissue Int* 60:148–154.
29. Munoz-Torres M, Jodar E, Escobar-Jimenez F, Lopez-Ibarra PJ, Luna JD (1996) Bone mineral density by dual X-ray absorptiometry in Spanish patients with insulin-dependent diabetes mellitus. *Calcif Tissue Int* 58:316–319.
30. Sosa M, Dominguez M, Navarro MC, Segarra MC, Hernandex D, de Pablos P, Betancor P (1996) Bone mineral metabolism is normal in non-insulin-dependent diabetes mellitus. *J Diabetes Complications* 10:201–205.
31. Barrett-Connor E, Kritz-Silverstein D (1996) Does hyperinsulinemia preserve bone? *Diabetes Care* 19:1388–1392.
32. Pouilles JM, Tremollieres F, Ribot C (1996) Variability of vertebral and femoral postmenopausal bone loss: a longitudinal study. *Osteoporosis Int* 6:320–324.
33. Bjarnason K, Hassager C, Ravn P, Christiansen C (1995) Early postmenopausal diminution of forearm and spinal bone mineral density: a cross-sectional study. *Osteoporosis Int* 5:35–38.

34. Mellstrom D, Johansson C, Johnell O, Lindstedt G, Lundberg P, Obrant K, et al. (1993) Osteoporosis, metabolic aberrations, and increased risk for vertebral fractures after partial gastrectomy. *Calcif Tissue Int* 53:370–377.
35. Pastores GM, Wallenstein S, Desnick RJ, Luckey MM (1996) Bone density in type 1 Gaucher disease. *J Bone Miner Res* 11:1801–1807.
36. Rude RK, Olerich M (1996) Magnesium deficiency: possible role in osteoporosis associated with gluten-sensitive enteropathy. *Osteoporosis Int* 6:453–461.
37. Walters JRF, Banks LM, Butcher GP, Fowler CR (1995) Detection of low bone mineral density by dual energy X-ray absorptiometry in unsuspected suboptimally treated coeliac disease. *Gut* 37:220–224.
38. Paton NIJ, Macallan DC, Griffin GE, Pazianas M (1997) Bone mineral density in patients with human immunodeficiency virus infection. *Calcif Tissue Int* 61:30–32.
39. Zanchetta JR, Rodriguez G, Negri AL, del Valle E, Spivacow FR (1996) Bone mineral density in patients with hypercalciuric nephrolithiasis. *Nephron* 73: 557–560.
40. Pietschmann F, Breslau NA, Pak CYC (1992) Reduced vertebral bone density in hypercalciuric nephrolithiasis. *J Bone Miner Res* 7:1383–1388.
41. Silverberg SJ, Locker FG, Bilezikian JP (1996) Vertebral osteopenia: a new indication for surgery in primary hyperparathyroidism. *J Clin Endocrinol Metab* 81: 4007–4012.
42. Grey AB, Stapleton JP, Evans MC, Tatnell MA, Reid IR (1996) Effect of hormone replacement therapy on bone mineral density in postmenopausal women with mild primary hyperparathyroidism. *Ann Intern Med* 125:360–368.
43. McDermott MT, Perloff JJ, Kidd GS (1994) Effects of mild asymptomatic primary hyperparathyroidism on bone mass in women with and without estrogen replacement therapy. *J Bone Miner Res* 9:509–514.
44. Koppelman MC, Kurtz DW, Morrish KA, Bou E, Susser JK, Shapiro JR, Loriaux DL (1984) Vertebral body mineral content in hyperprolactinemic women. *J Clin Endocrinol Metab* 59:1050–1053.
45. Schlechte J, Khoury G, Kathol M, Walker L (1987) Forearm and vertebral bone mineral in treated and untreated hyperprolactinemic amenorrhea. *J Clin Endocrinol Metab* 64:1021–1026.
46. Wakasugi M, Wakao R, Tawata M, Naoya G, Koizumi K, Onaya T (1993) Bone mineral density in patients with hyperthyroidism measured by dual energy X-ray absorptiometry. *Clin Endocrinol* 38:283–286.
47. Campos-Pastor MM, Munoz-Torres M, Escobar-Mimenez F, Ruiz del Almodovar M, Jodar Gimeno E (1993) Bone mass in females with different thyroid disorders: influence of menopausal status. *Bone Miner* 21:1–8.
48. Roux C, Abitbol V, Chaussade S, Kolta S, Guillemant S, Dougados M, Amor B, Couturier D (1995) Bone loss in patients with inflammatory bowel disease: a prospective study. *Osteoporosis Int* 5:156–160.
49. Bjarnason I, Macpherson A, Mackintosh C, Buxton-Thomas M (1997) Reduced bone density in patients with inflammatory bowel disease. *Gut* 40:228–233.
50. Jahnsen J, Falch JA, Aadland E, Mowinckel P (1997) Bone mineral density is reduced in patients with Crohn's disease but not in patients with ulcerative colitis: a population based study. *Gut* 40:313–319.
51. Villareal DR, Murphy WA, Teitelbaum SL, Arens MQ, Whyte MP (1992) Painful diffuse osteosclerosis after intravenous drug abuse. *Am J Med* 93:371–381.
52. Whyte MP, Teitelbaum SL, Reinus WR (1996) Doubling skeletal mass during adult life: the syndrome of diffuse osteosclerosis after intravenous drug abuse. *J Bone Miner Res* 11:554–558.

53. Luisetto G, Mastrogiacomo I, Bonanni G, Pozzan G, Botteon S, Tizian L, Galuppo P (1995) Bone mass and mineral metabolism in Klinefelter's syndrome. *Osteoporosis Int* 5:455–461.
54. Kohlmeier L, Gasner C, Bachrach LK, Marcus R (1995) The bone mineral status of patients with Marfan Syndrome. *J Bone Miner Res* 10:1550–1555.
55. Johansson C, Roupe G, Lindstedt G, Mellstrom D (1996) Bone density, bone markers and bone radiological features in mastocytosis. *Age Ageing* 25:1–7.
56. Travis WD, Li C, Bergstralh EJ, Yam LT, Swee RG (1988) Systemic mast cell disease: analysis of 58 cases and literature review. *Medicine* 67:345–368.
57. Abildgaard N, Brixen K, Kristensen JE, Vejlgaard T, Charles P, Nielsen JL (1996) Assessment of bone involvement in patients with multiple myeloma using bone densitometry. *Eur J Haematol* 57:370–376.
58. Holmes JA, Evans, WD, Coles RJ, Ramsahoye B, Whittaker JA (1994) Dual energy X-ray absorptiometry measurements of bone mineral density in myeloma. *Eur J Haematol* 53:309–311.
59. Formica CA, Cosman F, Nieves J, Herbert J, Lindsay R (1997) Reduced bone mass and fat-free mass in women with multiple sclerosis: effects of ambulatory status and glucocorticoid use. *Calcif Tissue Int* 61:129–133.
60. Nevitt MC, Lane NE, Scott JC, Hochberg MC, Pressman AR, Genant HK, Cummings SR (1995) Radiographic osteoarthritis of the hip and bone mineral density. *Arthritis Rheum* 38:907–916.
61. Preidler KW, White LS, Tashkin J, McDaniel CO, Brossman J, Andresen R, Sartoris D (1997) Dual-energy X-ray absorptiometric densitometry in osteoarthritis of the hip. Influence of secondary bone remodeling of the femoral neck. *Acta Radiol* 38:539–542.
62. Sato Y, Maruoka H, Oizumi K, Kikuyama M (1996) Vitamin D deficiency and osteopenia in the hemiplegic limbs of stroke patients. *Stroke* 27:2183–2187.
63. Sato Y, Maruoka H, Honda Y, Asoh T, Fujimatsu Y, Oizumi K (1996) Development of osteopenia in the hemiplegic finger in patients with stroke. *Eur Neurol* 36: 278–283.
64. Takamoto S, Masuyama T, Nakajima M, Sekiya K, Kosaka H, Morimoto S, Ogihara T, Onishi T (1995) Alterations of bone mineral density of the femurs in hemiplegia. *Calcif Tissue Int* 56:259–262.
65. Goemaere S, Van Laere M, De Neve P, Kaufman JM (1994) Bone mineral status in paraplegic patients who do or do not perform standing. *Osteoporosis Int* 4; 138–143.
66. Revilla M, de la Sierra G, Aguado F, Varela L, Jimenez-Jimenez FJ, Rico H (1996) Bone mass in Parkinson's disease: a study with three methods. *Calcif Tissue Int* 58:311–315.
67. Turc J, Pages M, Poulles JM, Billey T, Montastruc JL, Ribot C, Rascol A (1993) Bone changes in Parkinson's disease. Abstract. *Neurology* 43:A236.
68. Kao CH, Chen CC, Wang SJ, Chia LG, Yeh SH (1994) Bone mineral density in patients with Parkinson's disease measured by dual photon absorptiometry. *Nucl Med Commun* 15:173–177.
69. Khovidhunkit W, Epstein S (1996) Osteoporosis in pregnancy. *Osteoporosis Int* 6:345–354.
70. Yamamoto N, Takahashi HE, Tanizawa T, Kawashima T, Endo N (1994) Bone mineral density and bone histomorphometric assessments of postpregnancy osteoporosis: a report of five patients. *Calcif Tissue Int* 54:20–25.
71. Karantanas AH, Kalef-Ezra JA, Sferopoulos G, Siamopoulos KC (1996) Quantitative computed tomography for spinal bone mineral measurements in chronic renal failure. *Br J Radiol* 69:132–136.

72. Johnson DW, McIntyre HD, Brown A, Freeman J, Rigby RJ (1996) The role of DEXA bone densitometry in evaluating renal osteodystrophy in continuous ambulatory peritoneal dialysis patients. *Peritonial Dial Int* 16:34–40.
73. Toyoda T, Inokuchi S, Saito S, Horie Y, Tomita S (1996) Bone loss of the radius in rheumatoid arthritis. *Acta Orthop Scan* 67:269–273.
74. Martin JC, Munro R, Campbell MK, Reid DM (1997) Effects of disease and corticosteroids on appendicular bone mass in postmenopausal women with rheumatoid arthritis: comparison with axial measurements. *Br J Rheum* 36:43–49.
75. Devlin J, Lilley J, Gough A, Huissoon A, Holder R, Reece R, Perkins P, Emery P (1996) Clinical associations of dual-energy X-ray absorptiometry measurement of hand bone mass in rheumatoid arthritis. *Br J Rheum* 35:1256–1262.
76. Deodhar AA, Brabyn J, Jones PW, Davis MJ, Woolf AD (1994) Measurement of hand bone mineral content by dual energy x-ray absorptiometry: development of the method and its application in normal volunteers and in patients with rheumatoid arthritis. *Ann Rheum Dis* 53:685–590.
77. Deodhar AA, Brabyn J, Jones PW, Davis MJ, Woolf AD (1995) Longitudinal study of hand bone densitometry in rheumatoid arthritis. *Arthritis Rheum* 38:1204–1210.
78. Lane NE, Pressman AR, Star VL, Cummings SR, Nevitt MC and the Study of Osteoporotic Fractures Research Group (1995) Rheumatoid arthritis and bone mineral density in elderly women. *J Bone Miner Res* 10:257–263.
79. Deodhar AA, Woolf AD (1996) Bone mass measurement and bone metabolism in rheumatoid arthritis: a review. *Br J Rheum* 35:309–322.
80. Orvieto R, Leichter I, Rachmilewitz EA, Margulies JY (1992) Bone density, mineral content, and cortical index in patients with thalassemia major and the correlation to their bone fractures, blood transfusions, and treatment with desferrioxamine. *Calcif Tissue Int* 50:397–399.
81. Scialabba FA, DeLuca SA (1990) Transient osteoporosis of the hip. *AFP* 41:1759–1760.
82. Sambrook PN, Kelly PJ, Fontana D, Nguyen T, Keogh A, Macdonald P, Spratt P (1994) Mechanisms of rapid bone loss following cardiac transplantation. *Osteoporosis Int* 4:273–276.
83. Castaneda S, Carmona L, Carvajal I, Arranz R, Diaz A, Garcia-Vadillo A (1997) Reduction of bone mass in women after bone marrow transplant. *Calcif Tissue Int* 60:343–347.
84. Kelly PJ, Atkinson K, Ward RL, Sambrook PN, Biggs JC, Eisman JA (1990) Reduced bone mineral density in men and women with allogeneic bone marrow transplantation. *Transplantation* 50:881–883.
85. Horber FF, Casez JP, Steiger U, Czerniak A, Montandon A, Jaeger P (1994) Changes in bone mass early after kidney transplantation. *J Bone Miner Res* 9:1–9.
86. Liberman UR, Weiss SR, Broll J, Minne HW, Quan H, Bell NH, et al. (1995) Effect of oral alendronate on bone mineral density and the incidence of fractures in postmenopausal osteoporosis. *N Engl J Med* 333:1437–1443.
87. Chesnut CH, McClung MR, Ensrud KE, Bell NH, Genant HK, Harris ST, et al. (1995) Alendronate treatment of the postmenopausal osteoporotic woman: effect of multiple dosages on bone mass and bone remodeling. *Am J Med* 99:144–152.
88. Gallagher JC, Goldgar D (1990) Treatment of postmenopausal osteoporosis with high doses of synthetic calcitriol. A randomized, controlled study. *Ann Intern Med* 113:649–655.
89. Dawson-Hughes B, Harris SS, Krall EA, Dallal GE (1997) Effect of calcium and vitamin D supplementation on bone density in men and women 65 years of age or older. *N Engl J Med* 337:670–676.

90. Chapuy MC, Arlot ME, Duboeuf F, Brun J, Crouzet B, Arnaud S, Delmas PD, Meunier PJ (1992) Vitamin D3 and calcium to prevent hip fractures in elderly women. *N Engl J Med* 327:1637–1642.
91. Reid IR, Evans MC, Wattie DJ, Ames R, Cundy TF (1992) Bone mineral density of the proximal femur and lumbar spine in glucocorticoid-treated asthmatic patients. *Osteoporosis Int* 2:103–105.
92. Laan RFJM, van Riel PLCM, van de Putte LBA, van Erning LJTO, van't Hof MA, Lemmens JAM (1993) Low-dose prednisone induces rapid reversible axial bone loss in patients with rheumatoid arthritis. *Ann Intern Med* 119:963–968.
93. Sambrook P, Birmingham J, Kelly P, Kempler S, Nguyen T, Pocock N, Eisman J (1993) Prevention of corticosteroid osteoporosis: a comparison of calcium, calcitriol, and calcitonin. *N Engl J Med* 328:1747–1752.
94. Marystone JF, Barrett-Connor EL, Morton DJ (1995) Inhaled and oral corticosteroids: their effects on bone mineral density in older adults. *Am J Public Health* 85:1693–1695.
95. Packe GE, Robb O, Robins SP, Reid DM, Douglas JG (1996) Bone density in asthmatic patients taking inhaled corticosteroids: comparison of budesonide and beclomethasone dipropionate. *J R Coll Physicians Lond* 30:128–132.
96. Hillard TC, Whitecroft SJ, Marsh MS, Ellerington MC, Lees B, Whitehead MI, Stevenson JC (1994) Long-term effects of transdermal and oral hormone replacement therapy on postmenopausal bone loss. *Osteoporosis Int* 4:341–348.
97. Lees B, Pugh M, Siddle N, Stevenson JC (1995) Changes in bone density in women starting hormone replacement therapy compared with those in women already established on hormone replacement therapy. *Osteoporosis Int* 5:344–348.
98. Kohrt WM, Birge SJ (1995) Differential effects of estrogen treatment on bone mineral density of the spine, hip, wrist and total body in last postmenopausal women. *Osteoporosis Int* 5:150–155.
99. Genant HK, Cann CE, Ettinger B, Gorday GS (1982) Quantitative computed tomography of vertebral spongiosa: a sensitive method for detecting early bone loss after oophorectomy. *Ann Intern Med* 97:699–705.
100. Ettinger B, Genant HK, Steiger P, Madvig P (1992) Low-dosage micronized 17β-estradiol prevents bone loss in postmenopausal women. *Am J Obstet Gynecol* 166:479–488.
101. Harris ST, Genant HK, Baylink DJ, Gallagher C, Harp SK, McConnell MA, et al. (1991) The effects of estrone (Ogen) on spinal bone density of postmenopausal women. *Arch Intern Med* 151:1980–1984.
102. Field CS, Ory SJ, Wahner HW, et al. (1993) Preventive effects of transdermal 17β-estradiol on osteoporotic changes after surgical menopause. *Am J Obstet Gynecol* 168:114–121.
103. Christiansen C, Christensen MS, Transbol I (1981) Bone mass in postmenopausal women after withdrawal of oestrogen/gestagen replacement therapy. *Lancet* 1:459–461.
104. Watts NB, Harris ST, Genant HK, Wasnich RD, Miller PD, Jackson RD, et al. (1990) Intermittent cyclical etidronate treatment of postmenopausal osteoporosis. *N Engl J Med* 323:73–79.
105. Paoletti AM, Serra GG, Cagnacci A, Vacca AMB, Guerriero S, Solla E, Melis GB (1996) Spontaneous reversibility of bone loss induced by gonadotropin-releasing hormone analog treatment. *Fertil Steril* 65:707–710.
106. Stevenson JC, Lees B, Gardner R, Shaw RW (1989) Comparison of the skeletal effects of goserelin and danazol in premenopausal women with endometriosis. *Horm Res* 32:S161-S163.

107. Bianchi G, Costantini S, Anserini P, Rovetta G, Monteforte P, Menada MV, Faga L, De Cecco L (1989) Effects of gonadotrophin-releasing hormone agonist on uterine fibroids and bone density. *Maturitas* 11:179–185.
108. Johansen JS, Riis BJ, Hassager C, Moen M, Jacobson J, Christiansen C (1988) The effect of a gonadotropin-releasing hormone agonist analog (nafarelin) on bone metabolism. *J Clin Endocrinol Metab* 67:701–706.
109. Riis BJ, Christiansen C, Johansen JS, Jacobson J (1990) Is it possible to prevent bone loss in young women treated with luteinizing hormone-releasing hormone agonists? *J Clin Endocrinol Metab* 70:920–924.
110. Ginsberg JS, Kowalchuk G, Hirsh J, Brill-Edwards P, burrows R, Coates G, Webber C (1990) Heparin effect on bone density. *Thromb Haemost* 64:286–289.
111. Passeri M, Biondi M, Costi D, Bufalino L, Castiglione GN, Di Peppe C, Abate G (1992) Effect of ipriflavone on bone mass in elderly osteoporotic women. *Bone Miner* 19:S57–S62.
112. Adami S, Bufalino L, Cervetti R, Di Marco C, Di Munno O, Fantasia L, et al. (1997) Ipriflavone prevents radial bone loss in postmenopausal women with low bone mass over 2 years. *Osteoporosis Int* 7:119–125.
113. Cundy T, Evans M, Roberts H, Wattie D, Ames R, Reid IR (1991) Bone density in women receiving depot medroxyprogesterone acetate for contraception. *Br Med J* 303:13–16.
114. Gennari C, AgnusDei D, Gonnelli S, Nardi P (1989) Effects of nandrolone decanoate therapy on bone mass and calcium metabolism in women with established postmenopausal osteoporosis: a double-blind placebo-controlled study. *Maturitas* 11:187–197.
115. Lufkin EG, Whitaker MD, Argueta R, Caplan RH, Nickelsen T, Riggs BL (1997) Raloxifene treatment of postmenopausal osteoporosis. *J Bone Miner Res* 12; S150.
116. Delmas PD, Bjarnason NH, Mitlak BH, Ravoux A, Shah AS, Huster WJ, Draper M, Christiansen C (1997) *N Engl J Med* 337:1641–1647.
117. McClung MR, Bensen W, Bolognese MA, Bonnick SL, Ettinger MP, Harris ST, et al. (1997) Risedronate increases BMD at the hip, spine and radius in postmenopausal women with low bone mass. Abstract. *J Bone Miner Res* 12:S169.
118. Stock JL, Avioli LV, Baylink DJ, Chesnut C, Genant HK, Maricic MJ, et al. (1997) Calcitonin-salmon nasal spray reduces the incidence of new vertebral fractures in postmenopausal women: three-year interim results of the PROOF study. Abstract. *J Bone Miner Res* 12:S149.
119. Overgaard K, Hansen MA, Jensen SB, Christiansen C (1992) Effect of salcatonin given intranasally on bone mass and fracture rates in established osteoporosis: a dose-response study. *Br Med J* 305:556–561.
120. Reginster JY, Deroisy R, Lecart MP, Sarlet N, Zegels B, Jupsin I, et al. (1995) A double-blind, placebo-controlled, dose-finding trial of intermittent nasal salmon calcitonin for prevention of postmenopausal lumbar spine bone loss. *Am J Med* 98:452–458.
121. Riggs BL, Hodgson SF, O'Fallon WM, Chao EYS, Wahner HW, Muhs JM, et al. (1990) Effect of fluoride treatment on the fracture rate in postmenopausal women with osteoporosis. *N Engl J Med* 322:802–809.
122. Pak CYC, Sakhaee K, Piziak V, Peterson RD, Breslau NA, Boyd P, et al. (1994) Slow-release sodium fluoride in the management of postmenopausal osteoporosis. *Ann Intern Med* 120:625–632.
123. Ryan WG, Wolter J, Bagdade JD (1991) Apparent beneficial effects of tamoxifen on bone mineral content in patients with breast cancer: preliminary study. *Osteoporosis Int* 2:39–41.

124. Love RR, Mazess RB, Barden HS, Epstein S, Newcomb PA, Jordan C, Carbone PP, DeMets DL (1992) Effects of tamoxifen on bone mineral density in postmenopausal women with breast cancer. *N Engl J Med* 326:852–886.
125. Grant DJ, McMurdo MET, Mole PA, Paterson CR, Davies RR (1993) Suppressed TSH levels secondary to thyroxine replacement therapy are not associated with osteoporosis. *Clin Endocrinol* 39:529–533.
126. Affinito P, Sorrentino C, Farace JM, di Carlo C, Moccia G, Canciello P, Palomba S, Nappi C (1996) Effects of thyroxine therapy on bone metabolism in postmenopausal women with hypothyroidism. *Acta Obstet Gynecol Scand* 75:843–848.
127. Guo CY, Weetman AP, Eastell R (1997) Longitudinal changes of bone mineral density and bone turnover in postmenopausal women on thyroxine. *Clin Endocrinol* 46:301–307.
128. Ross DS (1993) Bone density is not reduced during the short-term administration of levothyroxine to postmenopausal women with subclinical hypothyroidism: a randomized, prospective study. *Am J Med* 95:385–388.
129. Lindsay R, Hart DM, Kraszewski A (1980) Prospective double-blind trial of synthetic steroid (Org OD 14) for preventing postmenopausal osteoporosis. *Br Med J* 280:1207–1209.
130. Rymer J, Chapman MG, Fogelman I (1994) Effect of tibolone on postmenopausal bone loss. *Osteoporosis Int* 4:314–319.
131. Lippuner K, Haenggi W, Birkhaeuser MH, Casez J, Jaeger P (1997) Prevention of postmenopausal bone loss using tibolone or conventional peroral or transdermal hormone replacement with 17β-estradiol and dydrogesterone. *J Bone Miner Res* 12:806–812.

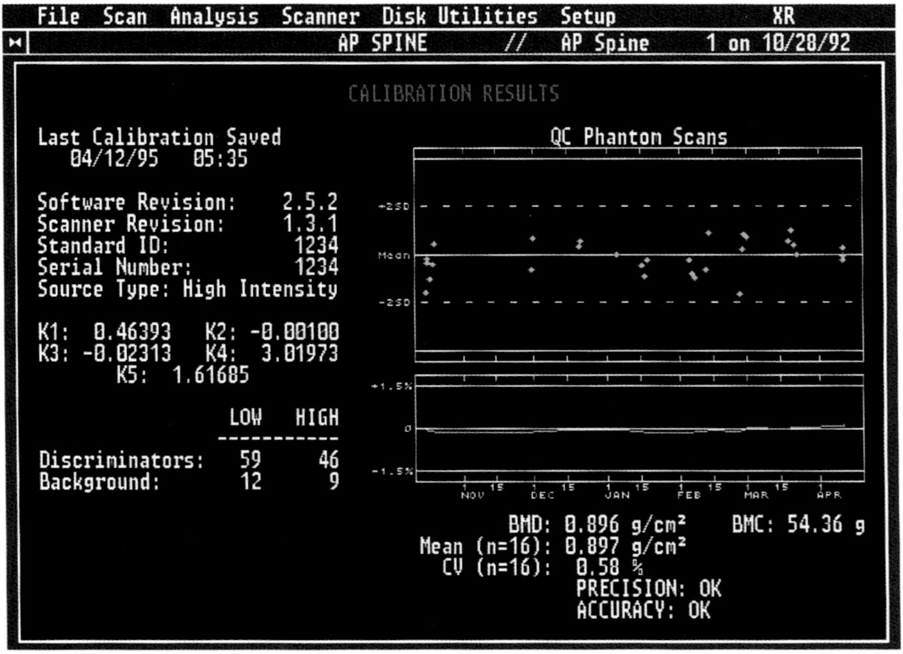

Plate 13 (Fig. 5-4; *see* full caption on p. 107 and discussion in Chapter 5).

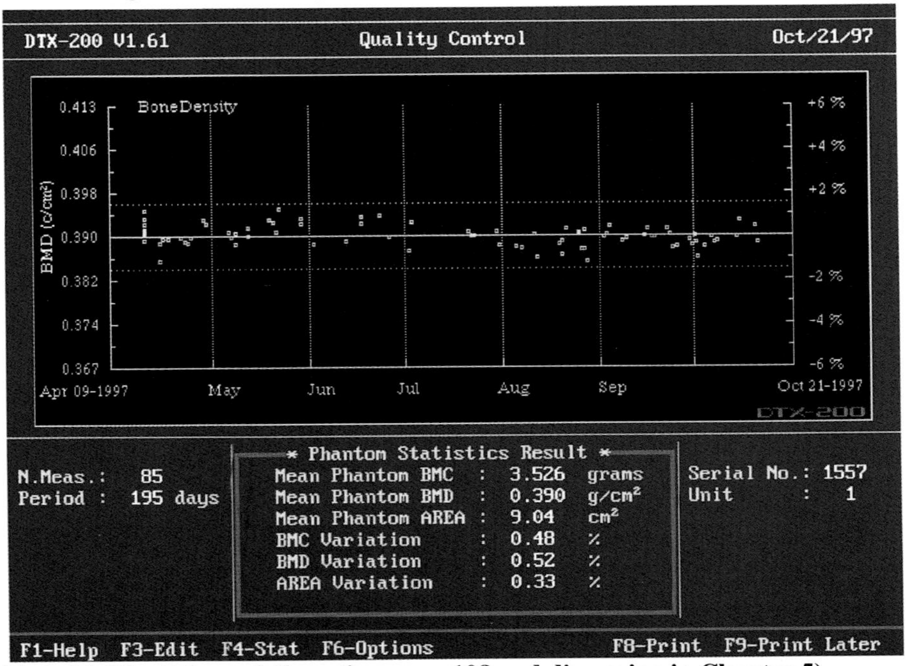

Plate 14 (Fig. 5-5; *see* full caption on p. 108 and discussion in Chapter 5).

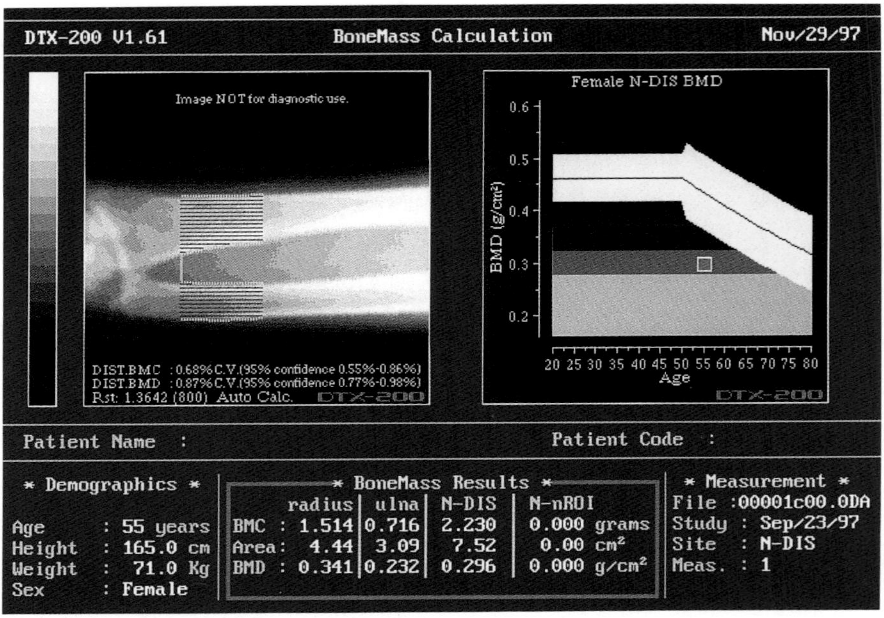

Plate 15 (Fig. 10-4; *see* full caption on p. 224 and discussion in Chapter 10).

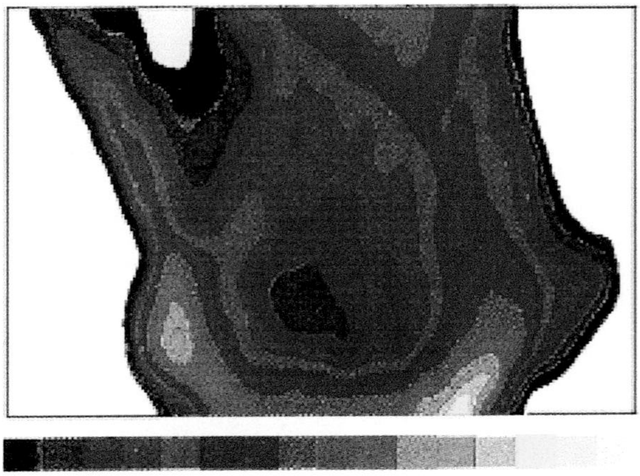

Plate 16 (Fig. 10-6; *see* full caption on p. 234 and discussion in Chapter 10).

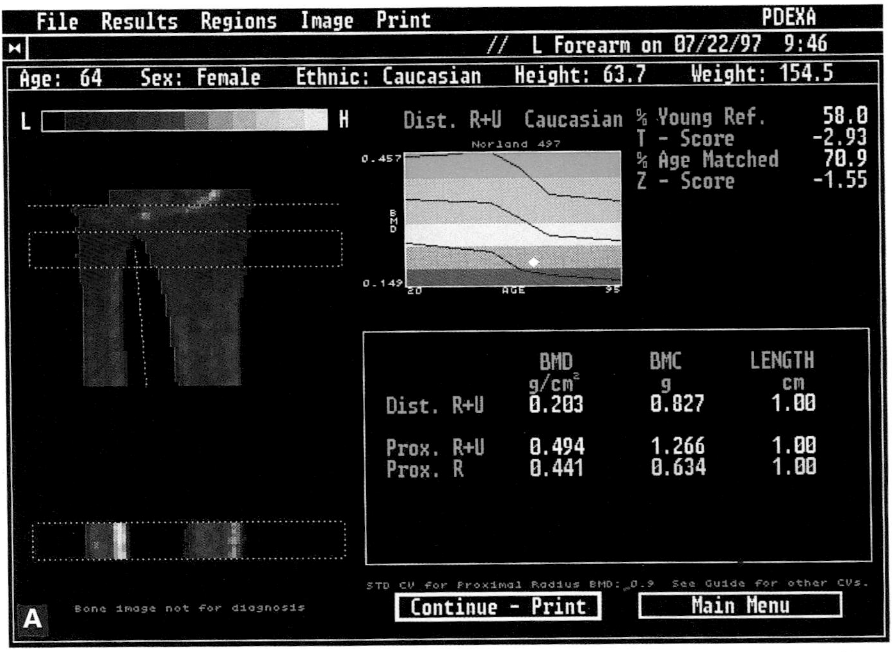

Plate 17 (Fig. 10-5A; *see* full caption on p. 228 and discussion in Chapter 10).

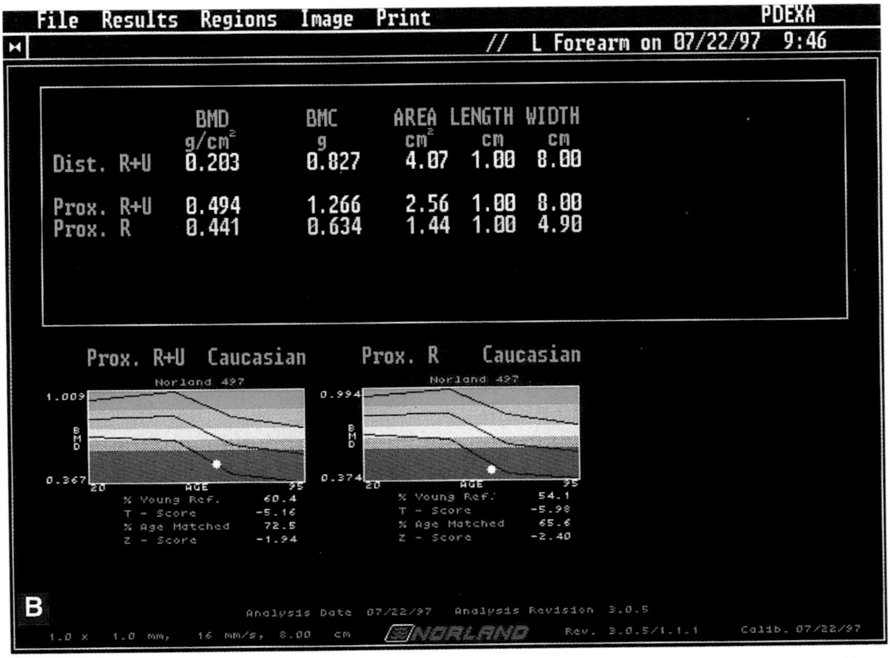

Plate 18 (Fig. 10-5B; *see* full caption on p. 229 and discussion in Chapter 10).

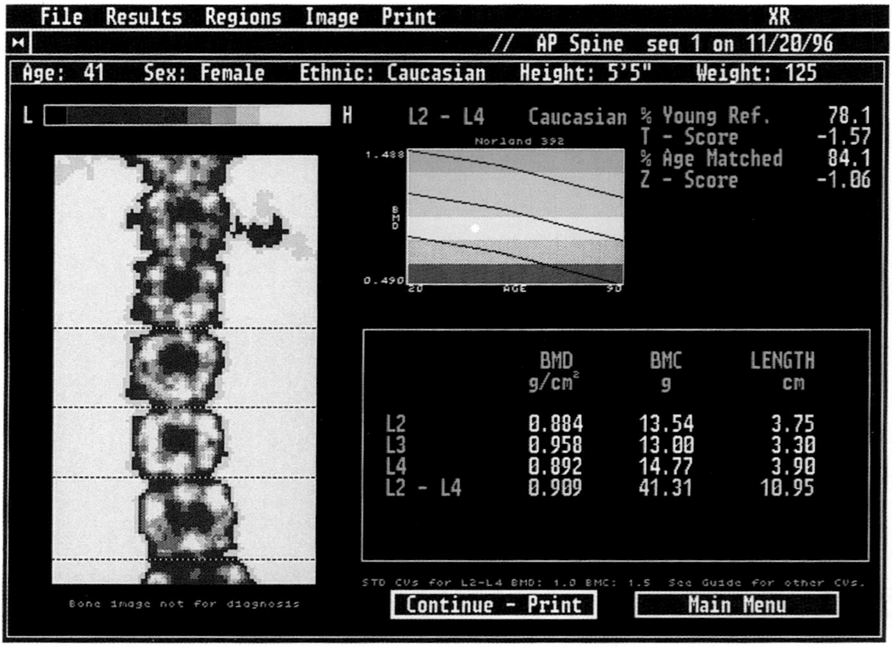

Plate 19 (Fig. 10-9; *see* full caption on p. 238 and discussion in Chapter 10).

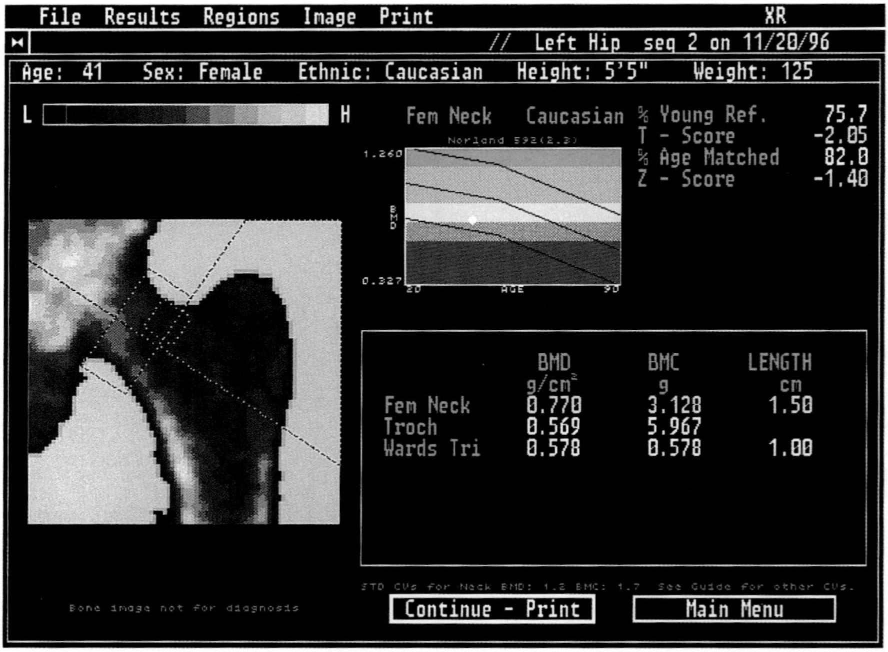

Plate 20 (Fig. 10-10; *see* full caption on p. 239 and discussion in Chapter 10).

8 Bone Density Data from DPA to DXA and Manufacturer to Manufacturer

CONTENTS

The extraordinary advances in bone-density technology over the past 30 years, enhancing the physician's ability to detect and manage metabolic bone disease, have also created a dilemma as physicians have attempted to compare results obtained on early dual-photon devices with today's dual-energy X-ray devices. As dual-energy X-ray technology has advanced, data from pencil-beam systems is now being compared with data from fan-array systems. Data from one manufacturer's pencil-beam DXA device may need to be compared to data from another manufacturer's pencil-beam device. This situation is not dissimilar to circumstances created during the evolution of other types of quantitative measurement techniques used in clinical medicine. For example, the measurement of some parameter in blood may have initially been performed using one type of assay, only to be later replaced by a different assay. There may be different ranges of normal, depending on the assay, and even depending on the laboratory. Although it would be ideal for a patient being followed with a quantitative measurement technique for any reason to return year after year to the same laboratory to be tested using the same assay, this is not a reasonable expectation. In the context of bone densitometry, it is useful to have some ability to compare measurements originally made with DPA to measurements being made with DXA. In addition, the differences between the values obtained on different manufacturers' DXA devices, with their respective reference ranges, must be appreciated.

FROM DPA TO DXA

When DXA was approved for clinical use in 1988, it was immediately apparent that these systems offered substantial advantages over ^{153}gadolinium-based DPA systems. It was just as clear, however, that, although the results obtained on any one patient with DXA were highly correlated with results from DPA, the BMD values were not identical.

Hologic DXA and Lunar DPA

Kelly et al. *(1)* evaluated the relationship between BMD values in the spine in 85 individuals ranging in age from 21 to 78 years, using the Lunar DP4 (Madison, WI), a ^{153}Gd DPA device, and the Hologic QDR-1000 (Waltham, MA), a pencil-beam DXA device. The correlation for the measurement of spine BMD between the two devices was extremely good, with $r = 0.98$. Of course, the two instruments did not give exactly the same results. Values obtained on the QDR-1000 were consistently lower than those obtained on the DP4. The equation that was derived to predict the DXA QDR-1000 values from the DPA values was:

$$QDR_{BMD} = (0.84 \times DPA_{BMD}) - 0.033$$

Pacifici et al. *(2)* evaluated lumbar spine BMD in 52 women, using the Hologic QDR-1000 and the Lunar DP4. Again, the results were correlated with a highly statistically significant r-value of 0.94. The values in the spine obtained with the QDR-1000 were approximately 6.8% lower than those obtained with the DP4. The equation for predicting the DP4 value from the measurement of the spine BMD with the QDR-1000 was:

$$DPA_{BMD} = 0.0242 + (1.0727 \times QDR_{BMD})$$

A larger comparison trial was performed by Holbrook et al. *(3)*, in which 176 individuals had lumbar spine bone-density studies, and 217 individuals had proximal femur bone-density studies on both the Hologic QDR-1000 and the Lunar DP3 (an early DPA device). Once again, the values obtained with the DXA device were consistently lower than those obtained with the DPA device for both the spine and proximal femur. The average difference in this study was 16%. Nevertheless, the BMDs, as measured with the two devices, were statistically correlated. In this study, equations were presented to allow the conversion of values obtained with the Hologic QDR-1000 to Lunar DP3 values. Equations for the BMDs in the spine were given for individual vertebrae, rather than an average. The equations were:

$$\text{L1 DP3}_{BMD} = 0.300 + (0.878 \times \text{L1 QDR}_{BMD})$$

$$\text{L2 DP3}_{BMD} = 0.239 + (0.944 \times \text{L2 QDR}_{BMD})$$

$$\text{L3 DP3}_{BMD} = 0.205 + (0.970 \times \text{L3 QDR}_{BMD})$$

$$\text{L4 DP3}_{BMD} = 0.152 + (1.005 \times \text{L4 QDR}_{BMD})$$

$$\text{Neck DP3}_{BMD} = 0.133 + (0.977 \times \text{Neck QDR}_{BMD})$$

$$\text{Ward's DP3}_{BMD} = 0.146 + (0.983 \times \text{Ward's QDR}_{BMD})$$

$$\text{Trochanter DP3}_{BMD} = 0.012 + (1.104 \times \text{Trochanter QDR}_{BMD})$$

Lunar DXA and Lunar DPA

BMD values in the spine, when obtained with the Lunar DPX, were originally reported as being approximately 3% lower than those that would be obtained with a Lunar DP3, based on an initial study of 41 subjects by Mazess et al. *(4)*.

Lees and Stevenson studied 70 subjects (2 men and 68 women), who underwent AP spine and proximal femur bone-density studies, using the Lunar DPX and Lunar DP3 *(5)*. The results between the two instruments were statistically significantly correlated. The *r*-value ranged from 0.96 at Ward's area in the proximal femur to 0.98 for the L2–L4 BMD. The BMD values in the lumbar spine were again lower when obtained on the DXA device than when obtained on the DPA device. The equation for predicting the L2–L4 BMD for the DPX from a measurement of L2–L4 on the DP3 was:

$$\text{L2–L4 DPX}_{BMD} = -0.110 + (1.052 \times \text{L2–L4 DP3}_{BMD})$$

There was less difference between the BMD values in the femoral neck, Ward's area, and the trochanter obtained on the DPX and DP3 than in the lumbar spine. At these sites in the proximal femur, however, the DPX values were slightly higher than the DP3 values. The equations for predicting the values that would be anticipated on the DPX from measurements of the proximal femur sites on the DP3 were:

$$\text{Neck DPX}_{BMD} = 0.028 + (1.002 \times \text{Neck DP3}_{BMD})$$

$$\text{Ward's DPX}_{BMD} = 0.004 + (1.031 \times \text{Ward's DP3}_{BMD})$$

$$\text{Trochanter DPX}_{BMD} = 0.043 + (0.955 \times \text{Trochanter DP3}_{BMD})$$

The general relationship between Lunar DP4 values and Hologic QDR-1000 and Lunar DPX values is summarized in a study from McClung and Roberts *(6)*. Ninety-three subjects underwent bone density measurements on all three machines at the AP spine and proximal femur. The ratio of mean values obtained for each combination of machines is shown in Table 8-1.

Table 8-1
Ratio of Values at the AP Lumbar Spine and Proximal Femur Obtained on 93 Subjects on the Lunar DP4, Lunar DPX, and Hologic QDR-1000

Site	*DPX/DP4*	*QDR/DP4*	*QDR/DPX*
AP Lumbar spine	0.89	0.78	0.87
Femoral neck	1.02	0.90	0.88
Trochanter	0.99	0.83	0.83
Ward's area	1.02	0.73	0.72

Calculated from data from ref. *6*.

Although these equations can be used to predict DXA values from earlier DPA measurements and vice versa, the margin of error in these equations limits their utility to exactly predict BMD. They can be used to approximate the BMD, however. This is often reassuring to the patient who has previously had a DPA study, and is now undergoing a DXA study. Even if there has been no change in the BMD over time, the spine BMD on the DXA study is expected to be lower. If the DXA device is a Hologic or Norland DXA (Fort Atkinson, WI) device, the BMDs in the proximal femur are also expected to be lower. If the DXA device is a Lunar device, the BMDs in the proximal femur may be slightly higher.

DXA: FROM LUNAR TO HOLOGIC TO NORLAND

All three manufacturers of central DXA devices produce machines with superior accuracy and precision in quantifying the bone density at virtually any skeletal site. The results obtained on any one machine, however, will not be identical to those obtained on either of the other two. Comparison studies using combinations of these machines can provide conversion equations for the measurement of bone density on one device to the anticipated measurement on another device.

The Hologic QDR-1000, the Lunar DPX, and the Norland XR-26 were compared in an in vitro study by Arai et al. *(7)*. Solutions of various concentrations of potassium phosphate, enclosed in an acrylic resin and then submerged in water, were used to simulate BMD. Each of the three machines was used to measure the various concentrations of potassium phosphate, to determine both the accuracy of the machines and the correlation between the BMDs as measured by each of the machines. Each machine accurately measured the BMD. The correlation between each pair of machines was highly statistically significant, with an r-value of 0.9999. The measured values were not identical, however. Values obtained with the DPX were 8.08% higher than those obtained with the XR-26, and

4.96% higher than those obtained with the QDR-1000. The QDR-1000 values were 2.96% higher than those obtained with the XR-26. An anthropomorphic Hologic spine phantom was also used in this study to compare the three DXA devices. The spine phantom was scanned 10 times on each manufacturer's machine. The BMD values obtained on the Lunar DPX were 16% higher than those obtained on the XR-26; the values obtained on the QDR-1000 were 1.5% lower than the XR-26.

Hologic DXA and Norland DXA

In vivo comparisons of spine measurements made using the Norland XR-26 and the Hologic QDR-1000 were conducted by Lai et al. *(8)* in 65 subjects. The correlation for BMD at the spine was 0.990, and was highly significant. BMDs obtained on the Norland XR-26 tended to be lower than those obtained on the QDR-1000. The equation for predicting the Hologic BMD from the measurement of BMD on the Norland XR-26 was:

$$\text{Hologic QDR 1000 Spine}_{\text{BMD}} = -0.1 + (1.09 \times \text{Norland XR-26 Spine}_{\text{BMD}})$$

Lunar DXA and Hologic DXA

The Lunar DPX and the Hologic QDR-1000 have also been compared in a study of 46 women by Pocock et al. *(9)*. These women underwent lumbar spine and proximal femur studies on both machines on the same day. The correlations were extremely good, with *r*-values of 0.98, 0.94, 0.96, and 0.96 for the lumbar spine, femoral neck, Ward's area, and the trochanter, respectively. The absolute BMD values were 16% lower on the QDR-1000 in the spine when compared to the DPX, and 17% lower in the femoral neck. The equation for predicting the QDR BMD in the femoral neck, based on a measurement of BMD in the femoral neck on the Lunar DPX, was:

$$\text{QDR Femoral neck}_{\text{BMD}} = 0.007 + (0.76 \times \text{DPX Femoral neck}_{\text{BMD}})$$

STANDARDIZATION OF ABSOLUTE BMD RESULTS

It is clear from the extremely good correlations between the measurements of BMD at the various sites, using the DXA devices from the three major manufacturers of central DXA devices in the United States, that these devices are indeed measuring the thing. But, because of differences in calibration and bone-edge detection algorithms, the absolute values obtained on the various machines can differ markedly. Because of this, there has been a great deal of interest in developing a standardized BMD to which all DXA results could be converted, regardless of which

Table 8-2
Conversion Formulas for BMDs of the AP Spine Between DXA Devices

Hologic QDR-2000 $Spine_{BMD}$ = (0.906 × Lunar DPX-L $Spine_{BMD}$) – 0.025
Hologic QDR-2000 $Spine_{BMD}$ = (0.912 × Norland XR 26 $Spine_{BMD}$) + 0.088
Lunar DPX-L $Spine_{BMD}$ = (1.074 × Hologic QDR 2000 $Spine_{BMD}$) + 0.054
Lunar DPX-L $Spine_{BMD}$ = (0.995 × Norland XR 26 $Spine_{BMD}$) + 0.135
Norland XR-26 $Spine_{BMD}$ = (0.983 × Lunar DPX-L $Spine_{BMD}$) – 0.112
Norland XR-26 $Spine_{BMD}$ = (1.068 × Hologic QDR 2000 $Spine_{BMD}$) – 0.070

Adapted from the *Journal of Bone and Mineral Research* 1994;9:1503–1514 with permission from the American Society for Bone and Mineral Research.

manufacturer's machine was used. In November 1990, the major manufacturers of DXA equipment agreed to work together in the area of standards, as part of the International Committee for Standards in Bone Measurement. Under the auspices of this committee, a study of 100 healthy women was performed, in which each of the women underwent AP spine and proximal femur studies on the Hologic QDR-2000, the Norland XR-26 Mark II, and the Lunar DPX-L *(10)*. The women ranged in age from 20 to 80, with an average age of 52.6 years. The difference in BMD in the spine was greatest between the Norland XR-26 and the Lunar DPX-L, averaging 0.118 g/cm^2, or 12.2%. The difference between the Lunar DPX-L and the Hologic QDR-2000 averaged 0.113 g/cm^2, or 11.7%. Between the Norland XR-26 and the Hologic QDR-2000, the average difference in BMD in the lumbar spine was only 0.012 g/cm^2, or 1.3%.

Based on this data, equations were derived for the conversion of lumbar spine BMD obtained on one manufacturer's machine to the BMD that would be expected to be obtained on each of the other two. These equations for each of the three pairs of scanners are shown in Table 8-2.

In order to convert each manufacturer's absolute BMD to a standardized BMD (sBMD), the European spine phantom (ESP) was scanned on each of the three devices. Based on those results, formulas for converting each manufacturer's absolute BMD in the spine to a standardized spine BMD were derived. These formulas are shown in Table 8-3.

The value for the sBMD is multiplied by 1000 to convert it to mg/cm^2, rather than reporting it as g/cm^2, in order to readily distinguish this value from the nonstandardized value. In other words, if the BMD obtained in the spine on a Lunar DPX-L is 0.985 g/cm^2, this value becomes 938 mg/cm^2 when reported as the sBMD (0.985 × 0.9522 = 0.9379 g/cm^2 × 1000 = 938 mg/cm^2). Using these formulas to convert the average spine BMD for the study population to the sBMD, the differences in BMD between the three machines was greatly reduced. Instead of an average difference of

Table 8-3
Formulas for Conversion of Manufacturer-Specific AP Spine BMDs to the Standardized BMD (sBMD)

$sBMD_{SPINE} = 1000\ (1.076 \times \text{Norland XR-26 } BMD_{SPINE})$
$sBMD_{SPINE} = 1000\ (0.9522 \times \text{Lunar DPX-L } BMD_{SPINE})$
$sBMD_{SPINE} = 1000\ (1.0755 \times \text{Hologic QDR-2000 } BMD_{SPINE})$

Adapted from the *Journal of Bone and Mineral Research* 1994; 9:1503–1514 with permission from the American Society for Bone and Mineral Research.

Table 8-4
Conversion Formulas for BMDs in Proximal Femur Between DXA Devices

$\text{Hologic QDR-2000 } Neck_{BMD} = (0.836 \times \text{Lunar DPX-L } Neck_{BMD}) - 0.008$
$\text{Hologic QDR-2000 } Neck_{BMD} = (0.836 \times \text{Norland XR 26 } Neck_{BMD}) + 0.051$
$\text{Lunar DPX-L } Neck_{BMD} = (1.013 \times \text{Hologic QDR 2000 } Neck_{BMD}) + 0.142$
$\text{Lunar DPX-L } Neck_{BMD} = (0.945 \times \text{Norland XR 26 } Neck_{BMD}) + 0.115$
$\text{Norland XR-26 } Neck_{BMD} = (0.961 \times \text{Lunar DPX-L } Neck_{BMD}) - 0.037$
$\text{Norland XR-26 } Neck_{BMD} = (1.030 \times \text{Hologic QDR 2000 } Neck_{BMD}) + 0.058$

Adapted from the *Journal of Bone and Mineral Research* 1994;9:1503–1514 with permission from the American Society for Bone and Mineral Research.

12.2% between the Norland and Lunar values, the difference using sBMD was only 2.8%. The difference between Hologic and Lunar was reduced to 2.2%, and the difference between Hologic and Norland was 2.7%.

Conversion formulas were also developed for the femoral neck for each pair of scanners. These formulas are shown in Table 8-4.

In December 1996, the International Committee for Standards in Bone Measurement approved the sBMD for the total femur region of interest *(11)*. The total femur region of interest includes the femoral neck, Ward's area, the trochanter, and the shaft of the proximal femur. This region appears to have equal diagnostic utility, but better precision than the femoral neck. The formulas for the sBMD for the total femur, shown in Table 8-5, were based on the work by Genant et al. *(10)*, from which the formulas for sBMD of the spine were also derived. The sBMD from any one of the three central DXA devices should fall within 3–6% of the sBMD on any of the other two.

FROM DXA MACHINE TO DXA MACHINE WITHIN MANUFACTURERS

It is not uncommon for patients to have had a DXA study at one facility that must be compared to a DXA study at a second facility. Even if the

Table 8-5
Formulas for Conversion of Manufacturer-Specific Total Femur BMD to Standardized BMD (sBMD)

$sBMD_{TOTAL\ FEMUR}$	$= 1000\ [(1.008 \times \text{Hologic BMD}_{TOTAL\ FEMUR}) + 0.006]$
$sBMD_{TOTAL\ FEMUR}$	$= 1000\ [(0.979 \times \text{Lunar BMD}_{TOTAL\ FEMUR}) - 0.031]$
$sBMD_{TOTAL\ FEMUR}$	$= 1000\ [(1.012 \times \text{Norland BMD}_{TOTAL\ FEMUR}) + 0.026]$

From ref. *11*.

studies have been performed on DXA machines from the same manufacturer, the results may vary slightly. If the machines have been properly calibrated and maintained, using good quality-control measures (*see* Chapter 5), the differences should be minimal. In a study performed at three different sites, three men and two women underwent total-body and lumbar spine bone-density studies in duplicate at each site *(12)*. The studies were performed on a Lunar DPX-L at one site, and on a Lunar DPX at the other two sites. The differences in total-body BMD between the three sites were <1.2%, and the differences in lumbar spine BMD among the three sites were <1.7%. When this is expressed as the percent coefficient of variation (%CV) between sites, the %CV for total-body BMD between sites was 0.7%, and for the lumbar spine, 1.4%. Two similar studies using the Hologic QDR-1000 also demonstrated good agreement between BMD studies performed at different sites on the Hologic DXA device. The %CV at the spine between 13 sites in one study was 1.4% for the spine and 2.1% for the hip *(13)*. In a second study, the %CV at the spine between eight sites for in vitro phantom measurements was 0.92%. For in vivo measurements on two subjects, the %CV at the spine was 3.68 and 1.85% at the femoral neck *(14)*. Although some of the intersite variation may be a result of differences in positioning or analysis, differences in machine calibration are also likely to be responsible. These types of differences between machines from the same manufacturer are not large enough to cause problems in the diagnosis of low bone mass, or the prediction of fracture risk, but they do present problems in the serial assessment of changes in BMD. Clearly, intersite variation between machines from the same manufacturers can be much larger than that indicated here, if strict quality-control procedures are not observed at densitometry sites.

FROM PENCIL-BEAM TO FAN-ARRAY DXA DATA

The latest generation of central DXA scanners are fan-array scanners, which were first introduced with the Hologic QDR-2000 *(15)*. The terminology reflects a change in design in these scanners, in which a fan-shaped beam is projected through an entire scan line and captured by an array of detectors. This is markedly different from the earlier pencil-beam devices, in which a very narrow X-ray beam was projected in a plane that was perpendicular to the region of interest. This narrowed beam moved in tandem with a single detector in a rectilinear path across the region of interest. Fan-array technology, such as found on the Hologic QDR-4500 and the Lunar Expert, has resulted in extraordinary skeletal image resolution and faster scan speeds. Extraordinary images, such as those seen in Fig. 1-16, are being utilized in a new application for densitometry: skeletal morphometry. The dimensions of the various regions of the skeleton can be accurately and precisely measured with fan-array technology and today's sophisticated computers.

The difference in design between pencil-beam systems and fan-array systems has introduced a confounding issue in comparing data generated on any manufacturer's pencil-beam device to data generated on the same manufacturer's fan-array device. Because the imaging geometry is different, there can be some magnification of the image that is dependent on the distance of the region of interest from the beam and detectors. BMC and area measurements can be affected. Because the BMC and area measurement should be altered to a similar degree, the effect on BMD theoretically should be minimal (because BMD is calculated by dividing BMC by area).

Using the Hologic spine phantom, Eiken et al. *(16)* compared the measurement of area, BMC, and BMD on the QDR-1000/W, a pencil-beam device, with that obtained on the QDR-2000, a fan-array device. As predicted, the BMC and area increased to a similar degree, leaving the BMD unchanged when measurements were obtained on the QDR-2000, compared to the QDR-1000/W. Blake et al. *(17)* confirmed these findings, using both spine phantom and spine and hip measurements on 20 subjects.

In a larger study, Faulkner et al. *(18)* evaluated the differences in BMD in the spine and proximal femur obtained using the Hologic QDR-1000/W and the Hologic QDR-2000. Sixty-nine women underwent AP spine and proximal femur studies on both devices. At the spine, there were no statistically significant differences observed in the BMC, area, or BMD between the pencil-beam and fan-array device, although the BMD obtained with the fan-array device was slightly higher. In the proximal femur, BMD values obtained with the fan-array device were again all slightly higher than those obtained with the pencil-beam device. Although the differences in BMD for all regions in the proximal femur, except the femoral neck, were statistically significant, the absolute differences were extremely small. Similarly, BMC and area measurements were all slightly increased when obtained on the fan-array device for all regions in the proximal femur, with the exception of the femoral neck. The differences in BMD between the pencil-beam device and the fan-array device were not large enough to be clinically significant, in terms of the accuracy of the measurement and comparisons to the reference databases developed using the pencil-beam device. This does introduce an additional source of error into serial measurements, however. The differences in BMD in the regions of the proximal femur between the pencil-beam and fan-array device ranged from 1.4 to 1.8%. This change in BMD, which is the result solely of changing from a pencil-beam to a fan-array device, must be kept in mind if the physician attempts to compare scans obtained on a patient over a period of time that were acquired using both devices.

REFERENCE DATABASES

Two of the most common applications of bone densitometry today are in the diagnosis of osteoporosis and the assessment of fracture risk. These applications depend on comparisons of the absolute BMD to the reference databases that are supplied by the manufacturers of bone densitometry equipment. The diagnosis of osteopenia or osteoporosis, using World Health Organization criteria, depend on comparing the patient's BMD to the average peak BMD of the young adult, and noting how many standard deviations (SDs) below this value the patient's value lies. In other words, this diagnosis is dependent on the young-adult *z*-score or *T*-score. Most fracture-risk data in the medical literature are presented as the increase in relative risk per SD decline in bone density. Fracture risk for an individual patient can then be calculated, based on the knowledge of the number of SDs below the peak young-adult BMD that the patient's BMD lies. These clinical applications depend, therefore, not only on the measurement of the BMD, but on the values that are calculated from comparisons to the reference databases. Each manufacturer of bone density equipment has independently created a reference database for their equipment.

It is logistically impossible to have every member a population in a given country undergo bone-density measurements in order to create a reference database. Therefore, a sample of the population is studied to create this reference population. From that sample, the average BMD value for the young-adult, and for each age group, can be calculated. Depending on the makeup of the individuals in the sample, a slightly different average or mean BMD will be obtained with each sample of the population that is studied. As was seen in Chapter 3, the SD (upon which the *T*-score and young-adult *z*-score are based), which is calculated for the values from any given sample, is dependent on the average value of the sample and the number of individuals that make up that sample. Thus, the SD will also vary from sample to sample. Once the data are collected, different statistical methods can be employed to create the reference curves for the population. In the creation of reference databases, each manufacturer has necessarily utilized a different sample of the population, and then applied the statistical methods that were most appropriate for that sample.

These statistical and design issues confound the recognized systematic differences in the measurement of bone mass and density between the different manufacturers' devices. The BMD values between machines can be converted using the calibration equations noted previously to another manufacturer's machine. The BMD values can also be converted to a standardized BMD. This does not solve the potential clinical dilemma posed by the practical necessity of different samples within a population being used to create the various databases.

Pocock et al. *(9)* observed the effect of differences in the reference databases between the Hologic QDR-1000 and the Lunar DPX on the percentage of young-adult and age-matched comparisons for the spine and femoral neck, after studying 46 women. The percentage comparisons for the spine tended to be very similar on the two devices. In the femoral neck, however, the % young-adult comparisons were 6.2% lower on the QDR-1000. The % age-matched comparisons were 3.3% lower on the QDR-1000.

Other authors have confirmed these observations. Laskey et al. *(19)* noted the effect of the differences in databases used for the Lunar DPX and the Hologic QDR-1000 for spine and proximal femur bone density. Fifty-three subjects underwent spine and proximal femur bone-density measurements on the same day on both devices. Laskey, like Pocock, found that the comparisons of the measured BMD to the reference database for the young adult or age-matched adult in the spine were similar. In the regions in the proximal femur, however, the differences were substantial. The magnitude of the difference approximated the magnitude of a 1 SD change. This is a sufficient difference to have profound clinical ramifications. For example, applying the WHO BMD criteria for the diagnosis of normalcy, osteopenia, or osteoporosis, a 1-SD difference could result in a different diagnosis, depending on which manufacturer's machine was used.

This problem was also studied by Faulkner et al. *(20)*. *T*-scores and young-adult *z*-scores at the spine were compared for 83 women, and in the proximal femur for 120 women who underwent bone-density studies on a Lunar DPX and Hologic QDR-1000/W. The difference between the *T*-scores in the spine on the QDR-1000/W and the young-adult *z*-scores on the Lunar DPX was not statistically or clinically significant, since it was <0.1 SD. In the femoral neck, however, there was a systematic difference of 0.9 SD.

Faulkner et al. *(20)* observed that these differences in the reference databases could be caused by a combination of factors: different inclusion criteria, relatively small numbers of individuals used to calculate the average and SD young-adult values, and different statistical methods employed in the calculation of the reference curves. Faulkner suggested correcting the proximal femur data from both manufacturers by employing proximal femur data that was obtained during the NHANES III study of the United States population. This is data that was collected between 1988 and 1991, using the Hologic QDR-1000 *(21)*. As originally reported, there were 194 non-Hispanic white women aged 20–29, whose data was used to calculate the young-adult mean BMD value and SD in five regions in the proximal femur. The average BMD in the femoral neck for these young adults from NHANES III was reported to be 0.849 g/cm^2, with a SD of 0.11 g/cm^2. These values were substituted for the average and SD values used in the QDR-1000 reference database of 0.895 and 0.10 g/cm^2, respectively. The equivalent Lunar DPX BMD young-adult BMD was then calculated using the cross-calibration equation from Genant et al. *(10)*. This resulted in a Lunar value of 1.000 g/cm^2 for the average young-adult BMD in the femoral neck, compared to the value of 0.980 g/cm^2 used in the manufacturer-supplied database prior to October 1997. The SD for the young-adult of 0.11 g/cm^2 from NHANES III was substituted for the Lunar-reported SD of 0.12 g/cm^2. When the *T*-scores and young-adult *z*-scores were recalculated for each machine using the corrected values based on the NHANES III data, the differences between the two manufacturer's databases largely disappeared.

NHANES III was conducted by the National Center for Health Statistics, Centers for Disease Control and Prevention. During the study, proximal femur bone density data was collected on 7116 men and women aged 20 and older *(21)*. There were a total of 3217 non-Hispanic whites, 1831 non-Hispanic blacks, and 1840 Mexican-Americans in this study population. There were no specific inclusion or exclusion criteria used to select individuals for bone-density measurements in this study, other than the presence of prior hip fracture or pregnancy, which were grounds for exclusion. The individuals who received bone-density measurements were otherwise part of a random sample of the population.

All three major manufacturer's of central DXA devices provide extensive reference databases for their machines. Methodological descriptions of the acquisition of these databases can be found in the operator's manuals for the devices *(22–24)*. Table 8-6 compares the young-adult peak BMD values and SDs for the L2–L4 AP spine and femoral neck for the reference databases of the three major manufacturers of central DXA devices (prior to the adoption of NHANES III femur data), and for NHANES III data *(25)*. Tables 8-7 through 8-23 provide more detailed information on each of the databases currently in use in the United States for Caucasian men and women.

Table 8-6
Mean and SDs for Peak BMD in g/cm^2 in Caucasian Women from Various Manufacturer's Reference Databases and NHANES III

Reference data	*AP Spine L2-4 (SD)*	*Femoral neck (SD)*
Hologic[a]	1.047 (0.110)	0.895 (0.100)
Lunar[b]	1.188 (0.120)	0.994 (0.120)
Norland US[c]	1.164 (0.162)	0.928 (0.131)
Norland Europe	1.085 (0.115)	0.900 (0.120)
NHANES III[d]	—	0.849 (0.109)

[a]Release date 11/91; femur data has now been replaced with NHANES III femur data.
[b]Reference data prior to 10/97.
[c]Release date 3/92.
[d]As acquired on a Hologic QDR device.

Adapted with permission from the publisher from Simmons A, et al. (1997) The effects of standardization and reference values on patient classification for spine and femur dual-energy X-ray absorptiometry. *Osteoporosis International* 7:200–206.

Table 8-7
Reference BMD Values in g/cm^2 for Caucasian Women on Norland XR-Series Bone Densitometer

Age	*L2–4 AP Spine (SD) n = 613*	*Femoral neck (SD) n = 613*	*Ward's (SD) n = 613*	*Trochanter (SD) n = 613*
20	1.164 (0.162)	0.928 (0.131)	1.030 (0.139)	0.787 (0.124)
50	1.050 (0.162)	0.796 (0.131)	0.803 (0.139)	0.708 (0.124)
90	0.814 (0.162)	0.616 (0.131)	0.439 (0.139)	0.481 (0.124)

Release date 3/92. Reproduced with permission from Norland Medical Systems, Ft. Atkinson, WI.

Table 8-8
Reference BMD Values in g/cm^2 for Caucasian Men on the Norland XR-Series Bone Densitometer

Age	*L2–4 AP Spine (SD)*	*Femoral neck (SD)*	*Trochanter (SD)*
20	1.109 (0.167)	1.048 (0.119)	0.884 (0.140)
80	0.947 (0.167)	0.652 (0.119)	0.638 (0.140)

Release date 3/92. Reproduced with permission from Norland Medical Systems, Ft. Atkinson, WI.

Table 8-9
Mean BMD Values for L2–L4
for Caucasian Men and Women on the Lunar DPX

	Women		*Men*	
Age	n	*Mean*	n	*Mean*
20–29	467	1.188	85	1.255
30–39	499	1.207	106	1.215
40–49	716	1.170	73	1.174
50–59	969	1.081	67	1.161
60–69	476	0.995	63	1.183
70–79	105	0.960	51	1.178
Totals	3232		445	

SD = 0.12 g/cm^2 (data in use prior to 10/97).
Reproduced with permission of Lunar, Madison WI.

Table 8-10
Mean BMD Values for Regions in Proximal Femur
for Caucasian Women on Lunar DPX

Age	N	*Neck*	*Ward's*	*Trochanter*
20–29	479	0.994	0.947	0.798
30–39	499	0.958	0.886	0.787
40–49	704	0.950	0.847	0.792
50–59	882	0.881	0.751	0.745
60–69	415	0.811	0.660	0.714
70–79	121	0.773	0.630	0.668
Totals	3100			

SD = 0.12 g/cm^2 (data in use prior to 10/97).
Reproduced with permission of Lunar, Madison WI.

Table 8-11
Mean BMD Values for Regions in Proximal Femur
for Caucasian Women on Lunar DPX

Age	N	*Neck*	*Ward's*	*Trochanter*
20–29	84	1.107	1.022	0.948
30–39	95	1.038	0.922	0.900
40–49	74	1.001	0.852	0.898
50–59	73	0.985	0.809	0.920
60–69	66	0.953	0.770	0.904
70–79	46	0.872	0.685	0.841
Totals	438			

SD = 0.12 g/cm^2 (data in use prior to 10/97).
Reproduced with permission of Lunar, Madison WI.

Table 8-12
Lunar Reference Data for Caucasian Women as of October 1997

Age	*AP Spine BMD*	*Lateral spine BMD*	*Femoral neck BMD*	*Total body BMD*
20–29	1.200	0.790	0.998	1.120
30–39	1.214	0.764	0.973	1.141
40–49	1.180	0.718	0.946	1.123
50–59	1.096	0.628	0.881	1.086
60–69	1.016	0.522	0.818	1.030
70–79	0.988	0.502	0.767	0.998
n	8905	1318	7811	2154

These values apply to the United States, Northern Europe, Australia, and South Africa. BMD values are in g/cm^2.

Reproduced with permission of Lunar, Madison, WI.

Table 8-13
Lunar Reference Data for Caucasian Men as of October 1997

Age	*AP Spine BMD*	*Lateral spine BMD*	*Femoral neck BMD*	*Total body BMD*
20–29	1.241	0.919	1.098	1.234
30–39	1.215	0.938	1.045	1.215
40–49	1.180	0.892	0.984	1.210
50–59	1.145	0.813	0.956	1.232
60–69	1.157	0.726	0.909	1.203
70–79	1.173	0.721	0.876	1.177
n	1460	392	1734	655

These values apply to the United States, Northern Europe, Australia, and South Africa. BMD values are in g/cm^2.

Reproduced with permission of Lunar, Madison, WI.

With the development of the cross-calibration equations between manufacturers, and the sBMD for the total femur, it became possible for the proximal femur data from NHANES III to be adopted as a common femur database for manufacturers, even though the data was obtained solely on Hologic DXA devices. Based on the equations for sBMD, the mean sBMD for U.S. white women aged 20–29 is 956 mg/cm^2, with a SD of 123 mg/cm^2 *(11)*. Age-specific reference data, using the sBMD for the total femur from NHANES III, is shown in Table 8-24. Standardized NHANES III proximal femur data are being offered as part of the reference databases by manu-

(text continued on p. 194)

Table 8-14
Hologic Reference Data for L1–L4 BMD for Caucasian Women (Release Date 11/91)

Age	*L1–L4 (g/cm^2)*
20	1.019
25	1.040
30	1.047
35	1.041
40	1.024
45	0.999
50	0.967
60	0.892
70	0.815
80	0.752
85	0.731

SD is 0.110 g/cm^2. Peak BMD is the value for the 30-year-old woman.

Reproduced courtesy of Hologic Inc., Waltham, MA.

Table 8-15
Hologic Reference Data for Five Regions of the Proximal Femur for Caucasian Women (Release Date 11/91; in use prior to the adoption of NHANES III data on 2/1/97)

Age	*Neck (g/cm^2)*	*Ward's (g/cm^2)*	*Trochanteric (g/cm^2)*	*Intertrochanteric (g/cm^2)*	*Total (g/cm^2)*
20	0.895	0.796	0.707	1.134	0.966
25	0.894	0.779	0.718	1.145	0.975
30	0.886	0.756	0.722	1.148	0.975
35	0.871	0.727	0.718	1.142	0.968
40	0.850	0.693	0.709	1.128	0.955
45	0.826	0.655	0.695	1.107	0.935
50	0.797	0.615	0.676	1.080	0.910
55	0.766	0.574	0.655	1.047	0.881
60	0.733	0.532	0.630	1.009	0.849
65	0.700	0.491	0.604	0.967	0.813
70	0.667	0.452	0.578	0.922	0.776
75	0.636	0.416	0.551	0.874	0.738
80	0.607	0.385	0.525	0.824	0.699
85	0.581	0.358	0.502	0.773	0.660
SD	0.100	0.110	0.090	0.140	0.120
Age at peak	22	20	30	29	28

Reproduced courtesy of Hologic Inc., Waltham, MA.

Table 8-16
Hologic Reference Data for L1–L4 BMD for Caucasian Men (Release Date 11/91)

Age	*L1–L4 (g/cm²)*
20	1.091
25	1.091
35	1.091
45	1.068
50	1.053
55	1.038
60	1.023
65	1.008
70	0.993
75	0.978
80	0.963
85	0.947

SD is 0.110 g/cm^2.
Reproduced courtesy of Hologic, Waltham, MA.

Table 8-17
Hologic Reference Data for Five Regions of Proximal Femur for Caucasian Men (Release Date 10/91; in use prior to the adoption of NHANES III data on 2/1/97)

Age	*Neck (g/cm²)*	*Ward's (g/cm²)*	*Trochanteric (g/cm²)*	*Intertrochanteric (g/cm²)*	*Total (g/cm²)*
20	0.979	0.832	0.797	1.243	1.072
25	0.958	0.801	0.788	1.228	1.058
30	0.936	0.769	0.779	1.212	1.043
35	0.915	0.737	0.770	1.197	1.029
40	0.894	0.706	0.761	1.181	1.015
45	0.873	0.674	0.752	1.166	1.001
50	0.851	0.642	0.743	1.150	0.986
55	0.830	0.611	0.734	1.135	0.972
60	0.809	0.579	0.725	1.119	0.958
65	0.788	0.547	0.716	1.103	0.944
70	0.766	0.516	0.707	1.088	0.929
75	0.745	0.484	0.699	1.072	0.915
80	0.724	0.452	0.690	1.057	0.901
85	0.703	0.421	0.681	1.041	0.887
SD	0.110	0.120	0.110	0.150	0.130
Age at peak	20	20	20	20	20

Reproduced courtesy of Hologic Inc., Waltham, MA.

Table 8-18
NHANES III Femoral Neck BMD Data
for Non-Hispanic White Women as Acquired on the Hologic QDR-1000

Age	N	*Mean BMD (g/cm²)*	*SD (g/cm²)*
20–29	194	0.849	0.109
30–39	243	0.831	0.117
40–49	215	0.803	0.127
50–59	200	0.732	0.111
60–69	239	0.682	0.114
70–79	232	0.618	0.099
80+	218	0.569	0.102

Adapted with permission of the publisher from Looker AC, et al. (1995) Proximal femur bone mineral levels of US adults. *Osteoporosis International* 5:389–409.

Table 8-19
NHANES III Femoral Neck BMD Data
for Non-Hispanic White Men as Acquired on the Hologic QDR-1000

Age	N	*Mean BMD (g/cm²)*	*SD (g/cm²)*
20–29	207	0.930	0.138
30–39	254	0.885	0.137
40–49	233	0.845	0.132
50–59	244	0.814	0.124
60–69	241	0.790	0.147
70–79	271	0.749	0.123
80+	226	0.698	0.149

Adapted with permission of the publisher from Looker AC, et al. (1995) Proximal femur bone mineral levels of US adults. *Osteoporosis International* 5:389–409.

Table 8-20
NHANES III Trochanter BMD Data
for Non-Hispanic White Women as Acquired on the Hologic QDR-1000

Age	N	*Mean BMD (g/cm²)*	*SD (g/cm²)*
20–29	194	0.703	0.090
30–39	243	0.703	0.104
40–49	215	0.681	0.108
50–59	200	0.635	0.099
60–69	239	0.594	0.103
70–79	232	0.546	0.094
80+	218	0.504	0.108

Adapted with permission of the publisher from Looker AC, et al. (1995) Proximal femur bone mineral levels of US adults. *Osteoporosis International* 5:389–409.

Table 8-21
NHANES III Trochanter BMD Data
for Non-Hispanic White Men as Acquired on the Hologic QDR-1000

Age	N	*Mean BMD (g/cm²)*	*SD (g/cm²)*
20–29	207	0.777	0.118
30–39	254	0.754	0.114
40–49	233	0.743	0.119
50–59	244	0.738	0.118
60–69	241	0.739	0.140
70–79	271	0.705	0.124
80+	226	0.667	0.147

Adapted with permission of the publisher from Looker AC, et al. (1995) Proximal femur bone mineral levels of US adults. *Osteoporosis International* 5:389–409.

Table 8-22
NHANES III Total Femur BMD Data
for Non-Hispanic White Women as Acquired on the Hologic QDR-1000

Age	N	*Mean BMD (g/cm²)*	*SD (g/cm²)*
20–29	194	0.934	0.108
30–39	243	0.936	0.128
40–49	215	0.913	0.139
50–59	200	0.863	0.130
60–69	239	0.799	0.132
70–79	232	0.728	0.114
80+	218	0.661	0.128

Adapted with permission of the publisher from Looker AC, et al. (1995) Proximal femur bone mineral levels of US adults. *Osteoporosis International* 5:389–409.

Table 8-23
NHANES III Total Femur BMD Data
for Non-Hispanic White Men as Acquired on the Hologic QDR-1000

Age	N	*Mean BMD (g/cm²)*	*SD (g/cm²)*
20–29	207	1.033	0.141
30–39	254	1.014	0.142
40–49	233	0.995	0.154
50–59	244	0.975	0.147
60–69	241	0.957	0.163
70–79	271	0.910	0.143
80+	226	0.842	0.167

Adapted with permission of the publisher from Looker AC, et al. (1995) Proximal femur bone mineral levels of US adults. *Osteoporosis International* 5:389–409.

Table 8-24
Standardized Total Femur Age-Specific Reference Data for U.S. White Women

Age (yr)	*sBMD for women mg/cm*^{2}
20–29	956
30–39	944
40–49	920
50–59	876
60–69	809
70–79	740
80+	679

Reproduced from the *Journal of Bone and Mineral Research* 1997; 12:1316–1317 with permission from the American Society for Bone and Mineral Research.

facturers, either in conjunction with the manufacturer-derived databases or as a replacement for the manufacturer-derived proximal femur data after September 1997.

REFERENCES

1. Kelly TL, Slovik DM, Schoenfeld DA, Neer RM (1988) Quantitative digital radiography *versus* dual photon absorptiometry of the lumbar spine. *J Clin Endocrinol Metab* 67:839–844.
2. Pacifici R, Rupich R, Vered I, Fischer KC, Griffin M, Susman N, Avioli LV (1988) Dual energy radiography (DER): a preliminary comparative study. *Calcif Tissue Int* 43:189–191.
3. Holbrook TL, Barrett-Connor E, Klauber M, Sartoris D (1991) A population-based comparison of quantitative dual-energy X-ray absorptiometry with dual-photon absorptiometry of the spine and hip. *Calcif Tissue Int* 49:305–307.
4. Mazess RB, Barden HS (1988) Measurement of bone by dual-photon absorptiometry (DPA) and dual-energy X-ray absorptiometry (DEXA). *Annal Chirurg Gynaecol* 77:197–203.
5. Lees B, Stevenson JC (1992) An evaluation of dual-energy X-ray absorptiometry and comparison with dual-photon absorptiometry. *Osteoporosis Int* 2:146–152.
6. McClung M, Roberts L (1989) Correlation of bone density measurements by 153-Gd and X-ray dual photon absorptiometry. Abstract. *J Bone Miner Res* 4:S368.
7. Arai H, Ito K, Nagao K, Furutachi M (1990) The evaluation of three different bone densitometry systems: XR-26, QDR-1000, and DPX. *Image Technol Inf Display* 22:1–6.
8. Lai KC, Goodsitt MM, Murano R, Chesnut CH (1992) A comparison of two dual-energy X-ray absorptiometry systems for spinal bone mineral measurement. *Calcif Tissue Int* 50:203–208.
9. Pocock NA, Sambrook PN, Nguyen T, Kelly P, Freund J, Eisman JA (1992) Assessment of spinal and femoral bone density by dual X-ray absorptiometry: comparison of Lunar and Hologic instruments. *J Bone Miner Res* 7:1081–1084.

10. Genant HK, Grampp S, Gluer CC, Faulkner KG, Jergas M, Engelke K, Hagiwara S, Van Kuijk C (1994) Universal standardization for dual X-ray absorptiometry: patient and phantom cross-calibration results. *J Bone Miner Res* 9:1503–1514.
11. Hanson J (1997) Standardization of femur BMD. *J Bone Miner Res* 12:1316,1317.
12. Economos CD, Nelson ME, Fiatarone MA, Dallal GE, Heymsfield SB, Wang J, et al. (1996) A multicenter comparison of dual-energy X-ray absorptiometers: in vivo and in vitro measurements of bone mineral content and density. *J Bone Miner Res* 11:275–285.
13. Blake GM, Tong CM, Fogelman I (1991) Intersite comparison of the Hologic QDR-1000 dual energy X-ray bone densitometer. *Br J Radiol* 64:440–446.
14. Orwoll E, Oviatt SK, and the Nafarelin Bone Study Group (1991) Longitudinal precision of dual-energy X-ray absorptiometry in a multicenter study. *J Bone Miner Res* 6:191–197.
15. Steiger P, von Stetten E, Weiss H, Stein JA (1991) Paired AP and lateral supine dual X-ray absorptiometry of the spine: initial results with a 32 detector system. *Osteoporosis Int* 1:190.
16. Eiken P, Barenholdt O, Bjorn Jensen L, Gram J, Pors Nielsen S (1994) Switching from DXA pencil-beam to fan-beam. I: studies in vitro at four centers. *Bone* 15:667–670.
17. Blake GM, Parker JC, Buxton FM, Fogelman I (1993) Dual X-ray absorptiometry: a comparison between fan beam and pencil beam scans. *Br J Radiol* 66:902–906.
18. Faulkner KG, Gluer CC, Estilo M, Genant HK (1993) Cross-calibration of DXA equipment: upgrading from a Hologic QDR 1000/W to a QDR 2000. *Calcif Tissue Int* 52:79–84.
19. Laskey MA, Crisp AJ, Cole TJ, Compston JE (1992) Comparison of the effect of different reference data on Lunar DPX and Hologic QDR-1000 dual-energy X-ray absorptiometers. *Br J Radiol* 65:1124–1129.
20. Faulkner KG, Roberts LA, McClung MR (1996) Discrepancies in normative data between Lunar and Hologic DXA systems. *Osteoporosis Int* 6:432–436.
21. Looker AC, Wahner HW, Dunn WL, Calvo MS, Harris TB, Heyse SP, Johnston CC, Lindsay RL (1995) Proximal femur bone mineral levels of US adults. *Osteoporosis Int* 5:389–409.
22. Hologic. Reference database and reports. *QDR 4500 Operator's Manual*. Waltham, MA, pp. 8-1–8-20.
23. Lunar. Comparison to reference population. *DPX-IQ User's Manual*. Madison, WI, pp. 5.1–5.19.
24. Norland. Patient comparison. *XR-Series X-ray Bone Densitometer Operator's Guide*. Ft. Atkinson, WI, pp. 12.1–12.30.
25. Simmons A, Simpson DE, O'Doherty MJ, Barrington S, Coakley AJ (1997) The effects of standardization and reference values on patient classification for spine and femur dual-energy X-ray absorptiometry. *Osteoporosis Int* 7:200–206.

9 Clinical Indications for Bone Densitometry

CONTENTS

There is no question that the variety of densitometry techniques available to the physician today can accurately and precisely quantify the bone density at virtually any skeletal site. But when should these technologies be used? In what clinical circumstances should physicians consider measuring the bone density? Four major organizations have published guidelines on the use of bone mass measurements. As practice guidelines, they are intended to help the physician determine when a bone mass measurement may be useful in the care of individual patients. A fifth major organization has published guidelines for the diagnosis of osteoporosis, based on the absolute level of the bone density or bone mass that is measured.

CLINICAL GUIDELINES

1988 National Osteoporosis Foundation Guidelines

Some of the very first guidelines or indications for bone mass measurements were developed in 1988 by the National Osteoporosis Foundation (NOF). These guidelines, or clinical indications, were developed in response to a report from the Office of Health Technology Assessment (OHTA) of the U.S. Public Health Service, which had been submitted to the Health Care Finance Administration (HCFA). The report from OHTA concluded that the role of DPA and SPA in clinical practice had not been defined. The clinical indications from the NOF, which were submitted to HCFA, were published in 1989 in the *Journal for Bone and Mineral Research (1)*. The NOF pointed out that the methods that were available to measure bone mass or density were safe, accurate, and precise. They also noted that important clinical decisions could be influenced by the results of the measurements. The clinical circumstances in which the NOF believed that sufficient experience existed to support the use of bone-mass measurements were four. These were based primarily on the experience with SPA and DPA, since DXA had only been approved for clinical use in 1988. The four clinical indications for bone-mass measurements were:

1. In estrogen-deficient women, to diagnose significantly low bone mass, in order to make decisions about hormone replacement therapy.
2. In patients with vertebral abnormalities or roentgenographic osteopenia, to diagnose spinal osteoporosis, in order to make decisions about further diagnostic evaluation and therapy.
3. In patients receiving long-term glucocorticoid therapy, to diagnose low bone mass, in order to adjust therapy.
4. In patients with primary asymptomatic hyperparathyroidism, to identity low bone mass, in order to identify those at risk of severe skeletal disease who may be candidates for surgical intervention.

The NOF indications also recommended that specific skeletal sites and techniques be used in these different circumstances. For an assessment of fracture risk in a postmenopausal woman, the NOF suggested that any site by any technique was appropriate. For the confirmation of spinal demineralization or the diagnosis of spinal osteoporosis, measuring the spine with DPA, DXA, or QCT was recommended. A measurement of the spine by DPA, DXA, or QCT was also recommended for the purposes of detecting bone loss from corticosteroids. The recommended assessment of the effects of hyperparathyroidism on the skeleton consisted of a measurement of the spine by DXA, DPA, or QCT, or a measurement of the radius by SPA.

DXA measurements of the forearm were not suggested as part of the evaluation of the patient with hyperparathyroidism, because this capability was not in clinical use at the time. The serial assessment of bone density for therapeutic efficacy or disease effect is not mentioned in these indications, because the indications were primarily based on the clinical experience with SPA and DPA. The precision of bone-density measurements of the spine or proximal femur with DPA was not sufficient to make serial assessments feasible in most cases. In the text of the document, however, it was observed that the changes in bone density in the spine might be so rapid in the setting of corticosteroid-induced osteoporosis that serial assessment of spine bone density with DPA could be considered. Measurements of the forearm with SPA were also not thought to be useful for serial assessments of therapeutic efficacy. Although the precision of SPA measurements of the forearm was excellent, the changes in BMD at the forearm sites were thought to be too small to be detected in a clinically useful period of time.

The assessment of the estrogen-deficient woman with bone-mass measurements specifically referred to making decisions about hormone replacement therapy. At the time of these indications, there were no prescription alternatives to estrogen that were FDA-approved for the prevention of osteoporosis.

Finally, the NOF emphasized that these measurements should not be done if intervention decisions would not be affected by the result of the test. They noted that women who were to receive long-term estrogen replacement for reasons other than the prevention or treatment of osteoporosis did not need a measurement. The NOF also observed that measurements should not be done if sufficient quality-control procedures were not in place to ensure the accuracy of the results.

Guidelines of the International Society for Clinical Densitometry

The guidelines from the International Society for Clinical Densitometry (ISCD) were developed in 1994, during a meeting of an international panel of experts in bone densitometry. There were 22 members of this panel from eight countries. The guidelines addressed both the use and interpretation of bone-mass measurements in the prevention, detection, and management of all diseases characterized by low bone mass, with an emphasis on osteoporosis *(2)*. The guidelines provided a broad overview of how bone mass measurements should be used, regardless of the specific clinical circumstances in which they were employed. There were six major points on which the panel reached a consensus. Those points are summarized in Table 9-1.

The ISCD Guidelines are best appreciated if the scientific climate of the 1980s and early 1990s is understood. In the 1980s, medical conferences were awash in the bone-mass measurement controversy. This controversy largely centered on whether a measurement of bone mass or bone density could be used to predict fracture risk. In a decade in which DPA and SPA were the predominant techniques, bone densitometry was also not seen as useful for monitoring therapy. Indeed, therapeutic choices were viewed (rightly or wrongly) as being so limited that early detection of disease with bone mass measurements was perceived as having little value. The situation was further compounded by a lack of agreement on the actual definition of osteoporosis itself. In the late 1980s and early 1990s, however, rapid developments in the field made most of these controversies moot.

In 1988, DXA was FDA-approved for clinical use. The enhanced precision of DXA, particularly at the spine, made monitoring of the effects of disease or therapy practical. In 1993, several major fracture trials were published and added to a growing body of literature, which effectively laid to rest the bone-mass measurement controversy *(3–5)*. In 1994, the World

Table 9-1
Consensus Points from the International Society for Clinical Densitometry on the Clinical Utility of Bone-Mass Measurements

1. Bone mass measurements predict a patient's future risk of fracture.
2. Osteoporosis can be diagnosed on the basis of bone mass measurements even in the absence of prevalent fractures.
3. Bone mass measurements provide information that can affect the management of patients.
4. The choice of the appropriate measurement site(s) for the assessment of bone mass or fracture risk may vary depending upon the specific circumstances of the patient.
5. The choice of the appropriate technique for bone mass measurements in any given clinical circumstance should be based on an understanding of the strengths and limitations of the different techniques.
6. Bone mass data should be accompanied by a clinical interpretation.

Adapted with permission of the publisher from Miller PD et al. (1996) Consensus of an international panel on the clinical utility of bone mass measurement in the detection of low bone mass in the adult population. *Calcified Tissue International* 58:207–214.

Health Organization (WHO) published its guidelines for the diagnosis of osteoporosis *(8)*. Alendronate sodium and nasal-spray salmon calcitonin, approved in 1995, were dramatic additions to the therapeutic armamentarium. These developments profoundly changed the field of densitometry and osteoporosis, but they had been poorly communicated to the practicing physician, the public, insurers, and politicians. The ISCD guidelines attempted to change that.

Another major goal of the ISCD guidelines was to point out that all bone-mass measurement techniques have value when they are properly used. The bone densitometry industry is intensely competitive. This competitiveness has, at times, been misinterpreted by those outside the industry as meaning that some technologies were inferior to others. ISCD wished to emphasize that the devices that are FDA-approved for the measurement of bone density do exactly what they purport to do. They can accurately and precisely measure the bone density. Assuming that all the techniques are available, the choice of which technique to use should be determined by the intent of the measurement. The intent of the measurement determines which site or sites should be measured, and whether the primary need is accuracy or precision at that site. Once these determinations have been made, a particular technique may be seen to be preferable to another in that specific circumstance, but not necessarily in every circumstance that may follow.

Another major emphasis of the ISCD guidelines was that the appropriate measurement site is determined by the intent of the measurement. One skeletal site is not appropriate for all of the potential uses of bone mass measurements. ISCD also strongly recognized the need for strict quality control of the machines, and for training for the operators. The guidelines also emphasized the need for an interpretation of the numeric data by a physician trained in densitometry.

1996 American Association of Clinical Endocrinologists' Guidelines

In 1996, the American Association of Clinical Endocrinologists (AACE) developed guidelines for the prevention and treatment of osteoporosis *(6)*. As part of these guidelines, BMD measurements were discussed. The specific clinical circumstances in which the AACE believed that bone-mass measurements were appropriate were virtually identical to the original guidelines from the National Osteoporosis Foundation published in 1988, although they were clearly updated to reflect the more precise measurements that could be made with DXA, and the increase in available therapies. The clinical circumstances in which the AACE believed that bone mass measurements were appropriate were:

1. For risk assessment in perimenopausal or postmenopausal women who are concerned about osteoporosis and willing to accept available intervention.
2. In women with X-ray findings that suggest the presence of osteoporosis.
3. In women beginning or receiving long-term glucocorticoid therapy, provided intervention is an option.
4. For perimenopausal or postmenopausal women with asymptomatic primary hyperparathyroidism, in whom evidence of skeletal loss would result in parathyroidectomy.
5. In women undergoing treatment for osteoporosis, as a tool for monitoring the therapeutic response.

These guidelines reflect the increase in available therapeutic options beyond hormone replacement therapy for the prevention or treatment of osteoporosis. With the availability of nasal-spray calcitonin and alendronate sodium, a woman's choices for the prevention or treatment of this disease were no longer limited to hormone replacement therapy. The superior precision of DXA measurements also offered the ability to follow therapeutic efficacy over time with bone-mass measurements.

Because these guidelines are for the prevention and treatment of postmenopausal osteoporosis only, the AACE guidelines for the use of densitometry deal only with women. There was also a concerted effort to emphasize in these guidelines that bone mass measurements should be done only if the outcome of the measurement would directly influence a clinical decision to intervene in some manner. Although this is a statement that could be made for any clinical test, the AACE chose to emphasize this in these guidelines.

The AACE also noted that a measurement of the spine, hip, radius, or calcaneus could be used for fracture-risk assessment. They did not note whether they were recommending a global or site-specific fracture risk assessment. Although it was observed that, under ideal circumstances, a measurement of both the spine and hip would be performed at a baseline evaluation, and, again, should follow-up be indicated, the AACE recommended a bone-density study of the hip as the preferred site for the first measurement.

Guidelines from the European Foundation for Osteoporosis and Bone Disease

Also in 1996, the European Foundation for Osteoporosis and Bone Disease (EFFO) published some of the most practical guidelines yet for the clinical application of bone-density measurements *(7)*. Some of the clinical circumstances in which the EFFO believed that bone mass measurements should be considered are shown in Table 9-2. Like the AACE, the EFFO was careful to emphasize that bone-mass measurements should not be done if the result would not affect the clinical decision-making process.

In contrast to the AACE, the EFFO guidelines do not direct the physician to perform a baseline measurement at the hip, regardless of the reason for the measurement. The EFFO guidelines, like the ISCD guidelines, note that the site of the measurement should be determined by the intent of the measurement. Although the EFFO observed that the hip site may be less affected by changes of osteoarthrosis in the elderly, and was the preferred site for a site-specific hip fracture-risk assessment, they also observed that changes in BMD from therapeutic interventions were more likely to be documented in the spine. The EFFO also noted that the hip, wrist, or spine sites could be used for global fracture-risk assessments in women around the time of menopause. The EFFO recommended scanning only one site initially, but they acknowledged that there may be clinical circumstances in which two sites are necessary, in order to assess sites that are predominantly cortical or predominantly trabecular bone.

The EFFO guidelines noted that the interval between BMD measurements for the detection of bone loss over time would vary with the anticipated rate of loss from the disease process. In some circumstances, the interval could be as short as 6 months. In others, the interval would be 2 to 3 years. In monitoring changes in BMD from a therapeutic intervention, the EFFO noted that the interval between measurements would again be determined by the agent being used, and the site being measured. This statement reflects the combined effect of the expected rate of change from a particular agent at a given site, and the precision of the measurement at

Table 9-2
Indications for Bone-Mass Measurements from the EFFO Guidelines

1. Presence of strong risk factors
   a. Premature menopause (<45 yr)
   b. Prolonged secondary amenorrhea
   c. Primary hypogonadism
   d. Corticosteroid therapy (>7.5 mg/d for 1 yr or more)
   e. Conditions associated with osteoporosis
      i. Anorexia nervosa
      ii. Malabsorption
      iii. Primary hyperparathyroidism
      iv. Posttransplantation
      v. Chronic renal failure
      vi. Osteogenesis imperfecta
      vii. Neoplasm
      viii. Hyperthyroidism
      ix. Prolonged immobilization
      x. Cushing's syndrome
2. Radiographic evidence of osteopenia and/or vertebral deformity
3. Previous fragility fracture, for example of the hip, spine, wrist, or upper humerus
4. Significant loss of height or thoracic kyphosis
5. Monitoring of treatment
   a. Hormone replacement treatment in patients with secondary osteoporosis
   b. Other agents, e.g. bisphosphonates, calcitonin, fluoride salts, and vitamin D and its metabolites

Reproduced with permission of the publisher from Kanis J, et al. (1996) Practical guide for the use of bone mineral measurements in the assessment of treatment of osteoporosis: a position paper of the European Foundation for Osteoporosis and Bone Disease. *Osteoporosis International* 6:256–261.

that site. They note that the usual interval for such measurements is 1 to 2 years. The monitoring of women on hormone replacement therapy that was prescribed for postmenopausal hormone replacement is not recommended, except in the case of complicating factors that might increase the woman's risk for secondary osteoporosis. If hormone replacement was prescribed specifically for the treatment of osteoporosis, the EFFO does recommend periodic monitoring, because of the variability in response to treatment.

Guidelines of the Study Group of the World Health Organization for the Diagnosis of Osteoporosis

In an extensive report published in 1994, a WHO study group, which was composed of 16 internationally known experts in the field of osteoporo-

Table 9-3
BMD and BMC Criteria for Diagnosis of Osteoporosis in Caucasian Women as Proposed by a Study Group of the World Health Organization

Diagnostic category	BMD or BMC compared to the average value for a healthy young Caucasian woman
Normal	$\leq$1 SD below the average
Osteopenia or low bone mass	>1 SD below but less than 2.5 SD below the average
Osteoporosis	2.5 SD or more below the average
Severe or established osteoporosis	2.5 SD or more below the average with fragility fracture(s)

From ref. *8*.

sis, proposed specific criteria for the diagnosis of osteoporosis, based on a specific level of bone density *(8)*. The panel noted that a cutoff value of bone density at more than 2.5 SDs below the average value for healthy young women for the diagnosis of osteoporosis would label 30% of all postmenopausal women as having osteoporosis at some skeletal site. Fifty percent or more of these women have sustained a fracture of the spine, femur, forearm, humerus, or pelvis. The diagnostic categories established by the WHO study group are shown in Table 9-3. Although the table refers to values of bone density in terms of the number of SDs below the average value for a healthy young adult, the values could also be expressed as the *T*-score or young-adult *z*-score, since these terms are used in a synonymous fashion. These guidelines for diagnosis were proposed for Caucasian women only. They were not originally intended to be applied to women of other races, or to men. This is being done in clinical practice, however, in the absence of any other diagnostic guidelines for these groups.

The WHO study group recognized that an individual might be categorized differently, depending on the site at which they are assessed. They also emphasized that the use of bone density measurements for the diagnosis of osteoporosis should not be confused with the use of the technology for the prognosis of fracture risk. They correctly pointed out that bone-density values are used as risk factors for fracture, as well as being used as criteria for the diagnosis of disease, but that these two uses of the values were really quite distinct. For example, the disease hypertension is defined as blood pressure exceeding a certain diagnostic level. At the same time, this quantity, that is, the level of blood pressure, is a risk factor for stroke, and is used to prognosticate that risk. Similar analogies can be made for hypercholesterolemia, coronary heart disease, and myocardial infarction, and hyperuricemia, gout, and arthritis.

Although no other authoritative body has published proposed diagnostic levels of bone density for osteoporosis, a slightly higher cutoff level has tended to be equated with the diagnosis of osteoporosis in the United States. In approving certain medications for the management or treatment of osteoporosis, the US Food and Drug Administration has recommended the use of these drugs in individuals with a bone density that is 2 SDs or more below that of the young adult. In essence, this equates a diagnosis of osteoporosis with a bone density that is 2 SDs or more below that of the young adult, in contrast to the lower cutoff proposed by the WHO of more than 2.5 SDs below that of the young adult.

HOW DO THE GUIDELINES COMPARE?

There is far more unanimity among the guidelines from the various societies than there are differences. The four clinical circumstances in which bone mass measurements might be performed, which were originally proposed to HCFA by the National Osteoporosis Foundation in 1988, are also found in the guidelines from ISCD, EFFO, and AACE. The later guidelines from ISCD, EFFO, and AACE also note the utility of the newer technologies, such as DXA, in the serial assessment of bone density. The NOF, ISCD, and EFFO have all noted the utility of multiple skeletal sites, with the choice of site being determined by the intent of the measurement. EFFO and ISCD guidelines note that measurements of the spine, hip, and radius can all be used for global fracture-risk assessments. There is general agreement that hip-fracture risk is best assessed at the hip, if the technology required to perform the hip measurement is available.

All of the guidelines emphasize to some degree that the measurement should not be performed, if a decision to intervene will not be affected by the measurement. Both the NOF and ISCD have emphasized the need for strict quality-control procedures in the performance of densitometry.

The most glaring contrast among the guidelines is found in the emphasis by the AACE on the proximal femur as the preferred baseline measurement site. This recommendation appears to be based on the ability of the hip bone-density measurement to predict both spine- and hip-fracture risk, and the relative lack of dystrophic changes at the hip that would affect the accuracy of the measurement. It is also noted, however, that the hip can be used for follow-up measurements to assess therapeutic efficacy. Strictly speaking, this is true, but it would not seem to be a clinically practical observation. The combination of the precision of proximal femur testing and the rates of change seen in the regions of interest in the proximal femur, with currently available therapies, would result in a minimum wait of at least 3 years before efficacy could be assessed. Guidelines from the EFFO note that the spine, because of the greater percentage of trabecular bone, is more likely to demonstrate a greater response to therapeutic intervention than other sites. The precision of AP spine testing is also generally superior to that of proximal femur testing. This combination of superior precision and a greater expected magnitude of change makes the spine the preferred site for serial assessment of therapeutic efficacy.

CLINICAL APPLICATIONS OF BONE-MASS MEASUREMENTS

There is general agreement on the clinical circumstances in which bone-mass measurements can provide useful information for patient management. The physician must still determine which site should be measured, in order to obtain the information that will be most relevant to the clinical circumstance. How is that site determined? As emphasized in the ISCD and EFFO guidelines, the site is determined by the intent of the measurement.

In a broad sense, there are four major clinical applications of densitometry in medicine today: the quantification of bone mass or density, the assessment of fracture risk, skeletal morphometry, and body-composition analysis.

These are distinct applications of bone densitometry technology. The quantification of the bone density and the assessment of fracture risk are the two most common applications.

In the context of quantifying the bone mass or density, there are four general circumstances in which this could be done: to confirm suspected demineralization from a plain skeletal X ray, to diagnose osteopenia or osteoporosis, to document the effects of a disease process that can cause changes in the BMC or BMD on some region of the skeleton, and to follow the effects of a disease process or therapy on the skeleton over time.

For fracture-risk assessments, either of two types of assessment may be done: a global fracture-risk assessment, or a site-specific fracture-risk assessment. A global fracture-risk assessment is used to predict the risk of having any and all types of osteoporotic fracture. A site-specific fracture-risk assessment is used to predict the risk of a specific type of fracture, such as spine fracture or hip fracture.

It is useful to decide what the actual intent of the measurement may be in any given clinical circumstance. For example, in the evaluation of the perimenopausal woman considering hormone replacement, a measurement could be done to assess global fracture risk, to assess site-specific fracture risk, or to quantify the bone density for the purpose of the diagnosis of normalcy, osteopenia, or osteoporosis.

Selection of Sites to Measure

Site selection for skeletal morphometry or body-composition analysis is straightforward. Total-body measurements are performed for body-composition analysis. Skeletal morphometry software currently exists only for lateral spine measurements. Site selection for the purposes of quantifying the bone mass or density, or for fracture-risk assessment, requires a more thorough evaluation of the specific intent or goal of the measurement.

Assessment of Fracture Risk

As noted above, fracture-risk assessments may be of two types: global or site-specific. Current data suggests that a global fracture-risk assessment may be obtained at any of several different sites by any of the techniques that will measure those sites *(4)*. Both the spine and the femoral neck appear to be equally good predictors of global fracture risk. The 33% radial site in older populations is an excellent predictor of nonspine fracture risk *(9)*. There also seems to be no question that regions in the proximal femur are the best sites to measure for a site-specific hip fracture risk prediction, with the os calcis having almost equal utility in this regard *(3)*. Less clear is which site is the best site to measure for a site-specific spine fracture-risk prediction. Although the spine bone density does predict fracture risk at the spine, studies suggest that the proximal femur and the midradius are equally good predictors of spine-fracture risk *(4)*. Although this might seem implausible at first, it is quite likely that the spine bone density's ability to indicate fracture risk at the spine has been tempered in the populations studied, because of the study population's age. Many of these studies have been done in individuals 65 years of age and older. Artifacts in the spine, such as arthritic change and facet sclerosis, which are more common in older populations, will elevate the bone density in the spine *(10,11)*. As a consequence, the bone density in this region will not necessarily be low, even in an individual who has fractured. In addition, the overall magnitude of bone loss in the various regions of the skeleton tends to equalize in the older populations *(12–15)*. This gives other regions of the skeleton, such as the radius and proximal femur, greater predictive power for spine fractures in the older age groups, even though the bone densities in the spine, femur, and radius may have been very different when the individual was in their forties or fifties. In younger individuals, the AP spine is generally used for spine fracture-risk assessment. In older individuals, particularly if arthritic changes are present in the spine, the proximal femur or 33% radial sites may be used.

Quantification of Bone Density

Confirmation of Suspected Demineralization or Skeletal Fragility. When demineralization is suspected from a plain radiograph, confirmation of this visual impression should be obtained with bone densitometry. Ideally, the site that should be assessed with densitometry is the site that was noted on the plain film to be demineralized. Similarly, if the patient presents with a fracture for which the etiology is unknown, or which is suspected to be on the basis of fragility, the bone density should be quantified in the same region, as long as the fractured area itself can be excluded. If the specific site cannot be measured, because either the technology or software to access that site is not available, a similar site should be measured. For example, if the patient presents with a fracture or apparent demineralization in the thoracic spine, the lumbar spine can be quantified to assess overall spinal fragility. If the patient presents with a fracture of the right femoral neck, the left femur should be measured, since the fracture in the right femoral neck would be expected to elevate the bone density there.

Diagnosis of Osteoporosis. The diagnostic criteria for normalcy, osteopenia, and osteoporosis in women that have been established by the World Health Organization require a measurement of bone density as shown in Table 9-3. The diagnosis may vary, however, depending on which skeletal site is measured. As an individual ages, there is a tendency for the magnitude of bone loss from the various regions of the skeleton to equalize. As a consequence, in patients over the age of 65, the spine, proximal femur, midradius, and os calcis are all likely to reflect similar levels of bone density. Any of these sites could reasonably be used in the older population to diagnose osteopenia or osteoporosis. Nevertheless, heterogeneity in the bone density in the various regions of the skeleton is commonly seen. The younger the individual, the more likely one is to encounter a disparity in the bone density in the various regions. In a recent study of 237 women ages 20 to 45, 24% of the 20- to 29-year-olds had spine and femur *z*-scores that differed by more than 1. This percentage increased in the 30- to 45-year-olds to 32 to 46% *(16)*. The choice of site, then, becomes critical in making the proper diagnosis, particularly when interventions, such as estrogen replacement for menopausal women, may be based on that diagnosis. In a study from Pouilles et al., 85 women, whose average age was 53 years, underwent DXA studies of the spine and proximal femur *(17)*. Twenty-six percent of these women had sufficiently disparate bone densities in the spine and proximal femur to result in a misdiagnosis of the nonmeasured site, if only one of the two sites had been measured. In a very similar study, Lai et al. *(18)* evaluated 85 women, whose average age was 52.5 years, with DXA studies of the spine and femoral neck *(18)*. In this study, 37% of the women had disparate values that were sufficiently great to result in the failure to diagnose osteopenia or osteoporosis, and the consequent implications for fracture risk, if only one of the two sites had been measured. Davis et al. *(19)* evaluated four different skeletal sites in 744 women whose average age was 66.6 years. When the women were divided into tertiles of bone density based on the assessment of the spine,

Davis et al. *(19)* found that heterogeneity in the bone density was quite common, particularly in women whose spine bone density was in the midtertile. Even in women who were classified as being in the highest tertile for their age at the spine, 15% were in the lowest tertile at one other site. As a consequence, many authorities advocate a measurement of both the spine and the proximal femur in women in their forties and fifties. Based on the data from Davis, it seems clear that even women in their mid-sixties who have spine bone densities in the mid- or upper tertile, may still have low bone densities at other skeletal sites. Some of this disparity may again be explained by the effect of age-related artifacts elevating the BMD in the AP spine. In a study of 120 women whose mean age was 70 years, 66% of the women were classified as osteoporotic when DXA studies of the spine were performed in the lateral projection, compared to only 29% when the spine study was performed in the AP projection *(20)*. In this same study, 55% of the women were classified as osteoporotic when the diagnosis was based on the BMD in the femoral neck, and 43% were similarly classified when a predominantly cortical measure of the radius was used.

If a physician must assess only one skeletal site for the diagnosis of osteoporosis or the assessment of fracture risk, the preferred site appears to be the proximal femur. The proximal femur is less likely to be affected by age-related skeletal artifacts that would affect the accuracy of the measurement, although it is certainly not immune.* It is less likely to be normal in the presence of low bone density at the spine than vice versa. The proximal femur is an excellent predictor of hip-fracture risk, the type of fracture that confers the greatest morbidity and mortality.

Assessment of the Effect of Disease Processes on the Skeleton. If a disease process that can cause demineralization is suspected, a clinician may wish to quantify the bone density, both to help confirm the diagnosis, and also to help determine a necessary treatment plan. The selection of skeletal site for this purpose requires a knowledge of the type of bone that the disease process tends to affect and the composition of the various skeletal sites that can be measured.

There are certain disease states that tend to have a predilection for cortical bone, such as hyperparathyroidism or hyperthyroidism in premenopausal women. These changes would be best identified with a measurement of the midradius or femoral neck, because of the high cortical content of these regions. Cushing's disease will rapidly deplete the trabecular bone of the spine, as will corticosteroid use. Estrogen deficient bone loss is generally seen first in the spine. Age-related bone loss, on the other hand, seems

**See* Chapter 2 for a discussion of the effects of arthritic change and artifacts on BMD in the proximal femur.

to begin much earlier in the proximal femur than in the spine. These issues are discussed in greater detail in Chapter 7.

Serial Assessment of Bone Density to Assess the Effects of Disease or Therapeutic Interventions. The bone density may also be quantified to assess the effectiveness of prescribed interventions. The combination of factors that directs the choice of skeletal site includes the expected magnitude of the change at a given site and the precision of testing at that site with available technologies. The spine is most often followed for two reasons. Because of the higher rate of bone turnover found in a predominantly trabecular site like the spine, the expected magnitude of any change tends to be the greatest in the spine. The precision of AP spine testing is also equal to, or better than, that of testing at other skeletal sites, particularly with DXA. This combination means that significant changes in bone density are more likely to be detected at the spine in the shortest period of time than at any other site.

General Considerations in Site Selection

As a practical matter, if there has been a prior fracture in the region of interest, the BMD value will be increased by the fracture. Consequently, another site should be selected. In the lumbar spine, dystrophic calcification will increase the BMD. The most severe elevations in bone density are often seen with facet sclerosis. Osteophytes, disk-space calcification, and aortic calcification will elevate the density. Any calcification or metal in the abdomen overlying the spine will also cause false elevations when the spine BMD is measured in the AP projection. Although the lumbar spine can be measured in the lateral projection with DXA, eliminating the effects of facet sclerosis and most other forms of dystrophic calcification, this measurement is often limited to a single vertebral body. This is because the pelvis will overlap L4 at least 15% of the time, if the lateral is performed in the supine position, and at least 50% of the time when the lateral is performed in the left lateral decubitus position. There is always rib overlap of L1, and, over 90% of the time, rib overlap of L2 as well *(21)*. When only a single vertebra can be studied, the precision and accuracy of the measurement deteriorate. As a consequence, lateral lumbar spine DXA studies may be used in conjunction with an AP spine study, but they are virtually never used alone. Most forms of dystrophic calcification do not affect QCT studies of the spine. Although any one of several skeletal sites may serve for global fracture-risk assessments, or even site-specific fracture-risk assessments, it is clear that the bone density at one site cannot be predicted with sufficient accuracy from the measurement of bone density at another site *(22)*. Although the bone densities at the various sites are statistically significantly correlated with one another, the margin of error in such predictions is simply too great to be clinically useful. When the intent of the measurement is to quantify the bone density at a specific site, rather than assess fracture risk, that site must be measured.

REFERENCES

1. Johnston CC, Melton LJ, Lindsay R, Eddy DM (1989) Clinical indications for bone mass measurements. A report from the scientific advisory board of the National Osteoporosis Foundation. *J Bone Miner Res* 4:S2.
2. Miller PD, Bonnick SL, Rosen CJ (1996) Consensus of an international panel on the clinical utility of bone mass measurement in the detection of low bone mass in the adult population. *Calcif Tissue Int* 58:207–214.
3. Cummings SR, Black DM, Nevitt MC, Browner W, Cauley J, Ensrud K, et al. (1993) Bone density at various sites for the prediction of hip fractures. *Lancet* 341:72–75.
4. Metlon LJ, Atkinson EJ, O'Fallon WM, Wahner HW, Riggs BL (1993) Long-term fracture prediction by bone mineral assessed at different skeletal sites. *J Bone Miner Res* 8:1227–1233.
5. Gardsell P, Johnell O, Nilsson BE, Gullberg B (1993) Predicting various fragility fractures in women by forearm bone densitometry: a follow-up study. *Calcif Tissue Int* 52:348–353.
6. Hodgson SF, Johnston CC (1996) AACE clinical practice guidelines for the prevention and treatment of postmenopausal osteoporosis. *Endocr Pract* 2:155–171.
7. Kanis J, Devogelaer J, Gennari C (1996) Practical guide for the use of bone mineral measurements in the assessment of treatment of osteoporosis: a position paper of the European Foundation for Osteoporosis and Bone Disease. *Osteoporosis Int* 6:256–261.
8. World Health Organization (1994) Assessment of fracture risk and its application to screening for postmenopausal osteoporosis. *WHO Technical Report Series*. Geneva: WHO.
9. Hui SL, Slemenda CW, Johnston CC (1989) Baseline measurement of bone mass predicts fracture in white women. *Ann Intern Med* 111:355–361.
10. Drinka PJ, DeSmet AA, Bauwens SF, Rogot A (1992) The effect of overlying calcification on lumbar bone densitometry. *Calcif Tissue Int* 50:507–510.
11. Frye MA, Melton LJ, Bryant SC, Fitzpatrick LA, Wahner HW, Schwartz RS, Riggs BL (1992) Osteoporosis and calcification of the aorta. *Bone Miner* 19:185–194.
12. Pouilles JM, Tremollieres F, Ribot C (1993) The effects of menopause on longitudinal bone loss from the spine. *Calcif Tissue Int* 52:340–343.
13. He YF, Davis JW, Ross PD, Wasnich RD (1993) Declining bone loss rate variability with increasing follow-up time. *Bone Miner* 21:119–128.
14. Riggs BL, Wahner HW, Melton LJ, Richelson LS, Judd HL, Offord KP (1986) Rates of bone loss in the appendicular and axial skeletons of women: evidence of substantial vertebral bone loss before menopause. *J Clin Invest* 77:1487–1491.
15. Mautalen C, Vega E, Ghiringhelli G, Fromm G (1990) Bone diminution of osteoporotic females at different skeletal sites. *Calcif Tissue Int* 46:217–221.
16. Bonnick SL, Nichols DL, Sanborn CF, Lloyd K, Payne SG, Lewis L, Reed CA (1997) Dissimilar spinal and femoral *z*-scores in premenopausal women. *Calcif Tissue Int* 61:263–265.
17. Pouilles JM, Tremollieres F, Ribot C (1993) Spine and femur densitometry at the menopause: are both sites necessary in the assessment of the risk of osteoporosis? *Calcif Tissue Int* 52:344–347.

18. Lai K, Rencken M, Drinkwater BL, Chesnut CH (1993) Site of bone density measurement may affect therapy decision. *Calcif Tissue Int* 53:225–228.
19. Davis JW, Ross PD, Wasnich RD (1994) Evidence for both generalized and regional low bone mass among elderly women. *J Bone Miner Res* 9:305–309.
20. Greenspan SL, Maitland-Ramsey L, Myers E (1996) Classification of osteoporosis in the elderly is dependent on site-specific analysis. *Calcif Tissue Int* 58:409–414.
21. Rupich RC, Griffin MG, Pacifici R, Avioli LV, Susman N (1992) Lateral dual-energy radiography: artifact error from rib and pelvic bone. *J Bone Miner Res* 7:97–101.
22. Mazess RB, Barden HS (1990) Interrelationships among bone densitometry sites in normal young women. *Bone Miner* 11:347–356.

10 Case Studies

Contents

The cases in this chapter have come from my own files, and from several of my colleagues who graciously provided the cases to me. The cases represent some of the more common clinical applications of bone densitometry, and illustrate a variety of different approaches to the interpretation of bone density data in different clinical circumstances.

CASE 1

Patient History

The patient was a 69-year-old Caucasian woman who was 12 years postmenopausal. She had never been on estrogen replacement. She was known to have had prior traumatic fractures of her right ankle in 1966, and of her left elbow in 1976. In 1997, after complaining of back pain without a history of trauma, she was found to have a compression fracture at T7. She was begun on calcium supplementation and vitamin D. She was referred by her physician for evaluation of her bone density to confirm suspected fragility of the skeleton.

The patient also had a history of psoriasis since 1967, and hypertension since 1995. She had smoked for 35 years, and quit 12 years ago. She rarely

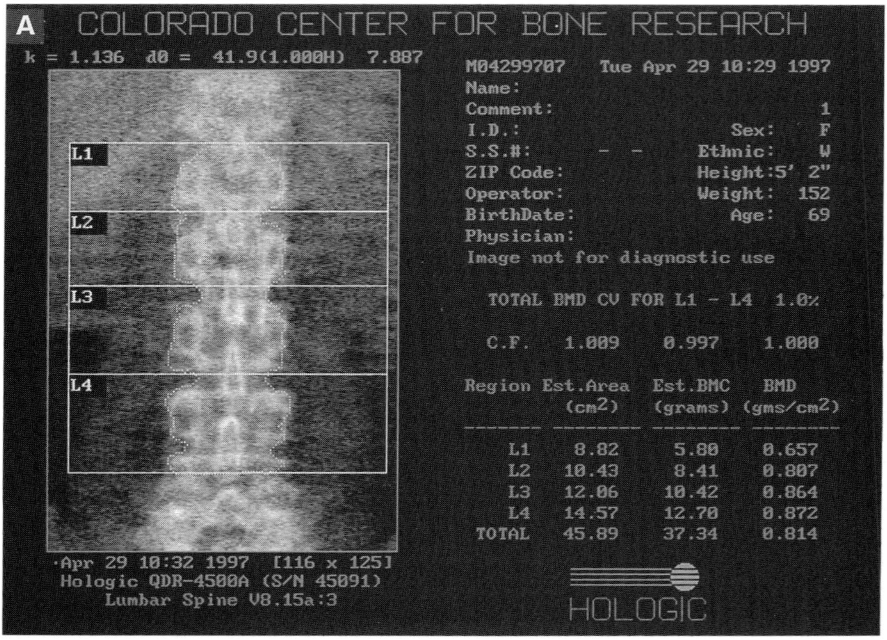

Fig. 10-1. (A) Case 1. AP Spine bone density data. Case courtesy of Dr. Paul Miller, Colorado Center for Bone Research, Lakewood, Colorado. The bone density data was acquired on the Hologic QDR-4500. The image should be reviewed for possible artifacts or structural changes that might affect the validity of the results. The individual BMC, area, and BMD values should be reviewed before reporting the average BMD. The labeling should be checked for accuracy.

drank alcoholic beverages, but did regularly consume caffeinated beverages, including coffee, tea, and diet colas. She walked 60 minutes per day for exercise, and continued to be able to perform her housework in spite of back pain. She took no oral prescription medications, although she used cortisone cream topically daily for her psoriasis.

Bone Density Studies

The patient underwent DXA studies of the AP spine and proximal femur on the Hologic QDR-4500 (Waltham, MA). These studies are shown in Figs. 10-1A,B and 10-2A,B. The average BMD for L1–L4 was 0.814 g/cm^2. This resulted in a T-score of –2.12. This means that the patient's average BMD at L1–L4 is 2.12 standard deviations (SDs) below the peak BMD of the young adult. Applying World Health Organization (WHO) criteria (*see* Chapter 9) to the lumbar spine BMD only, a diagnosis of osteopenia

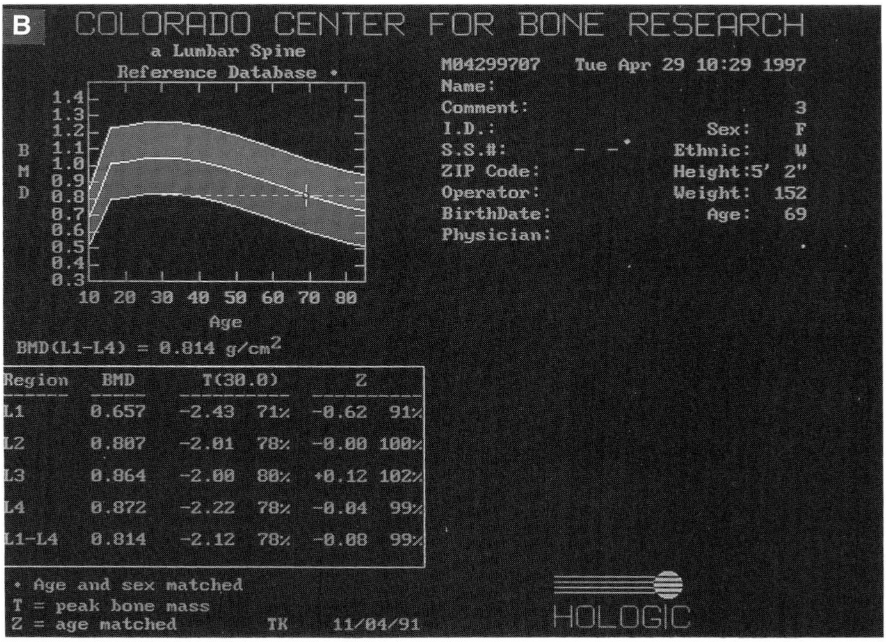

Fig. 10-1. (B) *(continued)* Case 1. AP Spine age-regression graph and reference database comparisons. Case courtesy of Dr. Paul Miller, Colorado Center for Bone Research, Lakewood, Colorado. The bone-density data was acquired on the Hologic QDR-4500. *T*- and *z*-scores and % comparisons to the manufacturer-supplied database are seen here for each vertebra and the average for L1–L4. The age-regression for BMD at the selected region ± 2 SDs is shown on the graph.

in the lumbar spine was appropriate. The *z*-score for the L1–L4 BMD average was –0.08. The patient's average BMD at L1–L4, therefore, was only 0.08 SDs below the value that was predicted for her age, sex, and race.

The femoral neck BMD was 0.624 g/cm^2. This resulted in a *T*-score of –2.71, indicating that the femoral neck BMD was 2.71 SDs below that of the peak BMD of the young adult. Applying WHO criteria to the femoral neck BMD, this BMD is compatible with a diagnosis of osteoporosis. The *z*-score for the femoral neck BMD was –0.49, indicating that the femoral neck BMD was 0.49 SDs below the value that would have been predicted on the basis of the patient's age, sex, and race.

The bone-density images were reviewed for the possible presence of artifacts that might affect the accuracy of the values, but none were seen. A review of the patient's plain spine films confirmed the fracture at T7, but no fractures or other obvious dystrophic calcification were seen that might

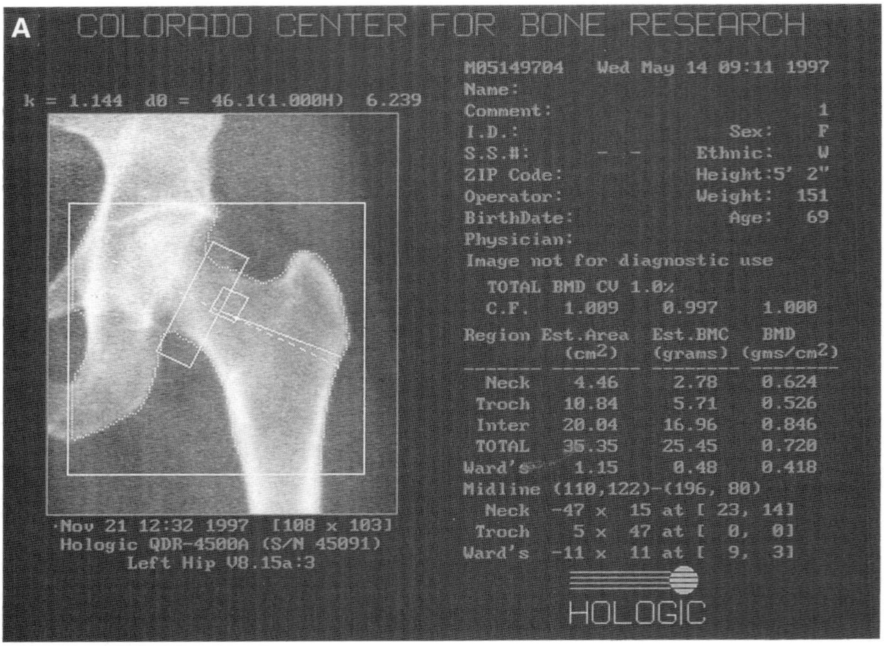

Fig. 10-2. (A) Case 1. Proximal femur bone density data. Case courtesy of Dr. Paul Miller, Colorado Center for Bone Research, Lakewood, Colorado. The bone density data was acquired on the Hologic QDR-4500. This study was performed 2 weeks after the spine study shown in Fig. 10-1A. Five regions of interest are displayed.

affect the spine BMD values.* Utilizing the lower of the two BMD values, and recognizing that the patient had already sustained a fragility fracture in the spine, the patient was considered to have severe or established osteoporosis, based on WHO criteria.

Laboratory Evaluation

The favorable comparison to her age-matched peers mitigated against the presence of secondary causes of bone loss (causes other than estrogen deficiency or age-related bone loss) in this woman. Nevertheless, since the patient's peak BMD was not known, and therefore the actual amount of any bone loss was not known, an evaluation to exclude the more common causes of secondary bone loss was deemed reasonable.

**See* Chapter 2 for a discussion of the effects of artifacts on BMD measurements in the spine.

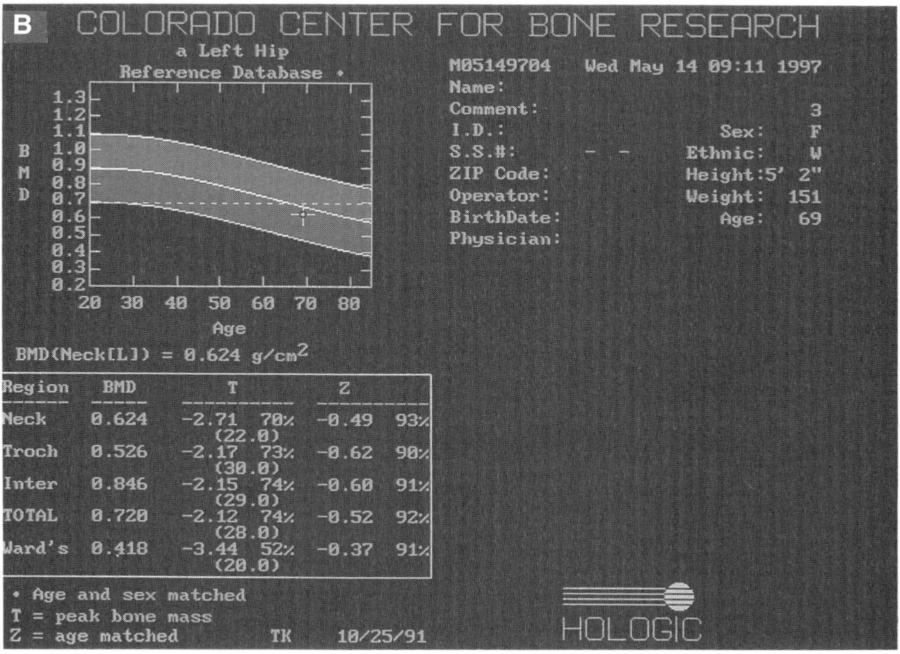

Fig. 10-2. *(continued)* **(B)** Case 1. Proximal femur age-regression graph and reference database comparisons. Case courtesy of Dr. Paul Miller, Colorado Center for Bone Research, Lakewood, Colorado. The bone-density data was acquired on the Hologic QDR-4500. The femoral neck BMD is plotted on the age-regression graph. *T*- and *z*-scores and % comparisons to the manufacturer-supplied database are seen in the table.

The patient's laboratory values are shown in Tables 10-1 and 10-2. A review of the patient's laboratory values did not suggest any secondary causes of metabolic bone disease, such as hyperparathyroidism, Paget's disease, or multiple myeloma.

Therapy and Follow-Up

The patient was begun on an oral bisphosphonate and her calcium supplementation and vitamin D were continued. She was cautioned to avoid activities that involved repeated or resisted trunk flexion, and to take reasonable precautions against falling. She was asked to modestly reduce her consumption of caffeinated beverages. Her use of topical cortisone was not thought to be sufficient to be of concern. No other modifiable risk factors were ascertained.

After 6 months, the patient reported that the therapy was well tolerated, and that she was pain-free, and continuing her usual activities. At the end

Table 10-1
Case 1 Complete Blood Count

Test	*Results*	*Reference range*
White cell count	9.7 THOU/MCL	3.8–10.8
Red cell count	4.5 MILL/MCL	3.6–5.1
Hemoglobin	14.0 G/DL	11.1–15.5
Hematocrit	42.7%	33.0–46.0
Platelet count	332,000	130.000–400,000
Neutrophil, segs	67.0%	40.0–75.0
Lymphocytes	21.0%	16.0–46.0
Monocytes	8.7%	0.0–12.0
Eosinophils	2.4%	0.0–7.0
Basophils	1.0%	0.0–2.0

All values are within normal limits.

Table 10-2
Case 1 Chemistry Panel

Test	*Results*	*Reference range*
SGPT	18 U/L	0–48
GGT	42 U/L	0–75
Alkaline phosphatase	75 U/L	20–125
Creatinine	1.2 MG/DL	0.7–1.8
Calcium	10.0 MG/DL	8.5–10.3
Phosphorus, inorganic	3.1 MG/DL	2.1–4.3
Sodium	137 MEQ/L	135–146
Potassium	3.9 MEQ/L	3.5–5.3
Chloride	101 MEQ/L	95–108

All values are within normal limits.

of 1 year of therapy, the AP spine bone-density study will be repeated to help assess therapeutic efficacy. The precision of AP spine bone-density testing at this facility was 1%. The average increase in lumbar spine bone density is approx 5% with the patient's current therapy. With a precision of 1%, a change from baseline of 2.77% must be seen to be 95% confident that a real change has occurred. Therefore, an interval of 1 year should provide sufficient time to document a significant increase in BMD.* If the therapy is ineffective in stopping bone loss, and a rate of loss of 1% per year

**See* Chapter 4 for a discussion of precision and its effect on the timing and interpretation of serial measurements.

results, definite bone loss may not be detectable for a period of 3 years at the 95% confidence level.

CASE 2

Patient History

The patient was a 72-year-old Caucasian woman who was 28 years postmenopausal. She had previously taken estrogen replacement for a period of 3 years only, but was not currently using estrogen replacement. She smoked for 15 years, but quit 30 years ago. She did not drink alcoholic beverages. She regularly consumed dairy products, and walked daily for 30–60 minutes. She took a calcium supplement in a dose of 1000 mg of elemental calcium, as well as 400 IU of vitamin D. There was a prior history of a traumatic left ankle fracture from a automobile accident in 1947. On a lateral chest film, the patient was found to have a compression fracture at T7, with no history of trauma to explain the fracture. She currently denied any back pain. She was evaluated with AP spine and proximal femur DXA studies, to confirm a suspected diagnosis of skeletal fragility resulting in spine fracture.

Bone-Density Studies

The patient underwent an AP spine study* on the Hologic QDR-4500. This is shown in Fig. 10-3A,B. A review of the AP spine bone-density image did not suggest any artifacts or technical problems that would invalidate the results of the study. The average BMD at L1–L4 was 0.681 g/cm^2, with a *T*-score of –3.33. This BMD, therefore, is 3.33 SDs below the peak BMD of the young adult. Applying WHO criteria, this woman has a BMD in the spine compatible with a diagnosis of osteoporosis. The presence of a presumed fragility fracture in the spine, combined with this low BMD, would change this diagnosis to severe osteoporosis.

The *z*-score for the L1–L4 average BMD is –1.07. The L1–L4 BMD is therefore 1.07 SDs below the BMD that would have been predicted for this 72-year-old woman on the basis of her age, sex, and race. Although this is not an extremely poor comparison to the patient's age-matched predicted value, the physician did evaluate the patient for possible secondary causes of metabolic bone disease, before concluding that estrogen deficiency and age-related bone loss were the only factors present here. This is reasonable,

*This image is acquired in the PA direction and is more appropriately called a PA spine study; however, it has become commonplace to refer to this study as an AP spine study.

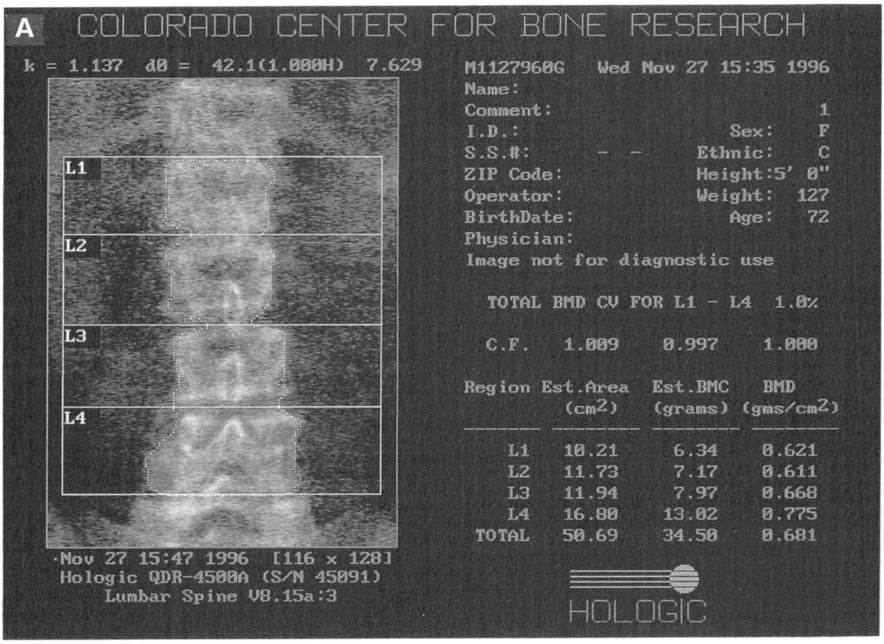

Fig. 10-3. (A) Case 2. AP Spine bone density data. Case courtesy of Dr. Paul Miller, Colorado Center for Bone Research, Lakewood, Colorado. The bone density data was acquired on the Hologic QDR-4500. An unusual finding here is a BMD that is higher at L1 than L2. The expected increase in area and BMC between L1 and L2 is seen, however, and the image does not suggest structural change or artifact at L1.

since the patient's peak BMD was unknown, and therefore the actual amount of any bone loss that this patient may have experienced was unknown.

Laboratory Evaluation

The patient's laboratory values are shown in Tables 10-3 and 10-4. All values are within normal limits.

Therapy and Follow-Up

The patient declined to resume hormone replacement for the treatment of osteoporosis. She was begun on alternative therapy that she tolerated well. After 1 year, the AP spine bone-density study was repeated to assess efficacy. The precision of AP spine bone density testing at this facility was 0.01 g/cm^2, or 1% (*see* Chapter 4). The L1–L4 BMD 1 year later was found to be 0.686 g/cm^2. This increase in BMD represents a change from baseline

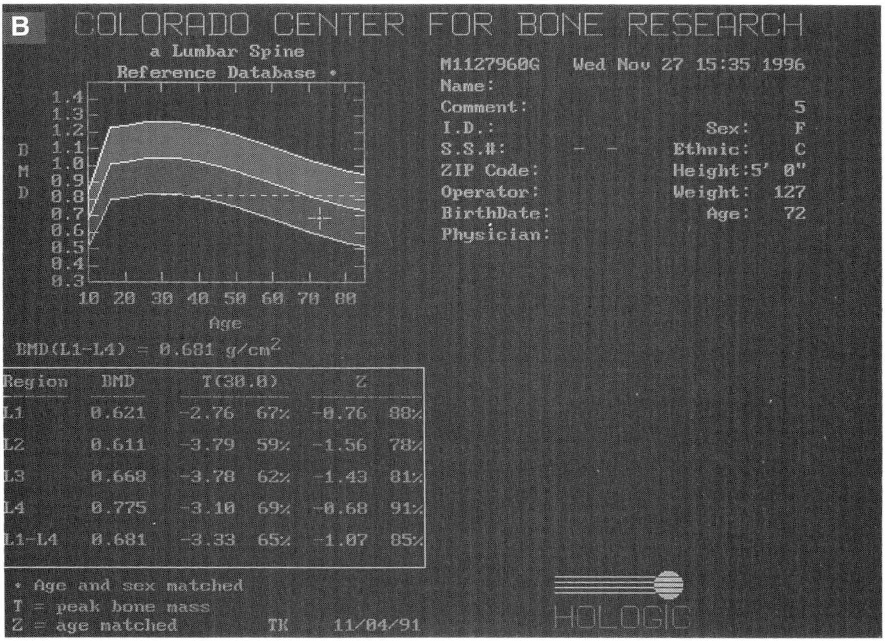

Fig. 10-3. *(continued)* **(B)** Case 2. AP Spine age-regression graph and reference database comparisons. Case courtesy of Dr. Paul Miller, Colorado Center for Bone Research, Lakewood, Colorado. The bone density data was acquired on the Hologic QDR-4500.

of 0.005 g/cm^2, or 0.7%.* Because a change from baseline of 2.77%, or 0.027 g/cm^2, was required for 95% statistical confidence that a real increase had occurred, the physician recognized that this change could not be considered significant at the 95% confidence level. How confident can the physician be that a real increase has occurred? Applying the values from Table 4-7, it can be seen that the physician can be only 28% confident that an increase has actually occurred.

CASE 3

Patient History

The patient was a 55-year-old woman who became menopausal at the age of 43. She never used hormone replacement. She took no prescription medications. There was a prior history of fracture of the left tibia and fibula

*[(0.686 – 0.681)/0.681] × 100 = 0.7%

Table 10-3
Case 2 Complete Blood Count

Test	*Results*	*Reference range*
White cell count	8.7 THOU/MCL	3.8–10.8
Red cell count	4.5 MILL/MCL	3.6–5.1
Hemoglobin	14.1 G/DL	11.1–15.5
Hematocrit	41.2%	33.0–46.0
Platelet count	301,000/CUMM	130,000–400,000
Neutrophils, segs	52.6%	40.0–75.0
Lymphocytes	35.7%	16.0–46.0
Monocytes	4.1%	0.0–12.0
Eosinophils	6.6%	0.0–7.0
Basophils	1.0%	0.0–2.0

All values are within normal limits.

Table 10-4
Case 2 Chemistry Panel

Test	*Results*	*Reference range*
SGPT	13 U/L	0–48
GGT	10 U/L	0–75
Alkaline phosphatase	68 U/L	10–125
Creatinine	1.1 MG/DL	0.7–1.8
Calcium	9.8 MG/DL	8.5–10.3
Phosphorus, inorganic	3.7 MG/DL	2.1–4.3
Sodium	138 MEQ/L	135–146
Potassium	4.1 MEQ/L	3.5–5.3
Chloride	105 MEQ/L	95–108

All values are within normal limits.

while snow skiing in 1983. There was no history of serious or chronic illness. The only surgical history was an appendectomy in 1950. She was referred for bone densitometry, to assess her risk for osteoporotic fracture in the absence of postmenopausal hormone replacement.

Laboratory Evaluation

Plain films of the thoracic and lumbar spine did not reveal any fractures. The laboratory values obtained by the patient's primary physician are shown in Tables 10-5 and 10-6. There was no evidence of secondary metabolic bone disease, based on the laboratory evaluation or the patient's medical history.

Table 10-5
Case 3 Complete Blood Count

Test	*Results*	*Reference range*
Hemoglobin	12.4 G/DL	12.0–15.5
Hematocrit	37%	34.9–44.5
Red cell count	4.16×10^{12}/L	3.90–5.03
White cell count	4.6×10^{9}/L	3.5–10.5
Neutrophils	2.25×10^{9}/L	1.70–7.00
Lymphocytes	1.73×10^{9}/L	0.90–2.90
Monocytes	0.32×10^{9}/L	0.30–0.90
Eosinophils	0.14×10^{9}/L	0.05–0.50
Basophils	0.20×10^{9}/L	0.0–0.3

All values are within normal limits.

Table 10-6
Case 3 Chemistry Panel

Test	*Results*	*Reference range*
Sodium	141 MEQ/L	135–145
Potassium	3.9 MEQ/L	3.6–4.8
Calcium	9.5 MG/DL	8.9–10.1
Phosphorus, inorganic	3.5 MG/DL	2.5–4.5
Protein, total	7.0 G/DL	6.3–7.9
Glucose	94 MG/DL	70–100
Alkaline phosphatase	203 U/L	90–234
SGOT (AST)	16 U/L	12–31
Bilirubin	0.7 MG/DL	0.1–1.1
Uric Acid	3.9 MG/DL	2.3–6.0
Creatinine	0.9 MG/DL	0.6–0.9
Albumin	4.5 G/DL	3.5–5.0
SGPT (ALT)	14 U/L	9–29
GGT	11 U/L	6–29
PTH	2.8 PMOL/L	1.0–5.2
TSH	4.0 MIU/L	0.3–5.0

The PTH, calcium, and phosphorus are evaluated to exclude hyperparathyroidism. The normal TSH excludes hyperthyroidism. The fasting glucose is normal, excluding diabetes and the creatinine suggests normal renal function. The alkaline phosphatase level is normal and not suggestive of Paget's disease. The normal protein and albumin levels, combined with the previously normal CBC mitigate against multiple myeloma.

Bone-Density Studies

The patient underwent a DXA study of the nondominant forearm, utilizing the DTX-200 (Osteometer MediTech, Roedovre, Denmark) shown

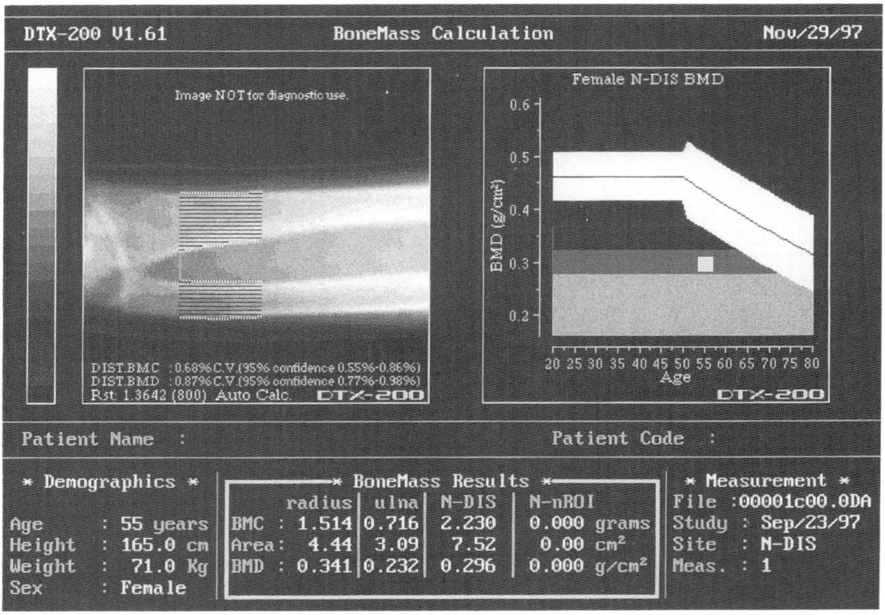

Fig. 10-4. Case 3. Forearm bone density study. The bone-density data was acquired on the Osteometer DTX-200. Results are given for the distal radius, ulna, and radius and ulna combined. The graph is a visual representation of the *T*-score of –3.6 and the *z*-score of –1.9. (*see* color plate 15 appearing after p. 174).

in Fig. 10-4. The DTX-200 measures BMD over a 2.4-cm region that begins at the 8-mm separation point. BMD is measured in both the radius and ulna. BMD, BMC, and area are presented for each bone, and as a combined distal measurement.

The BMD for the combined distal region of interest (ROI) in the nondominant forearm (N-DIS BMD) was 0.296 g/cm^2. This value can be seen on the graph shown in Fig. 10-4 to be more than 3 SDs below the peak value of the young adult, and more than 1 SD below her age-matched value. The actual *T*- and *z*-scores were –3.6 and –1.9, respectively. Based on the measurement of BMD at the distal radius and ulna, a global fracture-risk prediction was made by utilizing the *T*-score and an increase in relative risk per SD decline in BMD at the radius for any type of fracture of 1.42 (*see* Table 6-3). The relative risk for fracture was $1.42^{3.6}$, or 3.5. The densitometrist also noted that this distal BMD *T*-score of –3.6 was compatible with a diagnosis of osteoporosis based on WHO criteria. The findings and recommendations might be summarized as follows:

The patient is a 55-year-old Caucasian woman who is 12 years postmenopausal and has never utilized hormone replacement. She underwent a dual-energy X-ray study of the nondominant forearm (DTX-200) to quantify the bone density and assess her fracture risk. This study was performed on 09/23/97. The bone density was measured at the distal radius and ulna, a region that is approximately 25% trabecular and 75% cortical bone. The BMD was 0.296 g/cm^2. This value is 3.6 standard deviations below that of the young-adult. Utilizing WHO criteria for diagnosis in postmenopausal Caucasian women, this BMD is considered osteoporotic. Her risk for any type of osteoporotic fracture is increased 3.5-fold compared to an individual who has maintained an average peak bone density.

A review of the patient's medical history and laboratory evaluation does not suggest the presence of secondary causes of metabolic bone disease, leaving estrogen deficiency as the most likely contributing factor to any bone loss that may have occurred. It is not possible to quantify the magnitude of any presumed bone loss, since the patient's peak BMD is not known.

Therapeutic intervention to prevent bone loss and reduce the patient's risk of fracture should be considered. Non-prescription interventions would include calcium supplementation, vitamin D_3, and weight-bearing exercise. Prescription interventions that are currently FDA-approved for the management of osteoporosis include alendronate sodium, salmon calcitonin, and conjugated equine estrogen.

CASE 4

Medical History

The patient was a 64-year-old Caucasian woman with persistent complaints of upper- and midback pain, with no history of trauma. She became menopausal at the age of 49, and had never taken hormone replacement. She was being treated for hypertension with a long-acting beta blocker, but took no other prescription medications. There was no history of surgery other than a D&C at age 45. There was no prior fracture history. The patient previously smoked for 3 years only, quitting in 1958. There was a history of osteoporosis in her mother. On physical examination, no kyphosis or scoliosis was observed.

Laboratory Evaluation

Because of the persistent complaints of back pain, the primary physician requested plain spine films on this patient. No fractures were observed in the lumbar spine. In the thoracic spine, mild anterior wedging was observed at T7, T8, and T9, although the decreases in anterior height were insufficient to justify a diagnosis of fracture. Demineralization appeared to be present generally in the spine. The physician referred the patient for a bone density evaluation to quantify the bone density, and to confirm suspected demineralization.

Bone-Density Studies

The patient underwent a bone-density study of her nondominant forearm* using the Norland pDEXA (Fort Atkinson, WI), a DXA device dedicated to forearm measurements. This device will provide a measurement of bone density at the distal radius and ulna combined, at the proximal (33%) radius and ulna combined, and at the proximal (33%) radial site alone. The regions of interest are determined automatically by the computer, based on the forearm length entered by the operator, and determination of the location of the ulnar endplate during scan acquisition. The manufacturer's database to which the patient's values were compared was created by studying the nondominant forearm. The bone density study is shown in Fig. 10-5A.

The combined distal radial and ulnar BMD was 0.203 g/cm^2. This resulted in a T-score of –2.93. The T-score for the combined proximal radial and ulnar measurement and the proximal radial measurement are shown in Fig. 10-5B. The proximal sites have even lower T-scores of–5.16 in the combined region and –5.98 in the single region. Use of any of these three sites would result in a diagnosis of osteoporosis, applying WHO criteria, confirming the physician's visual impression of demineralization from plain films.

The bone-density data can also be used to predict lifetime hip fracture risk with the nomogram shown in Fig. 6-1 from Suman et al. *(1)*. This nomogram is based on comparisons of radial BMD to the average bone density of the 50-year-old woman. To use this nomogram, it is necessary to calculate the z-score for the patient's BMD, using the mean BMD for the 50-year-old woman as the average value upon which the z-score is based.** These values are available for the Norland pDEXA database, and are found in the operator's manual *(2)*. For Caucasian women in the 4/97 database, the mean BMD for the 50-year-old woman at the proximal radius is 0.824 g/cm^2. The SD for the 50-year-old woman is 0.085 g/cm^2. To calculate the z-score, the difference between the patient's BMD and the average BMD

**See* Chapter 2 for a discussion of the difference in BMC and BMD between dominant and nondominant forearms.

***See* Chapter 3 for a discussion of standard scores.

for the 50-year-old woman must be found. This is done by subtracting the patient's value from the mean value of the 50-year-old. The number of SDs contained in this difference is then found by dividing the difference by the SD for 50-year-old women. This results in a value of 4.5.*

A minus sign is placed in front of this value, because the patient's value is below the average value, making the *z*-score –4.5.** Utilizing this *z*-score and the patient's age and the nomogram in Fig. 6-1, the patient's lifetime risk of hip fracture can be seen to be at least 30%.

These results could be briefly summarized as follows:

The patient is a 64-year-old Caucasian woman who underwent a dual energy X-ray study of the nondominant forearm with the Norland pDEXA on 7/22/97. Bone mineral density was measured at the distal radius and ulna, proximal radius and ulna, and at the proximal radius alone. At all three sites, the bone mineral density is sufficiently low to warrant a diagnosis of osteoporosis based on WHO criteria. Based on the bone mineral density at the proximal radius, the patient's lifetime risk of hip fracture is estimated to be at least 30%.

CASE 5

Patient History

The patient was a 61-year-old woman at the time of her referral for a spine and proximal femur bone-density study in June of 1986. Menopause had occurred naturally at the age of 53. Hormone replacement had never been recommended to the patient, and she had not believed it to be necessary. The patient had never smoked. She had a 30-year history of hypothyroidism, treated with synthroid. Her current dosage was 0.2 mg daily. Her physician requested bone-density studies to evaluate her risk for osteoporotic fracture. Her initial studies were performed with dual-photon absorptiometry (DPA).

Bone-Density Studies

The results from her DPA studies are shown in Table 10-7. These results were obtained on a Lunar DP3 device (Madison, WI). Equivalent results on today's DXA devices would be expected to be lower in both the spine and proximal femur, if performed on a Hologic or Norland DXA device,

*(0.824 – 0.441)/0.085 = 4.5.

**It is important to note that this *z*-score compares the patient's BMD to the average BMD of the 50-year-old woman. The *z*-score for the proximal radius shown in Fig. 10-5B of –2.4 compares the patient's BMD to the average BMD of the 64-year-old woman.

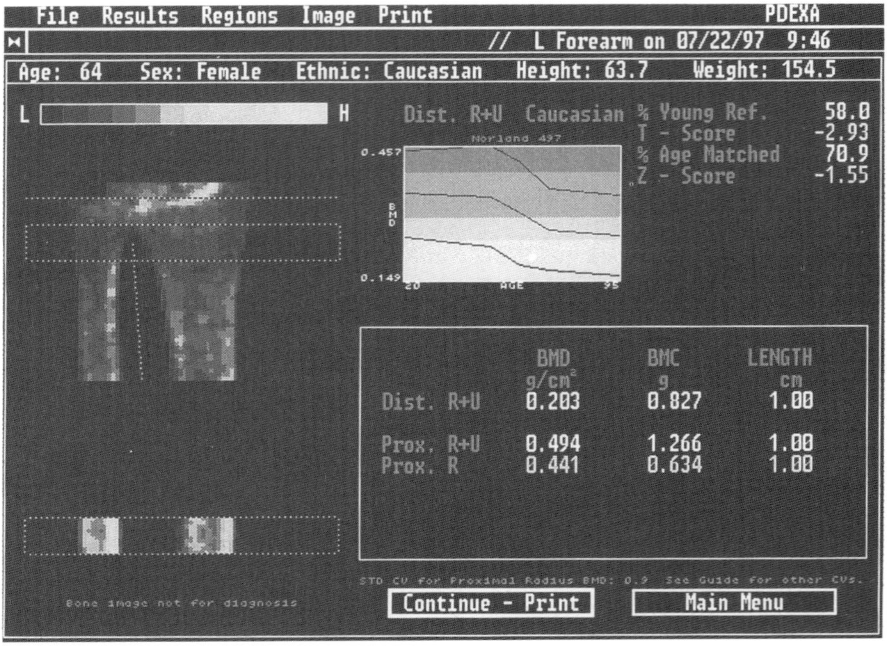

Fig. 10-5. (A) Case 4. Forearm bone density study. The bone-density data was acquired on the Norland pDEXA. The location of the distal region of interest on the pDEXA is not identical to the distal region of the DTX-200. The age-regression ± 2 SDs for the distal radius and ulna combined is shown in the graph. The narrow, horizontal, colored bars represent 1 SD changes in BMD from the peak BMD. (*see* color plate 17 appearing after p. 174).

and lower in the spine, if performed on a Lunar DXA device.* Very low bone densities were observed in both the spine and proximal femur on the DPA studies. In addition, the % age-matched comparisons were poor, suggesting the possibility of secondary metabolic bone disease. Because of this, laboratory studies were requested.

Laboratory Evaluation

Although the patient was clearly estrogen-deficient, the poor age-matched comparisons seen on her bone-density studies raised the possibility of other factors contributing to potential bone loss.** A major consideration at the time of the evaluation was excessive thyroid hormone

**See* Chapter 8 for a discussion of the conversion of DPA data to DXA data.

**It is actually not possible to immediately conclude that this patient has experienced any bone loss at all, since this is her initial bone density study and her actual peak bone density is unknown.

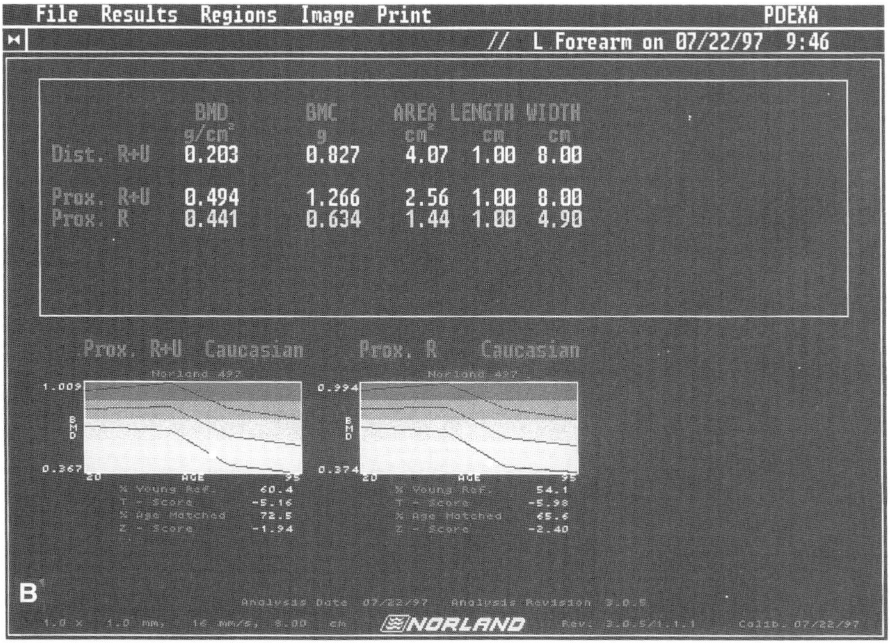

Fig. 10-5. *(continued)* **(B)** Case 4. Forearm bone density ancillary data. The bone density data was acquired on the Norland pDEXA. The age-regression graphs for the proximal radius and ulna combined and the proximal radius are shown here. (*see* color plate 18 appearing after p. 174).

Table 10-7
Case 5 Initial DPA Spine and Proximal Femur Results in 6/86

Site	*BMD g/cm^2*	*% Young adult*	*% Age-matched*
L2–L4	0.696	54.7	64.5
Femoral neck	0.57	56.4	69.5
Ward's	0.40	42.4	52.3
Trochanter	0.48	58.1	71.6

replacement.* Her laboratory studies are shown in Tables 10-8 and 10-9. The T4 was found to be markedly elevated. All other studies were within normal limits.

*See Chapter 7 for a discussion of the effects of thyroid hormone on bone density.

Table 10-8
Case 5 Complete Blood Count

Test	*Results*	*Reference range*
White cell count	5.1×10^3	7.8 ± 3
Red cell count	4.33×10^6	4.8 ± 0.6
Hemoglobin	13.4 G/DL	14.0 ± 2
Hematocrit	39.3%	42 ± 5
Segs	56%	42–81
Band	1%	0–6
Monocytes	3%	0–10%
Platelets	247×10^3	130–400

Therapy and Follow-Up

The patient's dose of synthroid was gradually reduced. She refused a recommendation of systemic hormone replacement. Instead, she was begun on a first-generation bisphosphonate in a cyclical fashion, combined with calcium supplementation and vitamin D. The patient was followed with serial measurements of spine bone density, as well as periodic measurements of T4, and later TSH, to adjust her dosage of synthroid. The spine bone density data is summarized in Table 10-10. By 4/21/87, her T4 and TSH were within normal limits on a dose of 0.1 mg daily. The BMD increased dramatically between her baseline study in June 1986 and her second study in April 1987. The increase in BMD from baseline was 23.6%.*

Although the precision of DPA spine testing was not as good as the precision obtainable today with DXA, this was clearly a significant increase. In September 1988, bone-density studies at this facility were being performed with a Lunar DPX. Based on cross-calibration studies, a decline in spine BMD was expected, if there had been no actual change in the patient's BMD from her prior DPA study. Unfortunately, it was not possible to perform both a DPA study and DXA study in September 1988 for the purposes of direct comparison. The expected DXA value was 0.793 g/cm^2, based on conversion equations from Lees and Stevenson *(3)*. The observed value was 0.746 g/cm^2. Subsequent DXA studies, however, confirmed continued small increases in spinal BMD. She continued on the cyclical bisphosphonate without difficulty, until she was lost to follow-up in 1991.

*$[(0.859 - 0.695)/0.695] \times 100 = 23.6\%$

Table 10-9
Case 5 Chemistry Panel

Test	*Results*	*Reference range*
Sodium	137 MMOL/L	134–147
Potassium	4.4 MMOL/L	3.5–5.5
Chloride	107 MMOL/L	96–110
Creatinine	0.9 MG/DL	0.5–1.7
Glucose	97 MG/DL	70–115
Calcium	9.2 MG/DL	8.3–10.5
Phosphate	3.2 MG/DL	2.5–4.6
Alkaline phosphatase	94 MU/ML	45–176
SGOT	28 MU/ML	0–72
SGPT	25 MU/ML	0–72
Protein, total	6.6 GM/DL	5.6–8.5
Albumin	4.5 GM/DL	3.0–5.5
PTH	97 PMOL/L	50–150
T4	16.16 MCG/ML	4.5–12

T4 is clearly elevated above the normal range.

Table 10-10
Case 5 Serial Spine BMD Values

Date	*L2–L4 BMD g/cm²*
6/26/86	0.695
4/21/87	0.859
9/21/88[a]	0.746
11/28/89	0.818
11/21/90	0.832

[a]This and subsequent studies were performed on a Lunar DPX instead of the Lunar DP3. The drop in spine BMD was expected with the change from DPA to DXA. It was not possible to perform both a DPA and DXA study on 9/21/88.

CASE 6

Patient History

The patient was a 68-year-old Caucasian woman who complained of loss of height and increasing curvature of the spine, with occasional backache. The patient reported that her maximum adult height was 5 ft 11 in. Her primary physician reported that her measured height was 5 ft 7 in. She experienced menopause at age 49, and had never utilized hormone replace-

Table 10-11
Case 6 Baseline and Serial BMD Studies

Date	*Region of interest*	*BMD g/cm^2*
9/14/90	L2–L4	0.566
9/14/90	Femoral neck	0.449
9/04/91	L2–L4	0.529
8/25/92	L2–L4	0.489

ment. She did not smoke, or drink alcohol. There was no family history of osteoporosis. She took no prescription medications. She had never had any type of surgery. There was a history of fracture of her right foot 25 years earlier. Plain films of the spine revealed compression fractures at T7, T11, and T12, and generalized demineralization. Bone-density studies were requested as a baseline prior to the initiation of therapy for presumed osteoporosis.

Bone-Density Studies

The patient's baseline and subsequent spine and proximal femur bone density studies are summarized in Table 10-11. These studies were performed on a Lunar DPX. The patient's L2–L4 BMD average of 0.566 g/cm^2 was only 47% of the average peak BMD of the young adult. This resulted in a young-adult *z*-score of –5.28. The femoral neck BMD at baseline was similarly very low, at 0.449 g/cm^2, resulting in a value of 46% of the peak BMD of the young adult, and a young-adult *z*-score of –4.43. Combined with the prevalent spine fractures, the patient was considered osteoporotic, confirming the referring physician's initial impression.* At both sites, the comparison to her age-matched peers was also very poor. The age-matched *z*-score for the L2–L4 BMD was –3.40, and, for the femoral neck, was –2.70. This suggested the possibility of secondary metabolic bone disease being present. The referring physician was encouraged to exclude causes of secondary metabolic bone disease.

Therapy and Follow-Up

The patient was begun on conjugated equine estrogen in a dose of 0.625 mg daily,** and was followed over the next 2 years with DXA measure-

*If the WHO criteria in use today were applied to this woman, she would be considered severely osteoporotic. WHO criteria were not in use in 1990. *See* Chapter 9 for a discussion of WHO criteria.

***See* Chapter 7 for a discussion of the minimum effective doses of estrogen replacement for skeletal preservation.

Table 10-12
Case 6 Complete Blood Count

Test	*Results*	*Reference range*
White cell count	4.6 TH/CUMM	4.0–11.0
Red cell count	4.07 MIL/CUMM	4.0–5.5
Hemoglobin	12.7 GM/DL	12.0–16.0
Hematocrit	37.8%	36–47
Platelet count	273 TH/CUMM	150–450
Granulocytes	66.9%	30–80
Lymphocytes	26.9%	15–45
Monocytes	5.1%	0–12
Eosinophils	0.6%	0–8
Basophils	0.5%	0–2

Table 10-13
Case 6 Chemistry Panel

Test	*Results*	*Reference range*
Sodium	143 MMOL/L	134–147
Potassium	4.7 MMOL/L	3.5–5.5
Chloride	107 MMOL/L	96–110
Creatinine	1.1 MG/DL	0.5–1.7
Glucose	68 MG/DL	70–117
Calcium	8.1 MG/DL	8.3–10.5
Phosphorus	4.4 MG/DL	2.5–4.6
Alkaline phosphatase	106 U/L	36–125
SGOT	53 U/L	1–40
SGPT	52 U/L	1–40
Bilirubin	0.5 MG/DL	0.1–1.7
Protein	5.6 GM/DL	6.0–8.5
Albumin	3.5 GM/DL	3.0–5.5
Cholesterol	154 MG/DL	174–200

ments of the spine, to assess the efficacy of hormone replacement in stabilizing the bone density. She also took calcium supplementation of 1000 mg daily and vitamin D 400 IU daily. Despite apparent excellent compliance, the patient demonstrated significant bone loss in the spine at 2 years follow-up. A review of medical records indicated a progressive weight loss of 24 lb during this period. On further questioning, the patient noted increased flatulence and intermittent diarrhea that she could not relate to any particular foods. Laboratory values obtained in August 1992 are shown in Tables 10-12 and 10-13.

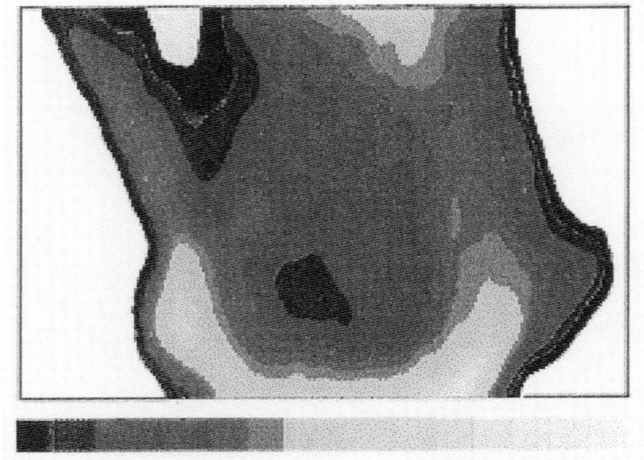

Fig. 10-6. Case 7. Contour image of the os calcis. The image was acquired on the Norland Medical Systems OsteoAnalyzer SXA3000. (*see* color plate 16 appearing after p. 174).

A review of the laboratory values was notable for the decreased calcium, protein, and cholesterol levels, along with slight elevations in SGOT and SGPT. The patient was referred to a gastroenterologist for additional evaluation. The patient underwent endoscopy and small bowel biopsy. The findings were compatible with sprue. She was placed on a gluten-free diet with resolution of her diarrhea and flatulence. In a 5-month period, she regained 19 lb, and noted a marked improvement in her energy and sense of well being.

Although estrogen deficiency is an expected cause of bone loss in a postmenopausal woman not on hormone replacement, the poor % age-matched comparison and age-matched *z*-score strongly suggested the presence of secondary metabolic bone disease. This patient's sprue required specific therapy before her osteoporosis could be successfully addressed.

CASE 7

Bone-Density Studies

The patient was a 46-year-old Caucasian woman who underwent a measurement of bone density of the right os calcis on the Norland Osteo-Analyzer SXA3000 (Ft. Atkinson, WI). The contour image of the os calcis is shown in Fig. 10-6. The BMD in the os calcis was reported to be 377.5 mg/cm^2. The remaining lifetime fracture probability (RLFP) projection is shown in Fig. 10-7.** The patient's *T*-score of –0.6 is plotted on the graph using the

**See* Chapter 6 for a discussion of remaining-lifetime fracture probability.
***See* Chapter 6 for a discussion of the fracture threshold.

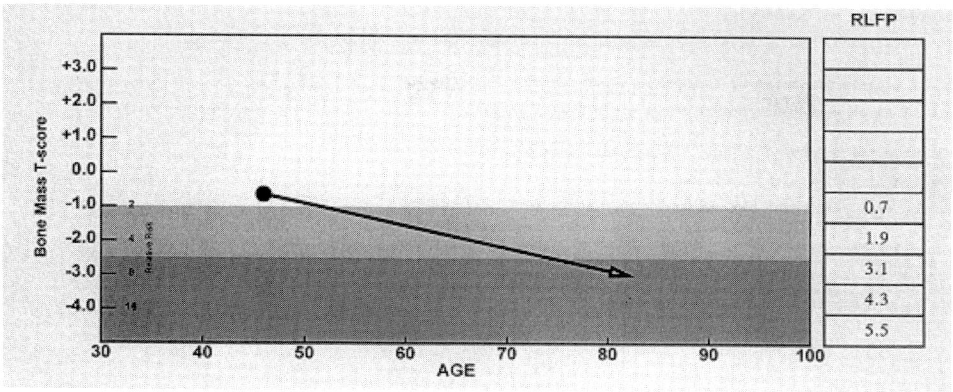

Fig. 10-7. Case 7. Remaining lifetime fracture probability (RLFP) prediction. Bone density data and RLFP analysis provided by Dr. Richard Wasnich, Hawaii Osteoporosis Center, Honolulu, Hawaii.

intersection of the *T*-score values on the *y*-axis and age on the *x*-axis. A global fracture risk prediction using relative risk can also be found using the inside scale on the *y*-axis. The arrow illustrates the decline in bone density that would result if the patient experienced a rate of bone loss of 1.5% per year. If this rate of bone loss is continued over the remaining period of the anticipated life span of the patient, her RLFP is predicted to be 3.1. In other words, the patient would be expected to experience 3.1 osteoporotic fractures in her remaining lifetime. The RLFP prediction can be modified by incorporating the expected effect of a therapy to prevent bone loss. In this case, the RLFP would be reduced to 0.3. This is not shown on the graph, but can be provided as part of the analysis. Rates of bone loss other than 1.5% can also be considered in the RLFP prediction if the clinical circumstances warrant. A brief summary of the findings, based on this study, might be as follows:

> *The patient is a 46-year-old Caucasian woman who underwent a single-energy X-ray study of the right os calcis on 11/6/96 on the OsteoAnalyzer SXA3000. The BMD was 377.5 mg/cm^2. This value is 89.9% of the average peak bone density of 420 mg/cm^2 in the 30-year-old Caucasian woman. Based on the T-score of –0.6 and applying WHO criteria for diagnosis in postmenopausal Caucasian women, this bone density is normal. Although the patient's current fracture risk is low, assuming a rate of bone loss of 1.5% and an average life span, she would be expected to experience 3.1 osteoporotic fractures in her lifetime. If bone loss is prevented, the number of osteoporotic fractures the patient would be expected to suffer would be reduced to 0.3.*

As noted in Chapter 6, RLFP is a future global fracture prediction. The exact type of anticipated fracture cannot be specified. Nevertheless, RLFP provides the most concrete explanation of fracture risk, and the potential benefit of therapy currently available.

Another approach to reporting the implications of bone loss and the benefits of therapy in this patient would be to utilize the concept of the fracture threshold.* For the os calcis, the fracture threshold has been defined as a BMD of 325 mg/cm^2. If the patient loses BMD at a rate of 1.5% per year, beginning at her current age of 46, how old will she be when she crosses the fracture threshold? If the rate of bone loss could be decreased to only 0.5% per year, what difference would this make? These values can be calculated utilizing her baseline os calcis BMD of 377.5 mg/cm^2. If bone loss progresses at a rate of 1.5% per year from a baseline level of 377.5 mg/cm^2, beginning at age 46, the patient will cross the fracture threshold at age 55. If bone loss is reduced to a rate of 0.5% per year by some intervention, she will not cross the fracture threshold until age 76. This interpretation might be summarized as follows:

If an average rate of bone loss of 1.5% is assumed, given the patient's current age and bone density, her bone density will fall below the fracture threshold at age 55. Interventions that reduce this rate of bone loss to 0.5% will delay reaching the fracture threshold until age 76.

CASE 8

Bone-Density Studies

This patient is a 54-year-old Japanese woman who underwent an SXA study of the os calcis on the Norland OsteoAnalyzer SXA3000. The BMD was 545.7 mg/cm^2. The patient's *T*-score (young-adult *z*-score) can be calculated using the peak BMD of the 30-year-old for the os calcis of 420 mg/cm^2 and SD of 67 mg/cm^2.** The difference between the peak BMD of 420 mg/cm^2 and the patient's BMD of 545.7 mg/cm^2 is 125.7 mg/cm^2. Since the magnitude of the SD is 67 mg/cm^2, the number of SDs contained in the difference between the peak BMD and the measured BMD is 1.9.† Thus, the patient's BMD is 1.9 SDs above the peak BMD. The *T*-score (or young-adult *z*-score) is +1.9.

The prediction of RLFP is shown in Fig. 10-8. Once again, the patient's *T*-score is plotted on the graph. If the patient lives an average life span, and a rate of bone loss of 1.5% per year is assumed, the RLFP for this patient

See Chapter 6 for a discussion of the fracture threshold.

***See* Chapter 3 for a discussion of standard scores.

†$(545.7 - 420.0)/67 = 1.9$

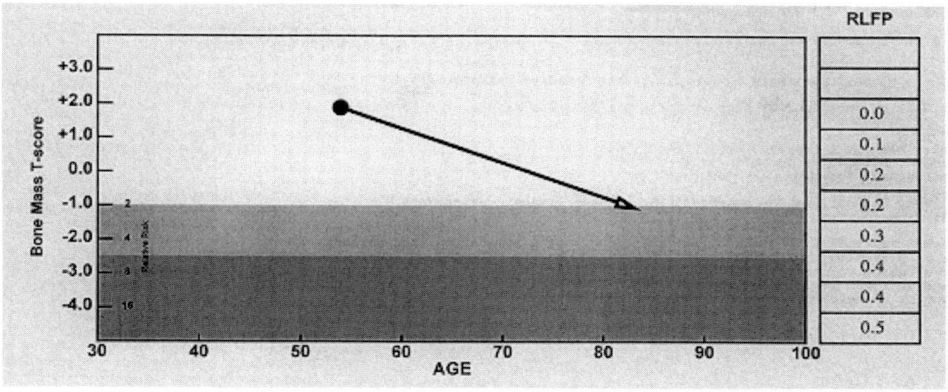

Fig. 10-8. Case 8. Remaining lifetime fracture probability (RLFP) prediction. Bone density data acquired on the Norland Medical Systems OsteoAnalyzer SXA3000. Bone density data and RLFP analysis provided by Dr. Richard Wasnich, Hawaii Osteoporosis Center, Honolulu, Hawaii.

is only 0.2. Not only is this patient's current fracture risk extremely low, her future global fracture-risk is also extremely low. The findings might be summarized as follows:

> *The patient is a 54-year-old Japanese woman who underwent an SXA study of the right os calcis. The os calcis is considered to be a predominantly trabecular, weight-bearing site in the appendicular skeleton.* The BMD was 545.7 mg/cm². This value is 1.9 standard deviations above the peak BMD of the 30-year-old woman. Her current risk for fracture is very low and even with a projected lifetime rate of bone loss of 1.5% per year, the number of osteoporotic fractures she would be expected to suffer is less than 1. Based on this bone density study, prescription intervention to prevent bone loss would not appear to be indicated. Nonprescription measures, such as calcium supplementation, daily consumption of 400 IU of vitamin D, and weight-bearing exercise, are appropriate as general preventive measures.*

CASE 9

Patient History

The patient is a 41-year-old Caucasian woman who underwent an AP spine and proximal femur study on the Norland XR-36. These studies are shown in Figs. 10-9 and 10-10. This woman had a history of breast cancer

**See* Chapter 2 for a discussion of skeleton site composition.

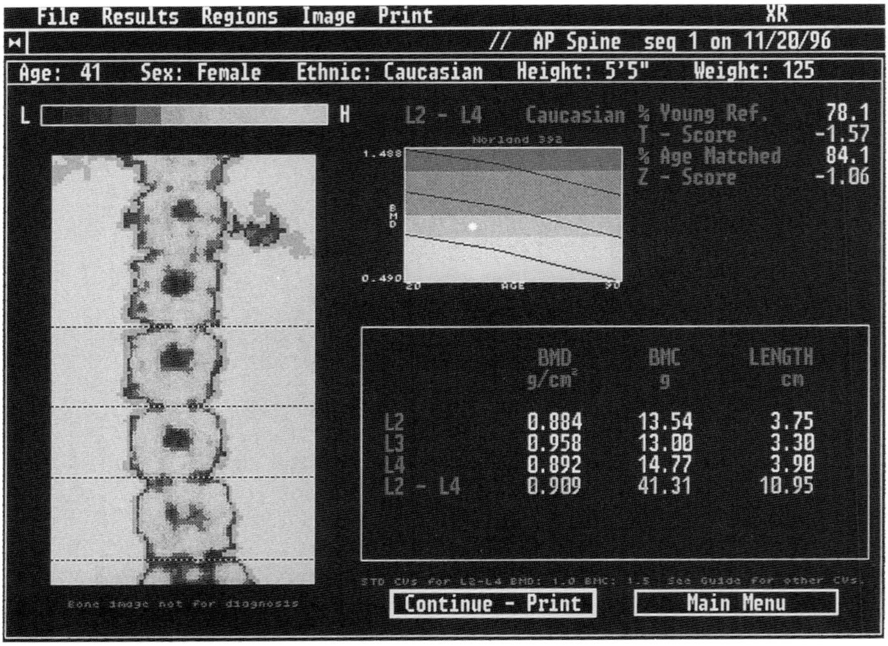

Fig. 10-9. Case 9. AP Spine bone density data. Bone-density data acquired on the Norland XR-36. The bone density image can be generated in color or as a gray-scale image. The graph shows the regression or change in BMD with advancing age ± 2 SDs. The narrow, horizontal bars represent 1 SD changes in BMD from the peak BMD. (*see* color plate 19 appearing after p. 174).

and subsequent ovarian failure as a result of chemotherapy. Because menopause had been induced at age 41, she was considered at high risk for osteoporosis. Bone density studies were requested to determine the patient's current bone density and need for prescription intervention to reduce her risk for fracture.

Bone-Density Studies

The L2–L4 average BMD was 0.909 g/cm^2, which was 78.1% of the average BMD of the young adult, and 84.1% of her age-matched peers. The L2–L4 *T*-score was –1.57. The BMD in the femoral neck was 0.770 g/cm^2, which was 75.7% of the average BMD in the femoral neck of the young adult, and 82% of her age-matched peers. The femoral neck *T*-score was –2.05. The findings and recommendations might be summarized as follows:

The patient is a 41-year-old Caucasian woman with a history of breast cancer and ovarian failure following chemotherapy. She was referred

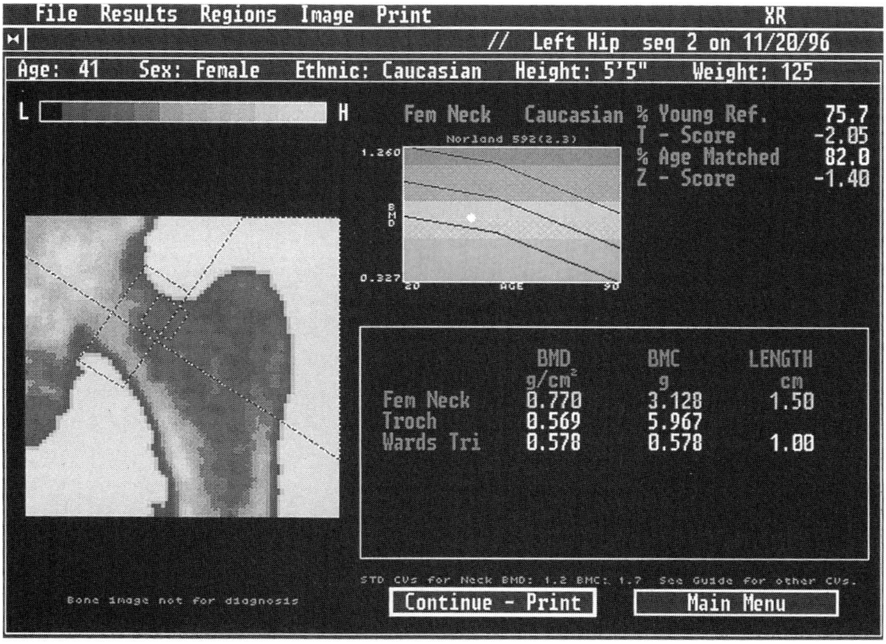

Fig. 10-10. Case 9. Proximal femur bone-density data. Bone-density data acquired on the Norland XR-36. *(see* color plate 20 appearing after p. 174).

for bone density testing of the AP spine and proximal femur to assess her need for prescription intervention to prevent bone loss and reduce her risk for osteoporotic fracture. These studies were performed on the Norland XR-36 dual-energy X-ray densitometer on 11/20/96. The effective radiation dose during each study was approximately 1 μSv. Review of the bone density images does not suggest the presence of fracture, degenerative calcification, or artifact that might affect the validity of the results. Very mild scoliosis is suggested on the spine bone density study. These impressions should be confirmed with plain films if necessary.*

Applying WHO criteria for diagnosis in postmenopausal Caucasian women, the average L2–L4 BMD and femoral neck BMD are considered osteopenic. Given the patient's young age at the time of chemically induced ovarian failure and the finding of osteopenia, prescription intervention to prevent bone loss appears to be warranted. Other non-prescription interventions to prevent bone loss, such as calcium supplementation and regular weight-bearing exercise, are also strongly recommended.

**See* Chapter 1 for a discussion of effective radiation dose during DXA studies.

This patient was begun on a bisphosphonate based on the bone-density studies performed in November 1996. Her AP spine bone density study was repeated in December 1997, to assess the efficacy of the intervention in preventing bone loss. Her L2–L4 BMD in December 1997 was 0.945 g/cm^2. Is this a significant increase?

At the testing facility, the precision of AP spine bone-density testing was reported to be 1%, or 0.011 g/cm^2, in individuals with an average BMD of 1.100 g/cm^2. If 1% is used as the precision value, a change of $2.77 \times 1\%$, or 2.77%, from baseline, is necessary to conclude that a real increase has occurred at the 95% confidence level, as seen in Table 4-4. If the value of 0.011 g/cm^2 is used as the precision value, a change of 2.77×0.011 g/cm^2, or 0.031 g/cm^2, is necessary to conclude that a real increase has occurred at the 95% confidence level. The measured change in BMD between 1996 and 1997 was actually 0.036 g/cm^2 ($0.945 - 0.909 = 0.036$), which was a change of 4.0% from baseline.* Clearly, whichever precision value is used for this calculation, the measured change exceeds the value necessary for significance at the 95% confidence level. But is the actual change from 1996 a 4% change? There is a range of values at the 95% confidence level for the actual change in BMD. This concept is illustrated in Table 4-8. This range is $4 \pm 2.77\%$, or a range of 1.23 to 6.77%. In other words, the physician can be 95% confident that a change of 1.23 to 6.77% has occurred. This information might be briefly summarized as follows:

*Over the last year, there has been a measured increase in the BMD of 0.036 gm/cm^2, or 4% of the baseline value. The precision at this facility in individuals with an average BMD of 1.100 g/cm^2 is 1%. This measured change in the patient is therefore considered to be a statistically significant increase in BMD at the 95% confidence level. Given the precision error that is inherent in the testing, the actual change may range from 1.23% to 6.77%.***

CASE 10

Patient History

This patient was a 62-year-old Caucasian woman with a complaint of low back pain. She was 10 years postmenopausal, and had been taking estrogen replacement for only 3 months. There was a history of osteoporo-

*$(0.036/0.909) \times 100 = 4\%$

**This last statement is not always necessary. It is more important to the physician to know that an actual increase has occurred, rather than the uncertainty in the absolute magnitude of that increase.

sis in her brother. Plain X rays performed prior to the bone density study did not reveal any spine fractures, but demineralization was suggested. Bone-density studies were performed to confirm the radiographic impression of demineralization. Other history obtained prior to the bone density study included a calcium intake of 1600 mg per day and a vitamin D_3 intake of 250 U per day. She did not smoke or drink alcohol at any time.

Bone-Density Studies

Her AP spine bone-density study is shown in Fig. 10-11. This study was performed on the Lunar DPX-L. In this case, the densitometrist had the advantage of knowing that no fractures were present on previously obtained plain films of the spine. There was also no apparent aortic calcification or facet sclerosis, or other degenerative changes that might affect the validity of the BMD results. A review of the bone density image also did not suggest any of these findings. The individual BMD values, and the average values for each possible combination of contiguous vertebrae, are shown in Table 10-14. The expected pattern of incremental change in BMD from level to level is seen in this study. L1 has the lowest BMD, as expected. There is an increase in BMD from L1 to L2, and again from L2 to L3. There is a decline in BMD from L3 to L4 that is not unusual, although the magnitude of the decline is greater than generally seen. A review of the individual BMC and area values for each level confirmed the expected increase in BMC and area at each level, except between L3 and L4. A review of the image to check the labeling of the vertebrae confirms the characteristic U or Y shape of L1, L2, and L3. The classic block H or X shape of L4 is not well seen here, but L5 illustrates the classic block I on its side appearance. The lowest set of ribs appears to be coming from T12. The location of the superior portion of the iliac crests is anticipated to be in the vicinity of the L4–5 disk space. In this study, it is apparently lower, because L5 is higher in the pelvis. With the knowledge that 83.5% of women age 50 and over have five lumbar vertebrae, with the lowest set of ribs on T12, combined with the finding of the characteristic shapes of L1, L2, L3, and L5, and the expected pattern of change of BMD, BMC, and area between the L1 to L3 vertebral levels, the densitometrist was confident that this labeling was correct.*

Because it is desirable, for reasons of statistical accuracy and precision, to use the average BMD of as many vertebrae as possible, and, concluding, after a preliminary review, that no levels needed to be excluded because of artifact, the densitometrist could choose either the L1–L4 or L2–L4

*See Chapter 2 for a discussion of the characteristic shapes of lumbar vertebrae as seen on DXA studies of the AP spine, and for a discussion of anomalous vertebral segmentation.

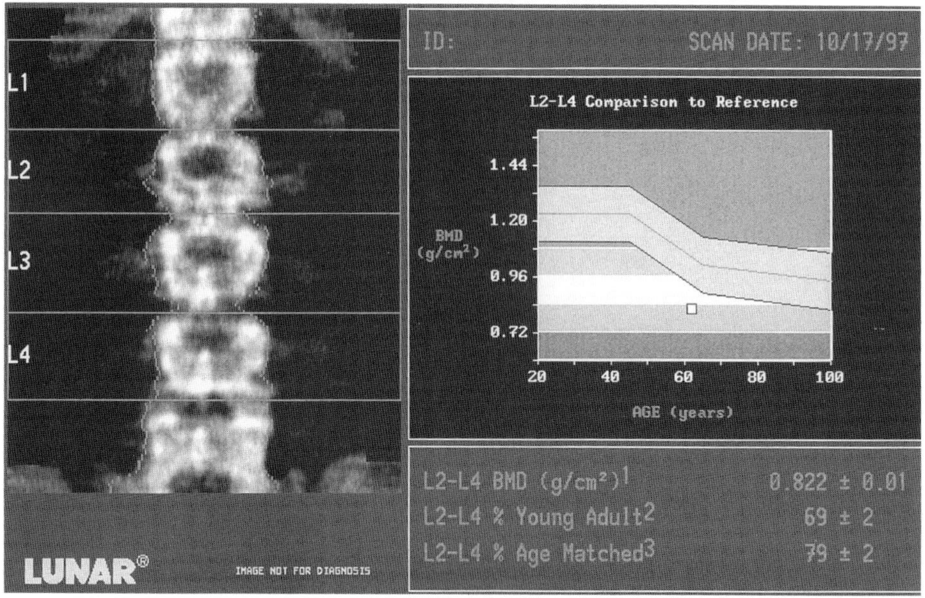

Fig. 10-11. Case 10. AP Spine bone density data. Case courtesy of Dr. Clifford Rosen, Maine Center for Osteoporosis Research and Education, Bangor, Maine. Bone-density data acquired on the Lunar DPX-L. The characteristic shapes of the vertebrae are reasonably well seen. The lowest set of ribs appears to be coming off T12. The iliac crests are lower than generally expected. The graph illustrates the regression of the L2–L4 BMD average against age ± 1 SD. The narrow, horizontal bars represent 1 SD changes in BMD from the peak BMD.

Table 10-14
Case 10 Ancillary Densitometry Data

				Young adult		Age-matched	
Region	*BMD g/cm²*	*BMC g*	*Area cm²*	%	T	%	z
L1	0.780	9.02	11.57	69	–2.92	80	–1.60
L2	0.797	9.52	11.94	66	–3.36	77	–2.04
L3	0.860	11.95	13.90	72	–2.83	83	–1.52
L4	0.805	10.66	13.25	67	–3.30	77	–1.98
L1–L2	0.789	18.55	23.52	69	–3.01	80	–1.69
L1–L3	0.815	30.50	37.41	70	–2.96	81	–1.64
L1–L4	0.813	41.16	50.66	69	–3.06	79	–1.75
L2–L3	0.831	21.48	25.84	69	–3.07	80	–1.76
L2–L4	**0.822**	**32.14**	**39.09**	**69**	**–3.15**	**79**	**–1.83**
L3–L4	0.833	22.16	27.14	69	–3.06	80	–1.74

The values for the default L2–L4 average are highlighted but the values for the individual vertebra should be reviewed before accepting the default average.

BMD average to interpret. The Lunar default average of L2–L4 was chosen. This value was 0.822 g/cm^2. As seen on the computer screen shown in Fig. 10-11, this value is 69% of the young adult, and 79% of her age-matched peers. The *T*-score and *z*-score for the L2–L4 average are seen in Table 10-14 (remember that the *T*-score is synonymous with the young-adult *z*-score, and that *z*-score is synonymous with age-matched z-score). The *T*-score was –3.1 and the *z*-score was –1.8.

A brief summary of the findings so far might be as follows:

This patient is a 62-year-old Caucasian woman who underwent an AP spine DXA study on 10/17/97 (Lunar, software version 4.3). A review of the bone density image does not suggest the presence of vertebral fracture or forms of dystrophic calcification that might affect the accuracy of the values and the validity of the interpretation. Effective radiation dose during the AP spine study was approximately 1 μSv.

The L2–L4 BMD average is 0.822 g/cm^2. This value is 69% of the peak BMD of the young adult and 79% of her age-matched peers. The patient's BMD is therefore 31% below the average peak BMD of the young adult and 21% below the BMD that would have been predicted on the basis of her age, sex, and race. The T-score of –3.1 indicates that the BMD of 0.822 g/cm^2 is 3.1 standard deviations below the average BMD of the young adult. Applying WHO criteria for diagnosis based on this T-score, the patient has a BMD in the spine compatible with a diagnosis of osteoporosis. The z-score of*

**See* Chapter 9 for a discussion of WHO criteria.

–1.8 indicates that the BMD of 0.822 g/cm² is 1.8 standard deviations below the BMD that would be predicted on the basis of her age, sex, and race. Although this is not an extremely poor comparison to the age-matched value that would suggest causes of bone loss other than estrogen deficiency, it is reasonable to exclude secondary causes clinically.

The densitometrist also chose to make an assessment of fracture risk, utilizing the *T*-score. Relative risk fracture data was utilized for this calculation. For measurements at the lumbar spine, a relative risk value of 2.2 and 1.6 per SD decline in BMD were utilized for site-specific fracture-risk predictions for the spine and hip, respectively. These relative risk values are shown in Table 6-4. Utilizing the *T*-score for the L2–L4 BMD average of –3.1, the calculation of the site-specific spine fracture risk is $2.2^{3.1}$.* The calculation of the site-specific hip-fracture risk is $1.6^{3.1}$. These calculations result in a relative risk for spine fracture of 11.5, and, for hip fracture, 4.3. This prediction of fracture risk can be summarized as follows:

Based on the measurement of BMD at the lumbar spine, the relative risk for spine fracture is 11.5, and for hip fracture is 4.3. This means that the patient has a risk for spine fracture that is 11.5 times greater and a risk for hip fracture that is 4.3 times greater than the individual who still has a lumbar spine bone density that is equal to the peak BMD of the young adult.

Another way of expressing risk that could be utilized would be to report the prevalence of either spine or hip fracture at this level of spine BMD.** As noted in Chapter 3, in this context, prevalence expresses how common fracture is at this level of BMD. The prevalence figures shown in Table 6-1 can be used for this expression of risk. The ranges of BMD shown in this table were derived using BMD measurements performed with DPA. To convert these values to equivalent DXA values (in this case, Lunar DXA values), the equation for converting Lunar DPA spine data to Lunar DXA spine data found in Chapter 8 can be used.† After making these conversions, the densitometrist might add:

The prevalence of spine fracture at this BMD has been shown to be 23.1% whereas the prevalence of hip fracture at this spine BMD is 9.7%.

**See* Chapter 3 for a discussion of the exponential relationship between absolute risk, relative risk, and the *T*-score.

***See* Chapter 3 for a discussion of different measures of risk.

†$\text{L2–L4 DPX}_{BMD} = -0.110 + (1.052 \times \text{L2–L4 DP3}_{BMD})$

The standardized BMD for the L2–L4 BMD of 0.822 g/cm^2 is also provided on the bone density printout.* The standardized BMD was reported to be 783 mg/cm^2. This value is not critical to the interpretation of the current test. It would become useful should the patient undergo bone density testing in the future, on another manufacturer's DXA device, in order to compare that study to the current study. Even if the value had not been given, the densitometrist could have calculated it, using the formula shown in Table 8-3.**

REFERENCES

1. Suman VJ, Atkinson EJ, O'Fallon WM, Black DM, Melton LJ (1993) A nomogram for predicting lifetime hip fracture risk from radius bone mineral density and age. *Bone* 14:843–846.
2. Norland Medical Systems (1996) Reference sets. *X-Ray Bone Densitometer Operator's Guide*. Ft. Atkinson, WI.
3. Lees B, Stevenson JC (1992) An evaluation of dual-energy X-ray absorptiometry and comparison with dual-photon absorptiometry. *Osteoporosis Int* 2:146–152.

**See* Chapter 8 for a discussion of the standardized BMD and its calculation.
**$sBMD_{SPINE}$ = 1000 (0.9522 × Lunar DPX-L BMD_{SPINE})

INDEX

M

N

ABOUT THE AUTHOR

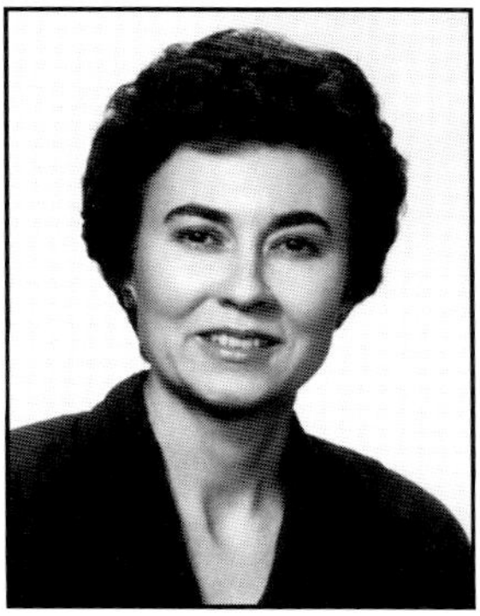

Dr. Bonnick is a native of Dallas, Texas. She is a graduate of Southern Methodist University of Texas Southwestern Medical School. She is board certified in internal medicine and a fellow in the American College of Physicians. She has worked in the field of women's health with an emphasis on osteoporosis and bone densitometry for over 15 years.

Dr. Bonnick is a member of the board of trustees of the International Society for Clinical Densitometry and a member of the teaching faculty for the Society's physician and technologist certification program in densitometry. She is also a member of the Bone Measurement Institute, the American Society for Bone and Mineral Research and the North American Menopause Society and a former member of the osteoporosis advisory committee for the Texas Department of Health.

She has served as a principal investigator in numerous research trials in the field of the prevention and treatment of osteoporosis and has published extensively. Dr. Bonnick is currently the Director of Osteoporosis Services and a research professor in the Center for Research on Women's Health at Texas Woman's University in Denton, Texas.